Abdul H. Sultan, Ranee Thakar and Dee E. Fenner (Eds)

Perineal and Anal Sphincter Trauma

Diagnosis and Clinical Management

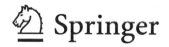 Springer

Abdul H. Sultan, MB ChB, MD, FRCOG
Consultant Obstetrician and Gynaecologist
Mayday University Hospital
Croydon, UK
and
Honorary Senior Lecturer
St George's Medical School
University of London
London, UK

Ranee Thakar, MB BS, MD, MRCOG
Consultant Obstetrician and Urogynaecologist
Mayday University Hospital
Croydon, UK
and
Honorary Senior Lecturer
St George's Medical School
University of London
London, UK

Dee E. Fenner, MD
Furlong Professor of Women's Health
Director of Gynecology
Department of Obstetrics and Gynecology
University of Michigan
Ann Arbor, MI, USA

British Library Cataloguing in Publication Data
A Catalogue record for this book is available from the British Library
Perineal and anal sphincter trauma
   1. Perineum – Wounds and injuries   2. Perineum – Surgery
   3. Anus – Wounds and injuries   4. Anus – Surgery
   I. Sultan, Abdul H.   II. Thakar, Ranee   III. Fenner, Dee E.
   617.5'55

ISBN 978-1-84800-996-7   e-ISBN 978-1-84628-503-5
DOI 10.1007/978-1-84628-503-5

Printed on acid-free paper.

Springer Science+Business Media
springer.com

Foreword

One of the rewards of medical teaching is to see the next generation advance the art and science of medicine beyond their forebears. We can be justifiably proud of this anthology on *Perineal and Anal Sphincter Trauma*, which owes so much to the endeavours of the editorial team. In addition to their own contributions, they have recruited a body of topic authors of international standing. The result is a book of wide breadth and depth, covering many aspects of disorders of the posterior pelvic compartment, which have hitherto not been found in one volume. The choice of topics is wide, and the description and illustrations are clear and concise. They cover both innovative and current practice, all founded on an evidence basis.

The intended readership is multidisciplinary, going beyond all those involved in "front line" obstetric care, to reach physicians, surgeons, radiologists and others, who deal with long term adverse effects of childbirth. This mirrors the professional background of the authorship. We are confident of its broad appeal and wish the book every success.

Christopher N. Hudson
Emeritus Professor of Obstetrics and Gynaecology
University of London
London, UK

Stuart L. Stanton
Emeritus Professor of Urogynaecology
University of London
London, UK

Bob L. Shull
Professor of Obstetrics and Gynecology
Vice-Chairman, Department of Obstetrics/Gynecology
Chief, Section of Female Pelvic Medicine and Reconstructive Pelvic Surgery
Scott and White Clinic
Texas A&M College of Medicine
Temple, USA

Preface

In the last two decades, there has been an increasing interest in obstetric perineal and anal sphincter trauma. This can be largely attributed to innovations in imaging, as it was the development of anal endosonography that led to the diagnosis of unrecognised anal sphincter trauma during childbirth. These sonographic injuries were initially considered to be occult, but it has now been established that the vast majority are in fact visible at the time of childbirth but remain undiagnosed. Consequently, attention is now focused on structured training programmes and hands-on workshops to improve understanding of anatomy and repair of perineal and anal sphincter trauma.

However, despite primary repair of anal sphincter injuries, the outcome is not universally optimal, and research on the ideal management continues. This highlights the need to identify risk factors in order to minimise the development of perineal and anal sphincter trauma.

This textbook aims not only to address these issues but also to provide in-depth information about anatomy and pathophysiology. In addition, other issues such as female genital mutilation, the management of faecal incontinence and medicolegal implications are also covered.

In producing this book, we would like to acknowledge our mentors for their teaching and inspiration, the patients who made us question our practice and the research fellows who contributed to the research. We would like to thank the multidisciplinary authors for their timely submission of chapters; last but not least we would like to extend our appreciation to our families for their perseverance and understanding.

Abdul H. Sultan
Ranee Thakar
Dee E. Fenner

Contents

Contributors

Clive Bartram, FRCS, FRCP, FRCR
Department of Radiology
St Mark's Hospital
Harrow, UK

Timothy J. Brown, BSc, MB, BS, MRCS
Physiology Unit
St Mark's Hospital
Harrow, UK

Susan M. Cera, MD
Department of Colorectal Surgery
Cleveland Clinic Florida
Weston, FL, USA

Erica Eason, MD
Division of General Obstetrics and Gynecology
Department of Obstetrics and Gynecology
University of Ottawa
The Ottawa Hospital
Ottawa, ON, Canada

Dee E. Fenner, MD
Division of Gynecology
Department of Obstetrics and Gynecology
University of Michigan
Ann Arbor, MI, USA

Harry Gordon, MBBS, FRCS (Edin), FRCOG
Consultant to the African Clinic
Central Middlesex Hospital London
London, UK

Kara Jennings, JD
Legal Services of South Central Michigan
Ann Arbor, MI, USA

Christine Kettle, PhD
Obstetric Department of Obstetrics and
  Gynaecology
University Hospital of North Staffordshire and
  Staffordshire University
Stoke-on-Trent, UK

Peter J. Lunniss, MS, FRCS
Centre for Academic Surgery and GI Physiology
  Unit
Barts and The London, Queen Mary's School of
  Medicine and Dentistry
The Royal London Hospital
London, UK, and
Academic Department of Medical and Surgical
  Gastroenterology
Homerton Hospital
London, UK

Christine Norton, PhD, MA, RN
Burdett Institute of Gastrointestinal Nursing
St Mark's Hospital
London, UK, and
Florence Nightingale School of Nursing
King's College London
London, UK

Nicholas A. Peacock, MA
Hailsham Chambers
London, UK

Robin K. S. Phillips, MBBS, FRCS
Department of Surgery
St Mark's Hospital
Harrow, UK

Rebecca G. Rogers, MD
University of New Mexico Health Sciences
    Center
Department of Obstetrics and Gynecology
Albuquerque, NM, USA

Kjell Erik Roxstrom, JD
AnnArbor, MI, USA

S. Mark Scott, PhD
Centre for Academic Surgery and GI Physiology
    Unit
Barts and The London, Queen Mary's School of
    Medicine and Dentistry
The Royal London Hospital
London, UK

Abdul H. Sultan, MB ChB, MD, FRCOG
Department of Obstetrics and Gynaecology
Mayday University Hospital
Croydon, UK

Ranee Thakar, MB BS, MD, MRCOG
Department of Obstetrics and Gynaecology
Mayday University Hospital
Croydon, UK

Steven D. Wexner, MD, FACS, FRCS, FRCS (Ed)
Department of Colorectal Surgery
Cleveland Clinic Florida
Weston, FL, USA

1
Anatomy of the Perineum and the Anal Sphincter

Ranee Thakar and Dee E. Fenner

1.1 Introduction

The anatomy of the pelvic floor, rectum and anal canal is a complex and surprisingly dynamic field with new insights, discoveries and controversies. The controversies arise as new and different tools are used to study anatomy for varying purposes. Anatomists, sprung through cadaveric dissections, propose a structure that may differ from a surgeon's depiction or understanding of the structure/function relationships of the pelvis as seen in the operating room. This controversy is best seen in describing the external anal sphincter (EAS) and the puborectalis muscle. Is the puborectalis a part of the EAS? Is the EAS a one, two, or three loop striated muscle? Perhaps all descriptions are correct, depending on the point of view and purpose of evaluation. The goal of this chapter is not to solve these controversies, but to describe the functional and structural anatomy as it is known from cadaveric dissections, radiological imaging and surgical repairs in order to improve the management of our patients.

1.2 Embryology

In the early embryo, the allantois and the hindgut open into a common cavity, the cloaca (Figure 1.1a). This is an endoderm-lined cavity that is in contact with the surface of the ectoderm. An ectodermal depression develops under the root of the tail of the fetus and sinks in towards the gut until only the thin cloacal membrane remains between the gut and the outside.[1] This ectodermal depression is called the proctodeum. The cloacal membrane is thus comprised of the cloacal endoderm and the ectoderm of the proctodeum or the anal pit. Partitioning of the cloacal membrane takes place during the fifth to seventh week of development when the urorectal septum, which is mesodermal in origin, grows down between the hindgut and the allantois to fuse with the cloacal membrane (Figure 1.1b). The area of fusion becomes the perineal body and separates the dorsal anal membrane from the larger ventral urogenital membrane. The anal membrane breaks down by the eighth week of gestation, establishing the anal canal. The urorectal septum also divides the cloacal musculature into anterior and posterior parts. The posterior portion develops into the EAS, while the anterior part becomes the superficial transverse perinei, the bulbospongiosus, the ischiocavernosus and the perineal membrane. This explains why one nerve, the pudendal nerve, supplies all musculature into which the cloacal membrane divides.[2]

Knowledge of embryology is also important to understand the differences in the linings, innervation, vascular supply and lymphatic drainage of the anal canal. The parts derived from the endoderm are lined by columnar epithelium, are innervated by autonomic nerves, and the lymphatics and veins drain towards the abdomen. The parts derived from the ectoderm are lined by stratified squamous epithelium, have a somatic nerve supply, and the veins drain towards the external iliac system, and the lymphatics to the inguinal lymph nodes.

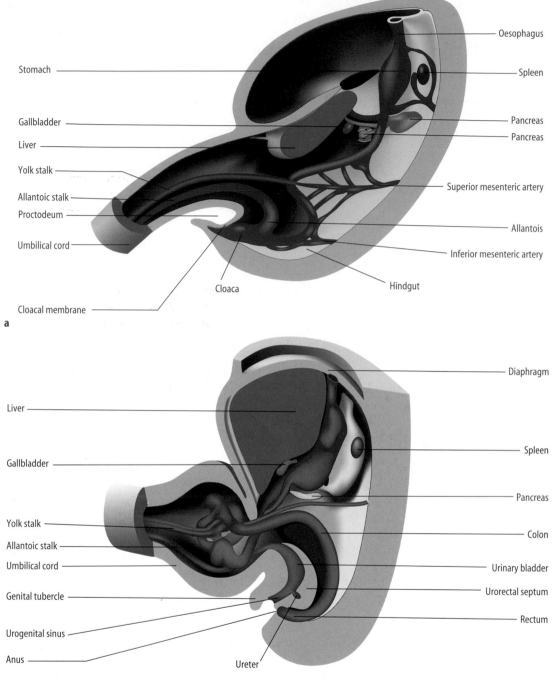

FIGURE 1.1. **a** Development of the gastrointestinal tract at about 5 weeks. **b** Fetus showing development of the anorectum after 5 weeks, demonstrating the growth of the urorectum towards the cloacal membrane.

The upper two-thirds (25 mm) of the anal canal is derived from the cloaca and the lower third (13 mm) develops from the proctodeum. This junction, about 2 cm from the anal verge, creates a demarcating line called the pectinate or dentate line. At this line the epithelium changes from stratified squamous to columnar cells.

Little is known about the development of the EAS and levator ani muscles. Although closely associated, embryo studies suggest the external sphincter and levator ani arise from two distinct primordia. The puborectalis muscle is a portion of the levator ani, and shares primordial with the ilio- and pubococcygeous muscles. The EAS is found after 8 weeks of gestation and is clearly distinct from the puborectalis at that time.[3]

1.3 Muscles of the Perineum

The perineum corresponds to the outlet of the pelvis and is somewhat lozenge shaped. Anteriorly, it is bound by the pubic arch, posteriorly by the coccyx, and laterally by the ischiopubic rami, ischial tubcrosities, and sacrotubcrous ligaments. The deep limit of the perineum is the inferior surface of the pelvic diaphragm and its superficial limit is the skin, which is continuous with that over the medial aspect of the thigh and the lower abdomen. The perineum can be divided into two triangular parts by drawing an arbitrary line transversely between the ischial tuberosities.[4] The anterior triangle, which contains the external urogenital organs, is known as the *urogenital triangle* and the posterior triangle, which contains the termination of the anal canal, is known as the *anal triangle*.

1.3.1 The Urogenital Triangle

The urogenital triangle (Figure 1.2a) is bound anteriorly and laterally by the pubic symphysis and the ischiopubic rami. Traditionally the urogenital triangle has been divided into two compartments: the superficial and deep perineal spaces, separated by the perineal membrane, which spans the space between the ischiopubic rami.[4] However, more recent studies of this region describe the perineal membrane as a complex structure with many parts. It is composed of two regions: one dorsal and one ventral. The dorsal region consists of bilateral transverse fibrous sheets that attach the lateral wall of the vagina and perineal body to the ischio-pubic ramus. The ventral region is a solid three-dimensional tissue mass in which several structures are embedded. It contains the compressor urethra and the urethrovaginal sphincter muscle of the distal urethra with the urethra and its surrounding connective tissue (Figure 1.3). The ventral margin of this mass is continuous with the insertion of the arcus tendineus fascia pelvis into the pubic bone. The levator ani muscles are attached to the cranial surface of the perineal membrane. The vestibular bulb and clitoral crus lie on the caudal surface of the membrane and are fused with it, there being no natural plane of cleavage between these erectile structures and the membrane. Therefore, the structure of the perineal membrane is not a trilaminar sheet with perforating viscera, but a complex three-dimensional structure with two distinctly different dorsal and ventral regions.[5]

Just beneath the skin of the anterior perineum lies the superficial perineal fascia (Colles' fascia). As described above, the erectile tissues are fused to the caudal surface of the perineal membrane complex. The erectile tissues are covered by the bulbospongiosus and the ischiocavernosus muscles. The superficial transverse perineal muscles attach the perineal body to the ischial tuberosities bilaterally. All of these perineal muscles are innervated by a branch of the pudendal nerve, which is a mixed motor and sensory nerve.

1.3.1.1 Superficial Transverse Perineal Muscle

The superficial transverse muscle is a narrow slip of a muscle, which arises from the inner and forepart of the ischial tuberosity and is inserted into the central tendinous part of the perineal body (Figure 1.2a). The muscle from the opposite side, the EAS from behind, and the bulbospongiosus in the front all attach to the central tendon of the perineal body.[4]

1.3.1.2 Bulbospongiosus Muscle

The bulbospongiosus muscle runs on either side of the vaginal orifice, covering the lateral aspects of the vestibular bulb anteriorly and the

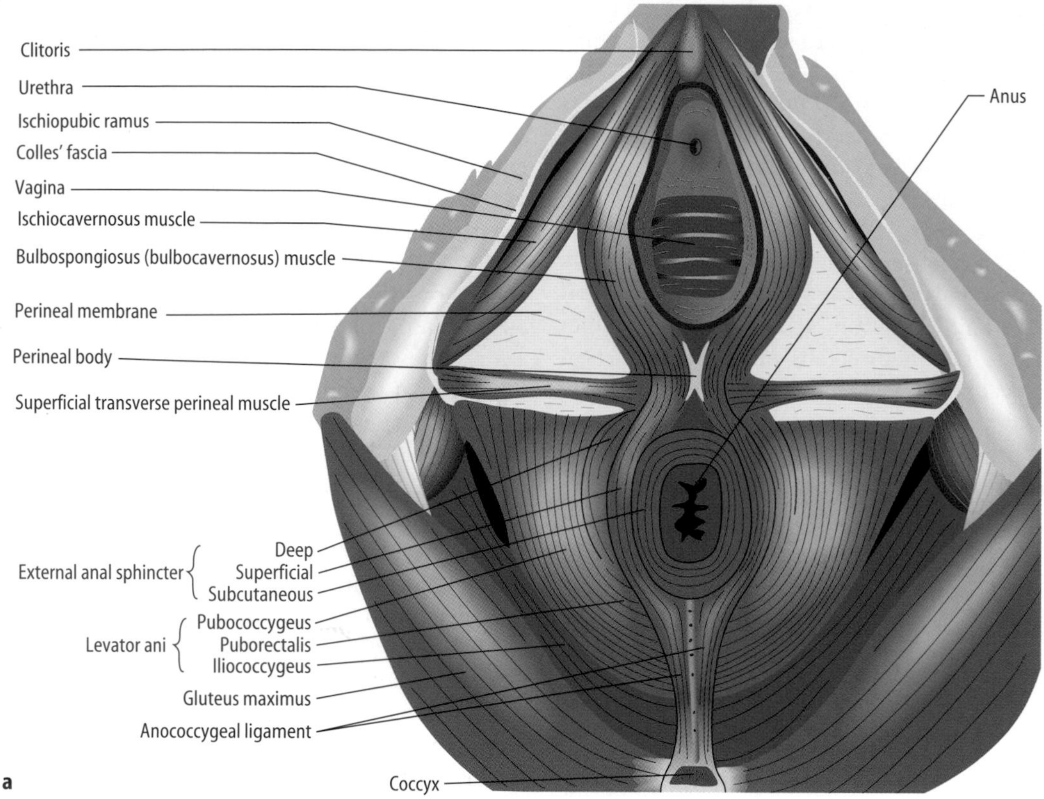

Clitoris

Urethra

Ischiopubic ramus

Colles' fascia

Vagina

Ischiocavernosus muscle

Bulbospongiosus (bulbocavernosus) muscle

Perineal membrane

Perineal body

Superficial transverse perineal muscle

Anus

External anal sphincter
{
Deep
Superficial
Subcutaneous
}

Levator ani
{
Pubococcygeus
Puborectalis
Iliococcygeus
}

Gluteus maximus

Anococcygeal ligament

a

Coccyx

Clitoris

Ischiopubic ramus

Bulbospongiosus muscle

Superficial perineal compartment

Ischial tuberosity

Vestibular bulb

Ischiocavernosus muscle

Perineal membrane

Bartholin's gland

Perineal body

External anal sphincter

Anococcygeal ligament

Coccyx

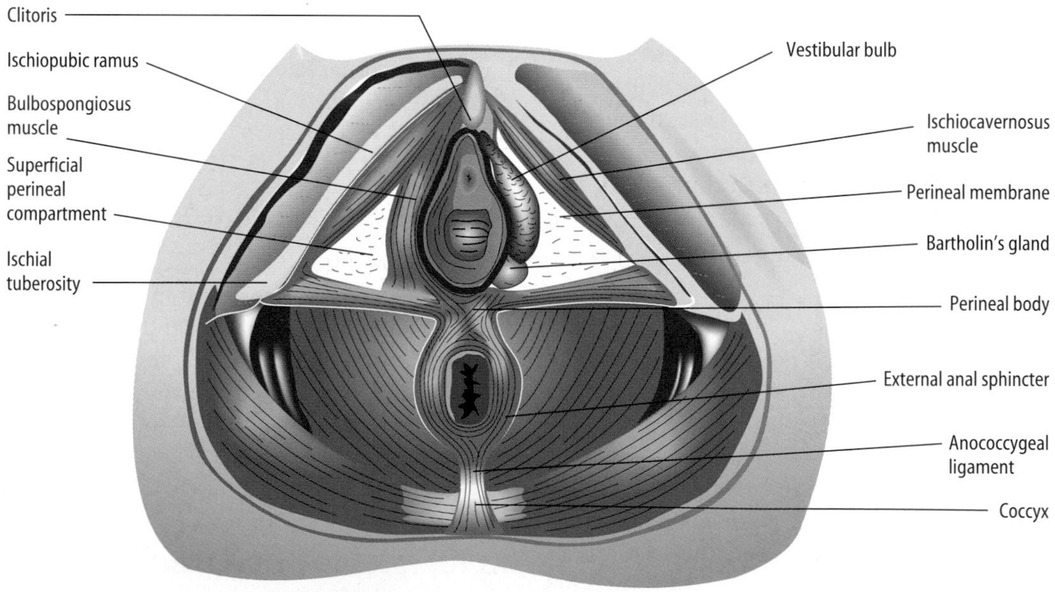

b

FIGURE 1.2. The superficial compartment contains the superficial transverse perineal muscle, the bulbospongiosus and the ischiocavernosus. These three muscles form a triangle on either side of the perineum, with a floor formed by the perineal membrane. (a) The left bulbospongiosus muscle has been removed to demonstrate the vestibular bulb and bartholin's gland (b).

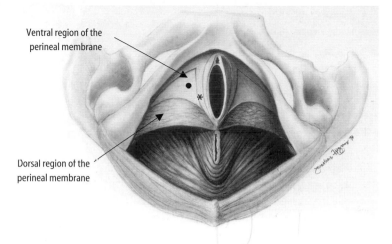

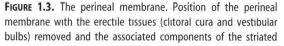

Ventral region of the
perineal membrane

Dorsal region of the
perineal membrane

FIGURE 1.3. The perineal membrane. Position of the perineal membrane with the erectile tissues (clitoral cura and vestibular bulbs) removed and the associated components of the striated urogenital sphincter and the urethrovaginal sphincter * and the compressor urethra •. (© Delancey, with permission.)

Bartholin's gland posteriorly (Figure 1.2b). Some fibres merge posteriorly with the superficial transverse perineal muscle and the EAS in the central fibromuscular perineal body. Anteriorly, its fibres pass forward on either side of the vagina and insert into the corpora cavernosa clitoridis, a fasciculus crossing over the body of the organ so as to compress the deep dorsal vein. This muscle diminishes the orifice of the vagina and contributes to the erection of the clitoris.

1.3.1.3 Ischiocavernosus Muscle

The ischiocavernosus muscle is elongated, broader at the middle than at either end, and is situated on the side of the lateral boundary of the perineum (Figure 1.2a). It arises by tendinous and fleshy fibres from the inner surface of the ischial tuberosity, behind the crus clitoridis, from the surface of the crus and from the adjacent portions of the ischial ramus. The ischiocavernosus compresses the crus clitoridis, retards blood flow through the veins, and thus serves to maintain erection of the clitoris.

1.3.2 The Anal Triangle

This area includes the anal canal, the anal sphincters, and ischioanal fossae.

1.3.2.1 Anal Canal

The rectum terminates in the anal canal (Figure 1.4a, b). Definitions of the anal canal vary among surgeons and anatomists.[6] The surgical anal canal is approximately 4 cm long and extends from the anal verge to the anorectal ring, which is defined as the proximal level of the levator–EAS complex.[7] This clinical description correlates with a digital or sonographic examination but does not correspond to the histological architecture.[8] The embryological anal canal extends from the anal valves (see below) to the anal margin and is approximately 2 cm long.[2]

The anal canal is attached posteriorly to the coccyx by the anococcygeal ligament, a midline fibromuscular structure, which runs between the posterior aspect of the EAS and the coccyx (Figure 1.2). The anus is surrounded laterally and posteriorly by loose adipose tissue within the ischioanal fossae, which is a potential pathway for spread of perianal sepsis from one side to the other. The pudendal nerves pass over the ischial spines at this point (Figure 1.5) and can be accessed digitally at this site for measurement of the pudendal nerve terminal motor latency using a modified electrode[9] (see Chapter 9). The perineum can also be anaesthetised by injection of local anaesthetic into the pudenal nerve at this site. Anteriorly, the perineal body separates the anal canal from the vagina.

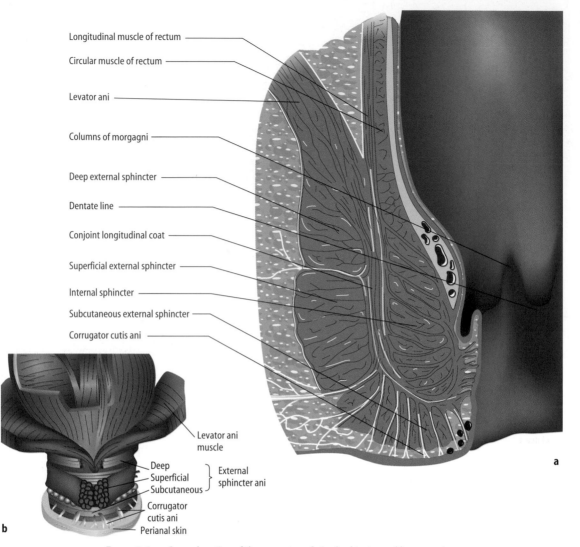

Longitudinal muscle of rectum

Circular muscle of rectum

Levator ani

Columns of morgagni

Deep external sphincter

Dentate line

Conjoint longitudinal coat

Superficial external sphincter

Internal sphincter

Subcutaneous external sphincter

Corrugator cutis ani

Levator ani muscle

Deep
Superficial   } External
Subcutaneous   sphincter ani

Corrugator cutis ani

Perianal skin

b

a

FIGURE 1.4. **a** Coronal section of the anorectum. **b** Anal sphincter and levator ani.

The anal canal is surrounded by an inner epithelial lining, a vascular subepithelium, internal anal sphincter (IAS), EAS and fibromuscular supporting tissue. The lining of the anal canal varies along its length due to its embryologic derivation. The proximal anal canal is lined with rectal mucosa (columnar epithelium) and is arranged in vertical mucosal folds called the columns of Morgagni (Figure 1.4a). Each column contains a terminal radical of the superior rectal artery and vein. The vessels are largest in the left-lateral, right-posterior and right-anterior quadrants of

the wall of the anal canal where the subepithelial tissues expand into three *anal cushions*. These cushions seal the anal canal and help maintain continence of flatus and liquid stools. The columns are joined together at their inferior margin by crescentic folds called anal valves.[2] About 2 cm from the anal verge, the anal valves create a demarcation called the dentate line. Anoderm covers the last 1–1.5 cm of the distal canal below the dentate line and consists of modified squamous epithelium that lacks skin adnexal tissues such as hair follicles and glands, but contains

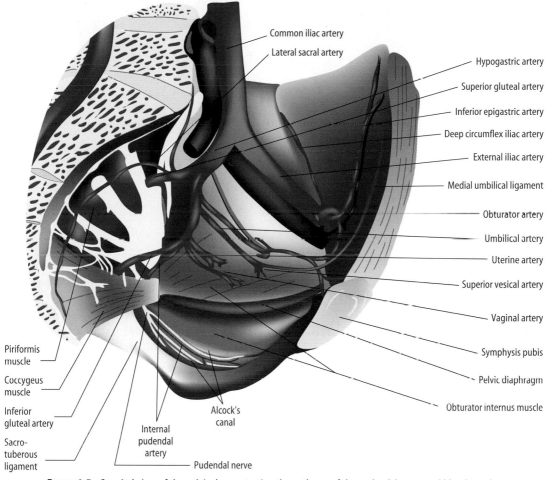

Common iliac artery
Lateral sacral artery
Hypogastric artery
Superior gluteal artery
Inferior epigastric artery
Deep circumflex iliac artery
External iliac artery
Medial umbilical ligament
Obturator artery
Umbilical artery
Uterine artery
Superior vesical artery
Vaginal artery
Symphysis pubis
Pelvic diaphragm
Obturator internus muscle

Piriformis muscle
Coccygeus muscle
Inferior gluteal artery
Sacro-tuberous ligament
Internal pudendal artery
Alcock's canal
Pudendal nerve

FIGURE 1.5. Saggital view of the pelvis demonstrating the pathway of the pudendal nerve and blood supply.

numerous somatic nerve endings. Since the epithelium in the lower canal is well supplied with sensory nerve endings, acute distension or invasive treatment of haemorrhoids in this area causes profuse discomfort, whereas treatment can be carried out with relatively few symptoms in the upper canal lined by insensate columnar epithelium.[9] As a result of tonic circumferential contraction of the sphincter, the skin is arranged in radiating folds around the anus and is called the anal margin.[8] These folds appear to be flat or ironed out when there is underlying sphincter damage. The junction between the columnar and squamous epithelia is referred to as the anal transitional zone, which is variable in height and position and often contains islands of squamous

epithelium extending into columnar epithelium. This zone probably has a role to play in continence by providing a highly specialised sampling mechanism (see Chapter 8).

1.3.2.2 Anal Sphincter Complex

The anal sphincter complex consists of the EAS and IAS separated by the conjoint longitudinal coat (Figure 1.4a). Although they form a single unit, they are distinct in structure and function.

External Anal Sphincter

Structurally, the EAS (Figure 1.4a) is subdivided into three parts: the subcutaneous, superficial and

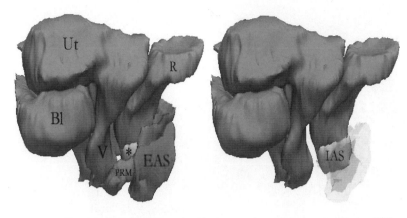

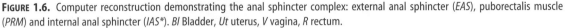

FIGURE 1.6. Computer reconstruction demonstrating the anal sphincter complex: external anal sphincter (*EAS*), puborectalis muscle (*PRM*) and internal anal sphincter (*IAS**). *Bl* Bladder, *Ut* uterus, *V* vagina, *R* rectum.

deep.[10] However, these subdivisions are not easily demonstrable during anatomical dissection or surgery, but may be of relevance during imaging (see Chapter 10). In females, the EAS is shorter anteriorly (Figure 1.6).[11] The deep EAS is intimately related to the puborectalis muscle and does not have posterior attachments.[12] The superficial EAS is attached posteriorly to the anococcygeal ligament, which is attached to the tip of the coccyx.[9] The subcutaneous part is circular but may have attachments to the perineal body anteriorly and the anococcygeal ligament posteriorly. In females, the bulbospongiosus and the transverse perineii fuse with the EAS in the lower part of the perineum.[9]

Internal Anal Sphincter

The IAS is a thickened continuation of the circular smooth muscle of the bowel and ends with a well-defined rounded edge 6–8 mm above the anal margin at the junction of the superficial and subcutaneous part of the EAS (Figure 1.4a). In contrast to the EAS, the IAS has a pale appearance to the naked eye.

The Longitudinal Layer and the Conjoint Longitudinal Coat

The longitudinal layer is situated between the EAS and IAS and consists of a fibromuscular layer, the conjoint longitudinal coat and the intersphincteric space with its connective tissue components[13] (Figure 1.4a). The longitudinal layer has a muscular and fibroelastic component. The muscular component is formed by the fusion of the striated muscle fibres from the puboanalis, the innermost part of the puborectalis with smooth muscle from the longitudinal muscle of the rectum.[9] Traced downwards, it separates opposite the lower border of the IAS and the fibrous septae fan out to pass through the EAS and ultimately attach to the skin of the lower anal canal and perianal region.[10]

1.3.2.3 Innervation of the Anal Sphincter Complex

As the IAS is a continuation of the circular fibres of the rectum, it shares the same innervation: sympathetic (L5) and parasympathetic nerves (S2–S4). It remains in a state of tonic contraction and accounts for 50–85% of the resting tone.[7] The conjoint longitudinal coat is innervated by autonomic fibres from the same origin. The EAS is innervated by the inferior rectal branch of the pudendal nerve. In contrast to the other striated muscles, the EAS contributes up to 30% of the unconscious resting tone through a reflex arc at the cauda equine level.

1.3.2.4 Vascular Supply

The anorectum receives its major blood supply from the superior (terminal branch of the inferior mesenteric artery) and inferior haemorrhoidal (branch of the pudendal artery) arteries, and to a lesser degree, from the middle haemorrhoidal artery (branch of the internal iliac), forming a wide intramural network of collaterals.[14] The venous drainage of the upper anal canal mucosa, IAS and conjoint longitudinal coat passes via the terminal branches of the superior rectal vein into the inferior mesenteric vein. The lower anal canal and the EAS drain via the inferior rectal branch of the pudendal vein into the internal iliac vein.[9]

1.3.2.5 Lymphatic Drainage

The anorectum has a rich network of lymphatic plexuses. The dentate line represents the interface between the two different systems of lymphatic drainage. Above the dentate line (the upper anal canal), the IAS and the conjoint longitudinal coat drain into the inferior mesenteric and internal iliac nodes. Lymphatic drainage below the dentate line, which consists of the lower anal canal epithelium and the EAS, proceeds to the external inguinal lymph nodes.

1.3.2.6 Ischioanal Fossa

The ischioanal fossa (previously known as the "ischiorectal fossa") extends around the anal canal and is bound anteriorly by the perineal membrane, superiorly by the fascia of the levator ani muscle and medially by the EAS complex at the level of the anal canal. The lateral border is formed by the obturator fascia and inferiorly by a thin transverse fascia, which separates it from the perianal space. The ischioanal fossa contains fat and neurovascular structures, including the pudendal nerve and the internal pudendal vessels, which enter through Alcocks's canal.[8]

1.4 Perineal Body

The perineal body is the central point between the urogenital and the anal triangles of the perineum (Figure 1.2). Its three-dimensional form has been likened to that of the cone of the red pine, with each "petal" representing an interlocking structure, such as an insertion site of fascia or a muscle of the perineum.[15] Within the perineal body there are interlacing muscle fibres from the bulbospongiosus, superficial transverse perineal, and EAS muscles. Above this level there is a contribution from the conjoint longitudinal coat and the medial fibres of the puborectalis muscle. Therefore, the

support of the pelvic structures, and to some extent the hiatus urogenitalis between the levator ani muscles, depends upon the integrity of the perineal body.

1.5 The Pelvic Floor

The pelvic floor (pelvic diaphragm) is a musculo-tendineous sheet that spans the pelvic outlet and consists mainly of the symmetrically paired levator ani (Figure 1.7). The fasciae investing the muscles are continuous with visceral pelvic fascia above, perineal fascia below, and obturator fascia laterally. The pelvic floor supports the urogenital organs and the anorectum, exiting the pelvis through their respective foramen. The muscles of the levator ani differ from most other skeletal muscles in that they: (1) maintain constant tone, except during voiding, defaecation and the Valsalva manoeuvre; (2) have the ability to contract quickly at the time of acute stress (such as a cough or sneeze) to maintain continence; and (3) distend considerably during parturition to allow the passage of the term infant and then contract after delivery to resume normal functioning.[16]

The levator ani (Figure 1.7) is a broad muscular sheet of variable thickness attached to the internal surface of the true pelvis and is subdivided into parts according to their attachments and pelvic viscera to which they are related, namely iliococcygeus, pubococcygeus and ischiococcygeus.[4] Although referred to as separate muscles, the boundaries between the different parts cannot be easily distinguished and they perform many similar physiological functions.

The ischiococcygeus part (sometimes named coccygeus) may be considered as a separate muscle. It is a narrow triangular sheet of muscular and tendinous fibres, its apex arising from the spine of the ischium and sacrospinous ligament, and its base inserting into the margin of the coccyx and into the side of the lowest piece of the sacrum. It assists the levator ani and piriformis in closing in the back of the pelvic outlet.

The iliococcygeus muscle is the lateral component of the levator ani muscle and arises from the ischial spine below and anterior to the attachment of the ischiococcygeus and to the obturator fascia as far forward as the obturator canal. The most

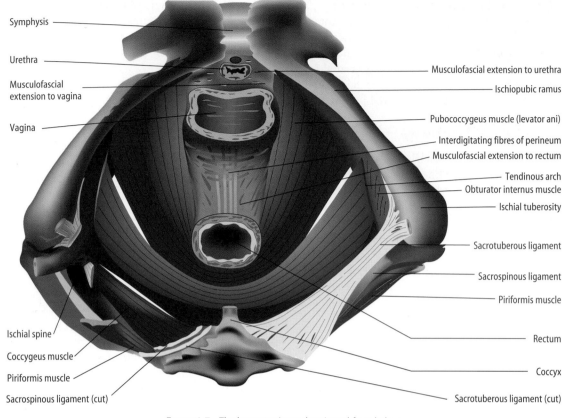

Symphysis

Urethra

Musculofascial
extension to vagina

Vagina

Musculofascial extension to urethra

Ischiopubic ramus

Pubococcygeus muscle (levator ani)

Interdigitating fibres of perineum
Musculofascial extension to rectum

Tendinous arch
Obturator internus muscle

Ischial tuberosity

Sacrotuberous ligament

Sacrospinous ligament

Piriformis muscle

Rectum

Coccyx

Ischial spine

Coccygeus muscle

Piriformis muscle

Sacrospinous ligament (cut)

Sacrotuberous ligament (cut)

FIGURE 1.7. The levator ani muscles viewed from below.

posterior fibres are attached to the coccyx and the sacrum, but most join with fibres from the opposite side to form a raphe, which is more or less continuous with the fibroelastic anococcygeal ligament, and is attached to the coccyx and anococcygeal raphe. The pubococcygeus arises from the back of the pubis and from the anterior part of the obturator fascia, and is directed backward almost horizontally along the side of the anal canal toward the coccyx and sacrum, to which it finds attachment. The greater part of this muscle is inserted into the coccyx and into the last one or two pieces of the sacrum. The pubococcygeus is often subdivided into separate parts according to the pelvic viscera to which they relate (i.e. pubourethralis and puborectalis in the male, pubovaginalis and puborectalis in the female). The most medial fibres of the pubococcygeus form a sling around the rectum and are named the puborectalis. The puborectalis is the most caudal component of the levator ani complex. It is situated cephalad to

the deep component of the EAS, from which it is almost inseparable (Figures 1.4a, b, 1.6). Thus the puborectalis serves both functions: as part of the sphincter mechanism and the pelvic floor. The U-shaped sling of striated muscle pulls the anorectal junction anteriorly to the posterior aspect of the pubis,[7] resulting in an angulation between the rectal and anal canal called the anorectal angle. There is considerable controversy as to the importance of this angle in the maintenance of continence.[17] Between the two arms of the puborectalis lies the levator hiatus, through which the rectum, vagina and urethra pass.

In the female, the anterior fibres of the levator ani descend upon the side of the vagina. These fibres have been called the puboperineal muscle and appear to undergo the greatest stretch during vaginal delivery. They have been found to be damaged in women with urinary incontinence and pelvic organ prolapse following delivery.[18]

1.5.1 Innervation of the Levator Ani

Although widely believed that the levator ani is supplied on its superior surface by the sacral nerve roots (S2–S4) and on its inferior surface by the perineal branch of the pudendal nerve, recent cadaveric dissections along with nerve staining studies have shown that the female levator ani is not innervated by the pudendal nerve, but rather by innervation that originates in the sacral nerve roots (S3–S5) and travels on the superior surface of the pelvic floor (levator ani nerve).[16]

The most common arrangement appears to be that the pubococcygeus is supplied by second and third sacral spinal segments via the pudendal nerve, and the ischiococcygeus and iliococcygeus by direct branches from third and fourth sacral spinal segments.[4]

1.5.2 Vascular Supply

The levator ani is supplied by branches of the inferior gluteal artery, the inferior vesical artery and the pudendal artery.

1.6 The Pudendal Nerve

The pudendal nerve derives its fibres from the ventral branches of the second, third and fourth sacral nerves and leaves the pelvis through the lower part of the greater sciatic foramen (Figure 1.5). It then crosses the ischial spine and re-enters the pelvis through the lesser sciatic foramen. It accompanies the internal pudendal vessels upward and forward along the lateral wall of the ischioanal fossa, contained in a sheath of the obturator fascia termed Alcock's canal (Figure 1.5). It is presumed that during a prolonged second stage of labour, the pudendal nerve is vulnerable to stretch injury due to its relative immobility at this site.

The inferior haemorrhoidal (rectal) nerve then branches off posteriorly from the pudendal nerve to innervate the EAS (Figure 1.8). The pudendal nerve then divides into two terminal branches: the perineal nerve and the dorsal nerve of the clitoris. The perineal nerve, the inferior and larger of the two terminal branches of the pudendal, is located

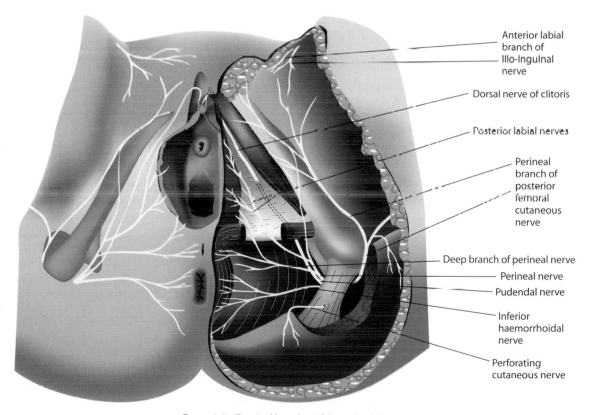

FIGURE 1.8. Terminal branches of the pudendal nerve.

below the internal pudendal artery. It divides into posterior labial and muscular branches. The posterior labial branches supply the labium majora. The muscular branches are distributed to the superficial transverse perineal, bulbospongiosus, ischiocavernosus and constrictor urethræ muscles. Branches from the perineal division frequently innervate the anterior EAS as well. The dorsal nerve of the clitoris, which supplies the clitoris, is the deepest division of the pudendal nerve (Figure 1.8).

1.7   Conclusion

An understanding of the anatomy of the pelvic floor, anal sphincters and perineum is essential for health care providers caring for women during and after vaginal delivery. Proper perineal and sphincter repair requires clear visualisation of the structures of the perineal body and sphincter muscles. When trauma occurs, the practitioner must be aware of the relationships between nerves, muscles and vessels in order to restore at best, normal anatomy and function.

References

1. Lunsman HH, Robertson EG. Evolution of the pelvic floor. In: Thomas Benson JT, ed. Female pelvic floor disorders. New York, London: Norton Medical Books, 1992, pp 3–18.
2. Cook TA, Mortenson N. Colon, rectum, anus, anal sphincters and the pelvic floor. The pelvic floor: its function and disorders. In: Pemberton AH, Swash M, Henry MM, eds. London: Harcourt Publishers Limited, 2002, pp 61–76.
3. The urogenital system. In: Moore K, ed. The developing human, 2nd edn. London: WB Saunders, 1977, pp 232–7.
4. True pelvis, pelvic floor and perineum. In: Standring S, ed. Grays's anatomy, 39th edn. London: Elsevier, Churchill Livingstone, 2005, pp 1357–71.
5. Stein TA, DeLancey JOL. Structure of the perineal membrane in females: histologic, anatomic, and MRI findings. Oral Presentation, American Urogynecologic Society Annual Meeting, San Diego, California, 28 July 2004.
6. Wendall-Smith CP. Anorectal nomenclature: fundamental terminology. Dis Colon Rectum 2000;43:1349–58.
7. Wexner SD, Jorge JMN. Anatomy and embryology of the anus, rectum and colon. In: Corman ML, ed. Colon and rectal surgery. Philadelphia: Lippincott-Raven, 1998, pp 1–26.
8. Kaiser AM, Ortega AE. Anorectal anatomy. Surg Clin N Am 2002;82:1125–38.
9. Anal canal. In: Standring S, ed. Grays's anatomy, 39th edn. London: Elsevier, Churchill Livingstone, 2005, pp 1205–11.
10. Milligan ETC, Morgan CN. Surgical anatomy of the anal canal with special reference to anorectal fistulae. Lancet 1934;2:150–6,1213–17.
11. Sultan AH, Kamm MA. Ultrasound of the anal sphincter. In: Schuster MM, ed. Atlas of gastrointestinal motility. Baltimore: William and Wilkins, 1993.
12. Bogduk N. Issues in anatomy: the EAS revisited. Aust N Z J Surg 1996;66:626–9.
13. Lunniss PJ, Phillips RKS. Anatomy and function of the anal longitudinal muscle. Br J Surg 1992;79:882–4.
14. Lund JN, Binch C, McGrath J et al. Topographical distribution of the blood supply to the anal canal. Br J Urol 1999;86:496–8.
15. Woodman P, Graney AO. Anatomy and physiology of the female perineal body with relevance to obstetrical injury and repair. Clin Anat 2002;15:321–34.
16. Barber MD, Bremer RE, Thor KB et al. Innervation of the female levator ani muscles. Am J Obstet Gynecol 2002;187:64–71.
17. Bartolo DCC, Macdonald ADH. Faecal incontinence and defecation. The pelvic floor: its function and disorders. In: Pemberton AH, Swash M, Henry MM, eds. London: Harcourt Publishers Limited, 2002, pp 77–83.
18. Kearney R, Sawhney R, Delancey JOL. Levator ani muscle anatomy evaluated by origin-insertion pairs. Obstet Gynecol 2004;104:168–73.

2
Diagnosis of Perineal Trauma

Abdul H. Sultan and Christine Kettle

2.1 Prevalence

More than 85% of women sustain some form of perineal trauma during vaginal delivery in the UK.[1] However, the prevalence is dependent on variations in obstetric practice, including rates of episiotomy, which vary not only between countries but also between individual practitioners within hospitals. In the Netherlands, the rate of episiotomy is 8% compared to 14% in England, 50% in the USA and 99% in East European countries.[2–4] Episiotomy rates also vary between hospitals in the same country: for example, in the USA the rates varied between 20% and 70% in individual units.[5]

2.2 Classification

Previous classifications of perineal trauma particularly in the UK have been inconsistent. Sultan and Thakar systematically reviewed all relevant obstetric text books in the library of The Royal College of Obstetricians & Gynaecologists (RCOG) and found that 17% did not mention any classification, while 22% classified anal sphincter injury as "second degree".[6]

Fernando et al.[7] surveyed 672 consultants in active obstetric practice and found that 33% classified a complete or partial external sphincter tear as "second degree". There was up to a tenfold regional variation in the "misclassification" and a distinct increasing trend towards the northern parts of the UK whereby a complete external anal sphincter tear was considered to be a second degree tear. This may reflect the teachings of Professor Ian Donald[8] from Glasgow, who defined a third degree tear as one in which both the anal sphincter and anal mucosa were torn.

In order to standardise the classification of perineal trauma, Sultan[9] proposed the classification shown in Figure 2.1, which has been adopted by the RCOG[10] and also internationally.[11] The classification is depicted in a schematic representation of the anal sphincter complex (Figure 2.2). The intact anal sphincter appears as a circular band of muscle (Figure 2.3a) that can be demonstrated by insertion of a finger in the anal canal (Figure 2.3b).

Isolated tears of the anal epithelium (buttonhole) and vagina but without involvement of the anal sphincters are rare[12] (Figure 2.4). In order to avoid confusion, such tears are not included in the above classification.

It is also possible to sustain a full-thickness third degree tear that only involves part of the length of the anal sphincter (Figure 2.5). In such circumstances or situations when the clinician is doubtful, the higher classification should be selected. For example, if there is uncertainty between a 3a and 3b tear, the tear should be classified as 3b.

Some refer to first and second degree tears as minor perineal trauma as opposed to major perineal trauma for third and fourth degree tears. However, as alluded to in Chapter 4, second degree tears can extend to become complex tears.

First degree: laceration of the vaginal epithelium or perineal skin only.

Second degree: involvement of the perineal muscles but not the anal sphincter.

Third degree: disruption of the anal sphincter muscles which should be further subdivided into:

> **3a:** <50% thickness of external sphincter torn.
> **3b:** >50% thickness of external sphincter torn.
> **3c:** internal sphincter also torn.

Fourth degree: a third degree tear with disruption of the anal epithelium as well.

FIGURE 2.1. Classification of perineal trauma.[9–11]

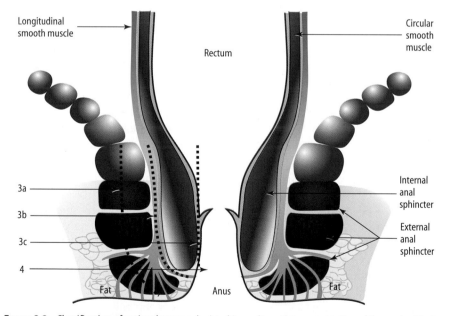

FIGURE 2.2. Classification of perineal trauma depicted in a schematic representation of the anal sphincters.

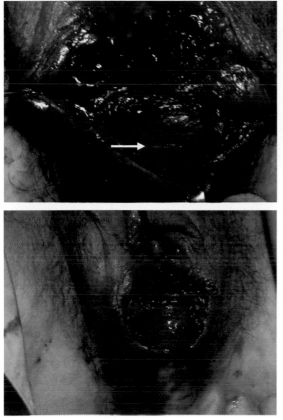

a

b

FIGURE 2.3. An intact anal sphincter (*arrow* in **a**) is demonstrated more clearly during a digital rectal examination (**b**).

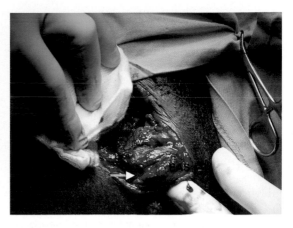

FIGURE 2.5. A partial tear (*arrow*) along the length of the external anal sphincter.

2.3 Objective Assessment of Perineal Trauma

The Birmingham Perineal Research Evaluation Group (BPREG) developed the Peri-Rule as part of their work to aid the assessment and objective measurement of second degree tears. The tool consists of a measuring device (Peri-Rule) and assessment proforma. The Peri-Rule is made of hollow, soft medical-grade plastic with a millimetre scale moulded on one side (105 mm long, 10 mm wide and 4 mm deep) and it can be sterilised; however, it is for single use only. The assessment proforma guides the midwife through each stage of the assessment procedure with clear diagrams illustrating the three measurements required (the depth of the tear from the fourchette into the greatest depth of the perineal body, the length of the tear from the fourchette to the apex of the tear of the vaginal wall and along the perineal skin towards the anus), in a specific order to reduce the risk of infection.

During the development phase, the inter-rater reliability of the Peri-Rule was assessed by requesting two midwives to measure the perineal tear, the second midwife being blinded to the results of the first midwife's assessment and measurements. There was a good level of agreement between the two raters (within 5 mm of each other) when measuring the three dimensions of perineal tears ($n = 130$), which were assessed using Cohen's Kappa (K) statistic (depth of tear $K = 0.67$

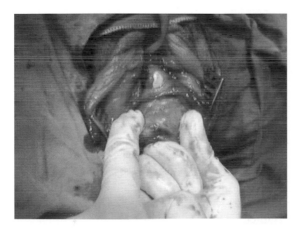

FIGURE 2.4. A "buttonhole" tear of the rectal mucosa (*arrow*) with an intact external anal sphincter demonstrated during a digital rectal examination (with permission).[12]

$[P < 0.05]$; vaginal wall length $K = 0.71$ $[P < 0.05]$ and perineal skin length $K = 0.75$ $[P < 0.05]$). The researchers also found that the mean size of second degree tears that were sutured was significantly higher than those that were left unsutured for all three measurements taken ($P < 0.001$ for depth, vaginal tear length and perineal tear length).[13]

The midwives who used the Peri-Rule found that it was easy and quick to use and that it assisted them in making a thorough assessment of the perineal trauma. Moreover, several experienced midwives reported that the Peri-Rule aided them in diagnosing third degree tears, which they had missed prior to assessment with the measuring tool. The Peri-Rule and proforma provides practitioners with an objective tool that encourages a standardised approach to perineal assessment and enables accurate measurement and documentation of second degree tears. The measurement tool is of particular value when recording objective baseline data for research or audit that is specifically related to the management of perineal trauma.

Further research work is currently underway to assess the use of Peri-Rule in relation to measuring more complex tears and episiotomies and to establish if the length of the perineum (from the fourchette to the anus) has any influence on the type and size of perineal trauma sustained. In addition, more work is planned to evaluate the efficacy of using the tool as part of routine perineal assessment compared to standard midwifery practice (S. Tohill, personal communication, 2005).

2.4 Making an Accurate Clinical Diagnosis

1. Informed consent should be obtained for a vaginal and rectal examination.

2. There must be good exposure of the perineal injury and, if this is not possible, the woman should be placed in lithotomy.

3. Good lighting is essential.

4. If the examination is restricted because of pain, adequate analgesia must be given prior to examination.

5. Following a visual examination of the genitalia, the labia should be parted and a vaginal examination performed to establish the full extent of the vaginal tear. When multiple or deep tears are present, it is best to examine and repair in lithotomy. The apex of the vaginal laceration should always be identified.

6. A rectal examination should then be performed (Figure 2.3b) to exclude injury to the anorectal mucosa and anal sphincter. The vagina should be exposed by parting the labia with the index and middle fingers of the other hand. We believe that every woman should have a rectal examination prior to suturing in order to avoid missing isolated tears such as "buttonhole" tears of the rectal mucosa (Figure 2.4). As can be seen in Figure 2.4, there is a rectal laceration with an intact anal sphincter. Furthermore, a third or fourth degree tear may be present beneath apparently intact perineal skin (Figure 2.6a, b, c), highlighting the need to perform a rectal examination in order to exclude obstetric anal sphincter injuries (OASIS).

7. In order to diagnose OASIS, clear visualisation is necessary and the injury should be confirmed by palpation. By inserting the index finger in the anal canal and the thumb in the vagina, the anal sphincter can be palpated by performing a pill-rolling motion. If there is still uncertainty, the woman should be asked to contract her anal sphincter and if the anal sphincter is disrupted, a distinct gap will be felt anteriorly. If the perineal skin is intact, there will be an absence of puckering on the perianal skin anteriorly. This may not be evident under regional or general anaesthesia. As the external anal sphincter (EAS) is in a state of tonic contraction, disruption results in retraction of the sphincter ends. Therefore, the sphincter ends need to be grasped and retrieved. The internal anal sphincter (IAS) should also be identified and repaired separately.

8. The IAS is a circular smooth muscle (Figure 2.7) that appears paler (similar to raw fish) than the striated EAS (similar to raw red meat). Under normal circumstances, the distal end of the IAS lies a few millimetres proximal to the distal end of the EAS. However, if the EAS is relaxed following regional or general anaesthesia, the distal end of the IAS will appear to be at a lower level. If the IAS or anal epithelium is torn, the EAS will invariably be torn.

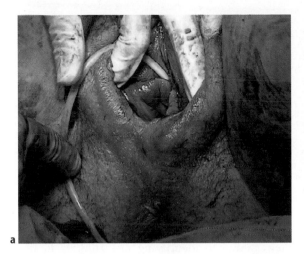

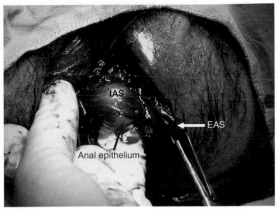

FIGURE 2.7. A grade 3b tear with an intact internal anal sphincter (*IAS*). The external sphincter (*EAS*) is being grasped with Allis forceps. Note the difference in appearance of the paler IAS and darker EAS.

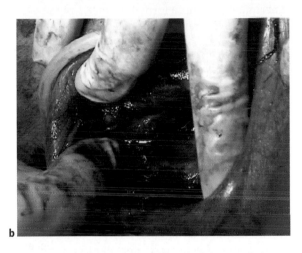

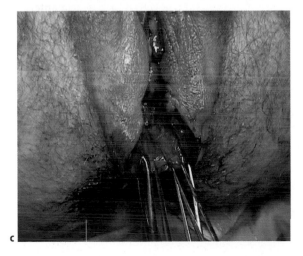

FIGURE 2.6. Third degree tear with an apparent intact perineum. (a) A "bucket handle" tear is demonstrated behind the intact perineal skin (b). The torn external sphincter is shown (c).

2.5 "Occult" OASIS

Following the advent of endoanal ultrasound (see Chapter 10), Sultan et al.[14] demonstrated that 33% of women sustained "occult" OASIS that were not identified at delivery (see Chapter 8 for pathophysiology). Prospective studies[11] have identified "occult" injuries ranging between 20[15] and 41%.[16] However, it remained to be established whether these injuries were truly occult or in fact unrecognised at delivery. Andrews et al.[17] reported a study in which 241 women having their first vaginal delivery had their perineum re-examined by an experienced research fellow and endoanal ultrasound was performed immediately after delivery and repeated 7 weeks postpartum. When OASIS were identified by the research fellow, the injuries were confirmed and repaired by the duty registrar or consultant. The prevalence of clinically diagnosed OASIS increased from 11% to 25% ($n = 59$). Every clinically diagnosed injury was identified by postpartum endoanal ultrasound. However, there were three women with sonographic defects in whom the injury was not identified clinically. Two of these had only small IAS defects with an intact EAS; one would not expect to detect these clinically. The other was a defect of both the IAS and

EAS and this could represent an occult but most probably an undiagnosed tear. At 7 weeks no de novo defects were identified by ultrasound. This study concluded that most sphincter defects that have previously been designated as "occult" injuries were in fact injuries that could have been recognisable at delivery but were not identified.

It was alarming to find that 87% and 27% of OASIS were not identified by midwives and doctors respectively. Although it is likely that some of these would have been detected at the time of suturing the tear, it is of some concern that clinical recognition of OASIS is suboptimal. This finding is not unique, as Groom and Paterson-Brown[18] found that the rate of third degree tears rose to 15% when all "second degree tears" were re-examined by a second experienced person.

These studies[17,18] suggest that there is a need for more focused and intensive training in the identification of OASIS. Sultan et al.[19] conducted an interview of 75 doctors and 75 midwives and reported that 91% and 60% respectively indicated inadequate training in perineal anatomy and 84% and 61% respectively reported inadequate training in identifying third degree tears.

However, there are also other possible reasons for underdiagnosis. Misclassification of OASIS as second degree has already been alluded to above. A further reason for under-reporting by the accoucheur is the stigma associated with OASIS. In many units, OASIS constitute a risk management trigger that may be regarded as punitive and it is therefore a disincentive to accurate reporting.

If OASIS are being missed, one would expect to see more women with anal incontinence, who apparently had only an episiotomy or a spontaneous second degree tear. Lal et al.[20] showed that significantly more women develop anal incontinence following a second degree tear than with an intact perineum (23% vs 3%, $P = 0.01$). Benifla et al.[21] identified a 16-fold increase in anal incontinence following a second degree tear ($P < 0.05$). Both these studies support the findings of Andrews et al. that a large number of OASIS were undiagnosed and wrongly classified as second degree tears.

2.6 Can Routine Anal Endosonography Immediately after Delivery Improve Accuracy in Detection of OASIS?

Faltin et al.[22] randomised 752 primiparous women with second degree lacerations to conventional examination (control group) and additional postpartum endoanal ultrasound (experimental group) and demonstrated that a considerable number of women have full-thickness OASIS that are not recognised at delivery. However, they excluded partial-thickness sphincter tears from their study. On identifying new injuries in the experimental group, a formal sphincter repair was performed. Overall, severe faecal incontinence was significantly reduced from 8.7% in the control group to 3.3% in the experimental group.

However, endoanal ultrasound is a technique that requires specific expertise, particularly in the immediate postpartum period when the anal canal is lax (even more with an epidural). Ultimately, the diagnosis rests on clinical assessment and a rectal examination because even if a defect is seen on ultrasound, it has to be clinically apparent to be repaired. As Faltin et al.[22] found in their study, when routine postpartum anal endosonography was used as the gold standard of diagnosing OASIS, five women had unnecessary intervention as the sonographic defect was not clinically visible despite exploration of the anal sphincter. As a result of this unnecessary exploration based on anal endosonography, 20% developed severe faecal incontinence. We therefore believe that with improvement in clinical diagnostic skills, detection of OASIS immediately after delivery can be significantly improved[17] and in practice, postpartum anal endosonography is of limited value. It would be prudent to divert resources towards clinical training (see Chapter 4) instead of attempting to teach new trainees the art of postpartum anal endosonography with its attendant limitations.[23]

2.7 Conclusions

We believe that current concepts need reappraisal and in particular, the stigma of causing OASIS needs to be removed. Causing a third or fourth degree tear is rarely culpable; missing it, however, is regarded as negligent. Postpartum endoanal ultrasound is an invasive and expensive alternative that requires expertise and may result in overdiagnosis of OASIS that cannot be identified clinically.[18] The keystone to diagnosis of OASIS lies in improved clinical training of doctors and midwives (see Chapter 4). To minimise the risk of undiagnosed OASIS, a digital anorectal examination should be performed in every woman following vaginal delivery and certainly prior to any suturing.[17,23]

References

1. McCandlish R, Bowler U, van Asten H et al. A randomised controlled trial of care of the perineum during second stage of normal labour. Br J Obstet Gynaecol 1998;105:1262–72.

2. Wagner M. Pursuing the birth machine: the search for appropriate technology. Camperdown: ACE Graphics, 1994, pp 165–74.

3. Statistical Bulletin – NHS Maternity Services. London: Department of Health, 2003.

4. Graves EJ, Kozak LJ. National hospital discharge survey: annual summary, 1996. Vital Health Stat 1999;13:1–46.

5. Webb DA, Culhane J. Hospital variation in episiotomy use and the risk of perineal trauma during childbirth. Birth 2002;29(2):132–6.

6. Sultan AH, Thakar R. Lower genital tract and anal sphincter trauma. Best Pract & Res – Clin Obstet Gynaecol 2002;16:99–116.

7. Fernando RJ, Sultan AH, Radley S, Jones PW, Johanson RB. Management of obstetric anal sphincter injury: a systematic review and national practice survey. BMC Health Serv Res 2002;2(1):9.

8. Donald I. Practical obstetric problems, 5th edn. London: Lloyd-Luke Ltd, 1979, pp 811–24.

9. Sultan AH. Obstetric perineal injury and anal incontinence. Clinical Risk 1999;5:193–6.

10. Royal College of Obstetricians & Gynaecologists. Management of third and fourth degree perineal tears following vaginal delivery. Guideline no 29. London: RCOG Press, 2001.

11. Norton C, Christensen J, Butler U et al. Anal incontinence. Incontinence, 2nd edn. Plymouth: Health Publications Ltd, 2005, pp 985–1044.

12. Sultan AH. Primary repair of obstetric anal sphincter injury. In: Staskin D, Cardozo L, eds. Textbook of female urology and urogynaecology. London: ISIS Medical Media, 2006 (in press).

13. Metcalfe A, Tohill S, Williams A, Haldon V, Brown L, Henry L. A pragmatic tool for the measurement of perineal tears. Br J Midwifery 2002;10(7):412–7.

14. Sultan AH, Kamm MA, Hudson CN, Thomas JM, Bartram CI. Anal sphincter disruption during vaginal delivery. N Engl J Med 1993;329:1905–11.

15. Zetterstrom J, Mellgren A, Jensen LJ, Wong WD, Kim DG, Lowry AC, Madoff RD, Congilosi SM. Effect of delivery on anal sphincter morphology and function. Dis Colon Rectum 1999;42:1253–60.

16. Rieger N, Schloithe A, Saccone G, Wattchow D. A prospective study of anal sphincter injury due to childbirth. Scand J Gastroenterol 1998;33:950–5.

17. Andrews V, Sultan AH, Thakar R, Jones P. Occult anal sphincter injuries – myth or reality? Br J Obstet Gynaecol 2006;113:195–200.

18. Groom KM, Paterson-Brown S. Can we improve on the diagnosis of third degree tears? Eur J Obstet Gynecol Reprod Biol 2002;101(1):19–21.

19. Sultan AH, Kamm MA, Hudson CN. Obstetric perineal tears: an audit of training. J Obstet Gynaecol 1995;15:19–23.

20. Lal M, Mann Ch, Callender R, Radley S. Does cesarean delivery prevent anal incontinence? Obstet Gynecol 2003;101:305–12.

21. Benifla JL, Abramowitz L, Sobhani I et al. Postpartum sphincter rupture and anal incontinence: prospective study with 259 patients. Gynecol Obstet Fertil 2000;28(1):15–22.

22. Faltin DL, Boulvain M, Floris LA, Irion O. Diagnosis of anal sphincter tears to prevent fecal incontinence: a randomized controlled trial. Obstet Gynecol 2005;106(1):6–13.

23. Sultan AH, Thakar R. Diagnosis of anal sphincter tears to prevent fecal incontinence: a randomized controlled trial. Obstet Gynecol 2005;106:1108–9.

3
Repair of Episiotomy, First and Second Degree Tears

Christine Kettle and Dee E. Fenner

3.1 Introduction

The morbidity associated with perineal injury related to childbirth constitutes a major health problem, affecting millions of women worldwide. The majority of women following vaginal delivery will suffer some degree of perineal pain or discomfort during the early postpartum period.[1] In the UK alone, approximately 1,000 women per day will require perineal repair following vaginal birth. Pain associated with perineal trauma can be very distressing for the new mother and may interfere with her ability to breast feed and cope with the daily tasks of motherhood.[2] It also appears to have a clear causal association with sexual dysfunction and ultimately may affect the woman's relationship with her partner.

In the UK, up to 44% of women will continue to have pain and discomfort for 10 days following birth[3] and 10% of women will continue to have long-term pain at 18 months postpartum.[4] Furthermore, 23% of women will experience superficial dyspareunia at 3 months postpartum;[5] up to 10% will report faecal incontinence[6] and approximately 19% will have urinary problems.[7] The rates of complications reported by women depend on the severity of perineal trauma and on the effectiveness of treatment.

A North American, randomised controlled trial (RCT) of restrictive versus routine or liberal use of median episiotomy was performed by Klein and colleagues.[8] They found that spontaneous tears were less painful than episiotomies, both immediately postpartum and at 3 months follow-up. At 3 months postpartum, 42% of women with an intact perineum versus 53% with a spontaneous tear, 54% with an episiotomy, and 79% with a third or fourth degree laceration experienced perineal pain. Nearly a quarter of the women with an episiotomy or third or fourth degree laceration described the pain as horrible and excruciating.[8]

Following a detailed review of the literature relating to this particular area, several key issues emerged, which may have a direct effect on the extent of morbidity experienced by women following perineal repair. These issues include: the extent of perineal damage, the technique and materials used for suturing and the skill of the person performing the procedure. If the suturing is performed perfunctorily it may have a major impact on women's health as well as significant implications for health service resources. It is important that practitioners ensure that routine procedures, such as perineal repair, are evidence-based in order to provide quality care that is effective, appropriate and cost-efficient, as set out in the UK's government consultation document *A first class service*.[9] However, it would appear that a dichotomy exists between some aspects of routine practice and the utilisation of research findings. There are a number of reasons given for this, some of which include lack of knowledge and skills, resistance to change, personal preference, tradition, restrictive local policies and lack of support.[10]

3.2   Prevalence

Despite the fact that maternity care has vastly improved over the past decade, women still sustain various degrees of perineal trauma following vaginal births. This is one aspect of childbirth that women appear to be unprepared for. Findings from a fairly recent large RCT indicate that 85% of women who have a vaginal birth will sustain some form of perineal trauma[11] and up to 69% of these will require stitches.[7,11] However, these rates vary considerably according to the policies of individuals, and institutions throughout the world. It is difficult to ascertain global rates of spontaneous perineal trauma requiring suturing due to classification inconsistencies and a lack of reporting perineal trauma.

3.3   Definition

Perineal trauma during vaginal birth may occur either spontaneously or when the midwife or obstetrician facilitates delivery by making a surgical incision (episiotomy) to increase the diameter of the vulval outlet. The term "episiotomy" actually refers to cutting the pudenda (external genitalia), whereas the term "perineotomy" is defined as an incision of the perineum and is the more accurate term.[12]

Anatomically, the perineum extends from the pubic arch to the coccyx and is divided into the anterior urogenital and posterior anal triangle. Anterior perineal trauma is defined as injury to the labia, anterior vagina, urethra or clitoris. Trauma in this area is associated with less morbidity. Little is known about the long-term effects of anterior perineal trauma. Posterior perineal trauma is defined as any injury to the posterior vaginal wall, perineal muscles or anal sphincters (external and internal) and may include disruption of the rectal mucosa.[13]

3.4   Classification of Perineal Trauma

Spontaneous perineal trauma can be subdivided into the following classifications according to the extent of the tissue damage:

1. First degree, which is very superficial and may involve:
   - skin and subcutaneous tissue of the anterior or posterior perineum
   - vaginal mucosa
   - a combination of the above resulting in multiple superficial lacerations.
2. Second degree, which is deeper and may involve:
   - superficial perineal muscles (bulbospongiosus, transverse perineal)
   - perineal body.

Second degree trauma usually extends downwards from the posterior and/or lateral vaginal walls, through the hymenal remnants, towards the anal margin and it usually occurs in the weakest part of the stretched perineum. If the trauma is very deep, the levator ani muscles (pubococcygeus) may be disrupted. Less frequently, the tear extends in a circular direction, behind the hymenal remnants, bilaterally upwards towards the clitoris, causing the lower third of the vagina to detach from underlying structures.[14] This type of complex trauma causes vast disruption to the perineal body and muscles but the perineal skin may remain intact, making it difficult to repair.

An episiotomy usually involves the same structures as a second degree tear but occasionally spontaneous trauma may occur simultaneously, resulting in more complex perineal injury.

3.5   Training

Prior to 1970, midwives in the UK were not permitted to perform perineal repairs and midwifery textbooks contained very little information relating to this particular area of childbirth. In fact, it was not until 1983 that perineal repair was included in the midwifery curriculum in the UK when the European Community Midwives Directives came into force and the CMB issued the following statement: "*Midwives may undertake repair of the perineum provided they have received instruction and are competent in this procedure*".

It is current practice in the UK for the attending midwife to suture perineal trauma, which has been sustained during a normal delivery, providing it is within her or his scope of practice.[15] There are wide variations between hospitals and practitioners in suturing techniques and materials chosen for perineal repair. Quite often the techniques used by individual practitioners originate from the way they were first taught, rather than being firmly based on clinical evidence.

A survey in London, carried out to assess the knowledge of trainee doctors ($n = 75$) and qualified midwives ($n = 75$) concerning perineal trauma and anatomy, found that only 20% of doctors and 48% of midwives considered their training satisfactory.[16] Indeed, many of the answers relating to anatomy and classification of perineal repair given by the respondents were incorrect. McClellan[17] surveyed senior obstetrics and gynaecology house officers in the USA concerning their experience and knowledge of perineal repairs. Representatives from one half of the programmes responded. Sixty per cent of residents reported receiving no didactics or formal training on episiotomy techniques. Only 7% had repaired more than 20 fourth degree lacerations and 40% reported repairing more than 20 third degree lacerations. This research highlights the discontent among trainee doctors and midwives with their training in perineal repair and recommends that more intense and focused training should be provided.

Consumers of midwifery services have also expressed dissatisfaction following their personal experiences of perineal repair. Most concerns were directly related to training issues, some of which include the operator being inexperienced and unsupervised or having to learn by trial and error.[18,19] A further consideration is that most practitioners have no means of observing the long-term effects of the perineal suturing in order to audit their own practice.[20] Furthermore, there are wide variations throughout the UK in the way the procedure is taught, supervised and assessed, as currently there are no national guidelines relating to the training of operators. Practitioners who are appropriately trained and assessed will be more likely to provide a consistently high standard of perineal repair, which might have a direct effect on the short- and long-term reduction of morbidity associated with this procedure.

In the USA, where more than 90% of deliveries are performed by physicians, midline episiotomy has been standard practice. Questions about the efficacy and benefit of episiotomy began to arise in the 1970s. Several studies found that midline episiotomies actually provide little benefit and in fact increase morbidity with higher third and fourth degree lacerations, greater blood loss, greater risk of infection and fistula, and increased postpartum pain.[21–23] Practitioners have been slow to respond to the evidence, but a significant decrease in the episiotomy rate has occurred over the past 20 years from 63.9 per 100 vaginal deliveries in 1980 to 39.2 per 100 vaginal deliveries in 1998 ($P < 0.05$).[24,25] The decreases have occurred for women of all ages, races, source of payment categories and in all regions of the USA. As a result, there has also been a steady decline in the number of third and fourth degree lacerations (Figure 3.1).[24,25]

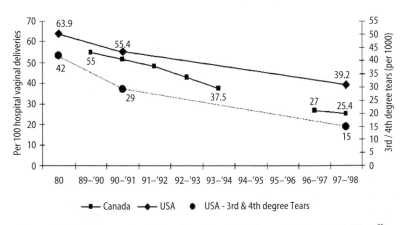

FIGURE 3.1. Episiotomy rates in Canada and the USA between 1980 and 1998. (Klein.[25])

3.6 Non-suturing of First and Second Degree Tears

The controversy regarding the best management of perineal trauma relating to suturing following childbirth has continued throughout the centuries. Some accoucheurs considered that perineal trauma should be left unsutured to facilitate subsequent deliveries, while others disputed that the woman and her partner would benefit if it were sutured. In the mid-twentieth century, Magdi[26] reported that the incidence of perineal trauma at the Kasr El Aini Hospital in Cairo was 24% in primiparous women as compared to 1.9% in multiparous women. He associated this remarkably low rate of perineal injury among multiparous women to the fact that many of them had sustained damage during previous deliveries, which was left unsutured by the attending midwife. Magdi[26] stated that it was deplorable that midwives were in the habit of ignoring perineal trauma and "neither practising nor calling for suturing to be performed." Indeed, it would appear that midwife advocacy of non-suturing perineal trauma following childbirth is not a new concept.

Non-suturing of first and second degree tears is becoming widespread in the UK despite the deficiency of reliable research evidence to support this practice.[27-29] Metcalfe and colleagues[30] reported that up to 50% of first and second degree tears were not sutured in some hospitals within the West Midlands, UK. Midwives who advocate this practice claim that women experience less pain and infection and the wound heals at a faster rate. However, those who support suturing question what subsequent effects non-suturing may have in relation to wound healing, aesthetics, sexual function, pelvic floor muscle strength, incontinence and prolapse. In the USA, suturing remains the primary management of perineal trauma following childbirth.

To date, there have been three small retrospective cohort studies carried out in the UK and two small RCTs in Sweden and Scotland to evaluate the effects of leaving first and second degree tears unsutured following childbirth.[28,31-34] The three retrospective studies (total $n = 212$ women) report no difference in morbidity or wound healing for women with perineal tears that were left unsutured. However, the results must be interpreted with caution due to their poor methodological quality.[28,31,32] The two RCTs compared the effects of non-suturing versus suturing of first and second degree tears.[33,34] The RCT ($n - 78$ primiparous women) carried out in Sweden found a non-significant increase in short-term discomfort (burning sensation and soreness) associated with non-suturing and no difference in rates of wound healing between groups; however, it is unclear how healing was defined and assessed.[33] The other RCT ($n = 74$ primiparous women), carried out in Scotland,[34] found no significant difference in McGill pain scores at 10 days and 6 weeks between non-suturing and suturing. Conversely, Fleming and colleagues[34] reported that significantly more women in the sutured group had good wound approximation at 6 weeks postpartum.

This dearth of research provides very little sound evidence of good methodological quality to support this controversial practice. Therefore, practitioners must be cautious about leaving trauma unsutured unless it is the explicit wish of the woman.[35]

3.7 Suture Methods

Perineal trauma is conventionally repaired in three layers (Figure 3.2). First, a continuous "locking" stitch is inserted to close the vaginal trauma, commencing at the apex of the wound and finishing at the level of the fourchette with a loop knot. A traditional "locking" stitch is used to repair the vaginal trauma, as a continuous "running" stitch may cause shortening of the vagina if it is pulled too tight, but no controlled studies have been carried out to investigate this theory. Next, the deep and superficial perineal muscles are re-approximated with three or four interrupted sutures, or sometimes a continuous running stitch is used. Finally, the skin is closed using continuous subcutaneous or interrupted transcutaneous techniques.[36]

3.7.1 Non-suturing of Perineal Skin

Pretorius[37] published his experience of using a simple technique for episiotomy repair, whereby

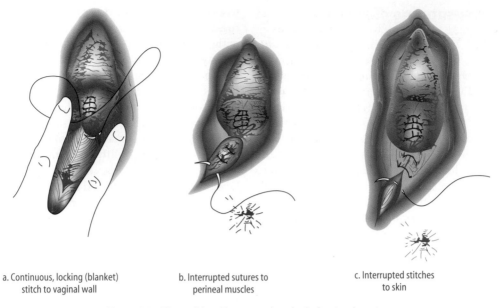

a. Continuous, locking (blanket)   b. Interrupted sutures to   c. Interrupted stitches
        stitch to vaginal wall   perineal muscles   to skin

FIGURE 3.2. The traditional interrupted method of perineal repair.

perineal trauma was re-approximated with a few catgut sutures and the vaginal mucosa and perineal skin were left unsutured. He found that although initially the separation of the skin edges looked "alarming", the wound healed rapidly with minimal scarring and very few problems. In addition, the women were able to move in and out of bed freely without the use of analgesics or ice packs.

More recently, two RCTs that compared leaving the perineal skin unsutured but apposed (the vagina and perineal muscle were sutured) versus suturing all three layers (a more conventional repair) found conflicting results relating to perineal pain.[38,39] The first RCT ($n = 1,780$ primiparous and multiparous women with first and second degree tears or episiotomies after spontaneous or assisted vaginal delivery) was carried out in a single UK centre and reported no significant difference between groups in perineal pain at 10 days postpartum.[38] The second multicentre RCT carried out in Nigeria[39] ($n = 823$ women who sustained a second degree tear or episiotomy) found that leaving the perineal skin unsutured significantly reduced the proportion of women with perineal pain up to 3 months after delivery.[39] Both trials reported a significant increase in wound gaping at 2 days postpartum in the unsutured perineal skin groups, which persisted up to 10 days but did not reach statistical significance in the Nigeria trial. The UK[38] and Nigeria[39] trials found that leaving the perineal skin unsutured significantly reduced superficial dyspareunia at 3 months after birth.

3.7.2 Perineal Skin Closure

A Cochrane systematic review of four European and one UK RCTs ($n = 1,864$ primiparous and multiparous women) found that a continuous subcuticular technique of perineal skin closure, when compared to interrupted transcutaneous stitches, was associated with less perineal pain up to 10 days postpartum.[40] However, only three of the trials[41–43] presented data on short-term pain in a suitable format for inclusion in the analysis and only one study[42] actually demonstrated statistical significance between the two intervention groups. No clear differences were seen in the need for analgesia, resuturing of the wound or dyspareunia between groups. Based on one trial ($n = 916$ women), sutures were removed less frequently in the continuous subcuticular group, but there were no significant differences in long-term pain.[43]

3.7.3 Continuous Repair of All Layers

Although researchers have suggested for over 70 years that continuous repair techniques are superior to interrupted suture methods in terms of reducing perineal discomfort during the early postpartum period, these techniques have not been widely used.[42,44–51] This may be due to lack of sound scientific evidence to support this practice, as most of the earlier findings were based on comparative case series or observational studies. Christhilf and Monias[46] suggest that another reason why continuous techniques are not received more favourably is that the lack of knots engenders some insecurity for the obstetrician. Similarly, Fleming[50] stated that even though researchers advocate the continuous technique in terms of reducing perineal pain and increasing mobility, practitioners admit personal uneasiness when first exposed to non-traditional repairs.

More recently, based on the observational study by Fleming,[50] Kettle and colleagues[36] conducted a large factorial design RCT ($n = 1,542$ women) to compare the effects of using a loose continuous suturing technique throughout the repair with the more traditional interrupted method. The study found that the continuous technique significantly reduced perineal pain at 10 days, which persisted up to 12 months after childbirth but did not reach statistical significance. Indeed, for every six women who were sutured with the continuous technique, there was one less who complained of pain at 10 days compared to those sutured with the interrupted method. Kettle and colleagues[36] reported no significant difference in rates of superficial dyspareunia between groups at 3 or 12

months postpartum. However, suture removal was significantly reduced up to 3 months postpartum in the continuous suture group.

Indeed, the findings of this study now provide scientific evidence to support earlier research, which suggested the loose continuous suturing technique was associated with a reduction in perineal pain. The results of the RCT carried out by Kettle and colleagues[36] relating to pain at 10 days postpartum accord with the findings of the Cochrane systematic review, which compared continuous subcutaneous and interrupted transcutaneous methods used for perineal skin closure.[52] Data were presented in a suitable format for meta-analysis in only three of the trials included in the systematic review[41–43] (Figure 3.3). It is interesting to note that the suturing technique used in the experimental group of the Isager-Sally et al. trial,[42] which demonstrates statistical significance between groups, was very similar to the continuous technique described by Kettle and colleagues.[36]

The difference in pain between suturing methods is thought to be due to increasing suture tension caused by oedema. With the continuous technique of repair, tension is transferred throughout the whole length of the single knotless suture in comparison to interrupted stitches, which are placed transversely across the wound. Another important factor, which could also contribute to this reduction in pain, is that the continuous skin sutures are inserted into the subcutaneous tissue,

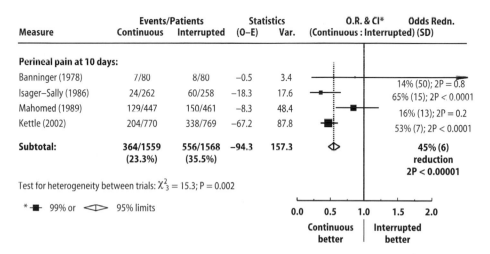

FIGURE 3.3. Meta-analysis of trials – perineal pain at 10 days postpartum.

thus avoiding nerve endings in the skin surface, whereas interrupted transcutaneous sutures are inserted through the skin. Given that the benefits are apparent by 2 days, this explanation seems most plausible.[36] Another advantage of the continuous technique is that only one packet of suture material is usually required to complete the repair, as compared to two or three packets used for the interrupted method, thus reducing the overall expenditure for hospitals.

3.8 Suture Materials

Throughout the ages many techniques have been utilised to close wounds. Between 50,000 and 30,000 BC, "eyed" needles were invented.[53] Other references indicate that linen strips coated with an adhesive mixture of honey and flour (similar to steri-strips) were used to close wounds. In the late nineteenth and twentieth centuries, catgut was favoured to repair perineal tears because stitches dissolved, whereas silkworm gut sutures usually had to be removed on the seventh day. Other materials that have been used for perineal repair over the past 50 years include, nylon, polyamide Supramid, prolene, chromic catgut, softgut and tissue adhesive.

Sutures are inserted to maintain wound closure, control bleeding, minimise the risk of infection and expedite healing. Well-aligned perineal wounds heal by primary intention with minimal complications, usually within 2 weeks of suturing. Wound edges must be re-approximated without tension, otherwise the tissue may become devascularised, resulting in disruption of the healing process.[54] Suture materials should cause minimal tissue reaction and be absorbed once the wound has healed.[55] Most skin requires suture support for approximately 8–14 days to achieve adequate healing. If sutures are placed transcutaneously and are left in situ longer than this period, they may become infected or cause "tram line" scars. Taylor and Karran[55] suggest that the use of synthetic absorbable suture material will avoid this problem.

Polyglycolic acid (Dexon®, Davis & Geck Ltd, UK) and polyglactin 910 (Vicryl®, Ethicon Ltd, Edinburgh, UK), introduced in 1970 and 1974 respectively, are the two most common absorb-able synthetic suture materials used for perineal repair. Standard polyglactin 910 (Vicryl) sutures are prepared from a copolymer of glycolide and lactide in a ratio of 90/10 and the substances are derived from glycolic and lactic acids.[56] The material is braided to improve handling and is coated with a mixture of a copolymer of lactide and glycolide in the ratio of 65/35 and an equal ratio of calcium stearate to reduce bacterial adherence and tissue drag.[56,57] During the manufacturing process, the material is dyed a bright violet colour to improve visualisation during surgical procedures.[58] It is attached to various sized stainless steel needles and sterilised by ethylene oxide gas. Polyglycolic acid sutures (Dexon) are produced from a homopolymer of glycolide and no dye is added, so the resulting material is a light tan colour. The polymer is converted into a braided suture material, which is very similar in composition to standard polyglactin 910.[57] This material is designed to maintain wound support for up to 30 days and is not totally absorbed from the tissue until approximately 90–120 days.[59] The long absorption period means that the suture material is retained in the tissue beyond the required healing time, whereby it becomes a potential source of infection, defeating the purpose of using absorbable stitches.[57]

3.8.1 Absorbable Synthetic Versus Catgut Suture and Material

A Cochrane systematic review of eight RCTs conducted in Europe and the USA ($n = 3,642$ primiparous and multiparous women) compared absorbable synthetic (standard polyglactin 910 or polyglycolic acid) versus catgut suture material for perineal repair.[52] The systematic review found that absorbable synthetic material significantly reduced short-term perineal pain, analgesia use within 10 days, rates of suture dehiscence and resuturing compared with catgut. At 3 months, there was no significant difference in perineal pain or dyspareunia between absorbable synthetic sutures and catgut. Fewer wounds needed resuturing in the absorbable synthetic groups up to 3 months postpartum, but there was no clear difference in terms of long-term pain and dyspareunia. Two of the trials ($n = 2,129$ women) found that absorbable synthetic suture material was associated with an increased risk of suture removal up to 3 months postpartum.[43,60]

3.8.2 Rapidly Absorbed Polyglactin 910 Suture Material

More recently, a new absorbable polyglactin 910 material (Vicryl Rapide®) has appeared on the market. It was first released to the German market in 1987 but it was not available in the UK until after the introduction of CE (Conformité Européene) marketing in 1994. The new, more rapidly absorbable polyglactin 910 material was not actually licensed for use in the UK until 1996 but has been available in the USA since 1995 (data on file at Ethicon Research Foundation). The new suture material is identical to standard polyglactin 910 (coated Vicryl) in chemical composition but it is undyed and due to a change in the manufacturing process, is absorbed in less time. Its tensile strength is reduced in 10–14 days and it is completely absorbed by the tissue in 42 days.[61] The more rapid absorption characteristics are achieved by exposing the material to gamma irradiation during the sterilisation process, resulting in a suture with a lower molecular weight than standard polyglactin 910 (coated Vicryl), which is more readily hydrolysed.[61] Hydrolysis is the absorption mechanism whereby water penetrates the implanted sutures and causes breakdown of the fibres polymer chain with minimal inflammatory response. The degraded lactide and glycolide acid material is then eliminated from the body mainly in urine and faeces (data on file at Ethicon Research Foundation).

Three RCTs ($n = 2,003$ women) have been carried out in Denmark, Northern Ireland and the UK to compare the effects of the new, more rapidly absorbed polyglactin 910 (Vicryl Rapide) with standard polyglactin 910 suture material.[36,62,63] The three trials found no clear difference in short-term pain between groups. However, two of the RCTs ($n = 1,850$ women) carried out by Gemynthe et al.[62] and Kettle et al.[36] found a significant reduction in "pain when walking" at 10–14 days postpartum. Only one of the trials ($n = 153$ women) reported by McElhinney et al.[63] found a reduction in superficial dyspareunia at 3 months postpar-

tum. All three RCTs[36,62,63] found that the new, more rapidly absorbed polyglactin 910 compared to standard polyglactin 910 suture material was associated with a significant reduction in the need for suture removal up to 3 months following childbirth. Therefore, in the light of current evidence, the new, more rapidly absorbed polyglactin 910 (Vicryl Rapide) is the most appropriate suture material for perineal repair.[13]

3.9 Management of Perineal Trauma

3.9.1 Assessment of Perineal Trauma: Basic Surgical Principles

Perineal trauma following childbirth, which has been carefully sutured, generally heals very rapidly within 2 weeks of the repair by primary intention. This is probably due to the fact that the perineal area, immediately after parturition, provides optimal conditions that are necessary for the promotion of quality healing. Some of these include moisture, warmth, increased vascularity, reduced exposure, and a favourable pH of approximately 4.5 (acid), in which organisms are usually unable to grow. Indeed, probably the most common local factor associated with delayed perineal wound healing and dehiscence is infection, which causes reduced collagen synthesis. This adversely causes the wound edges to be softened, which may result in sutures "cutting out" of the tissue with subsequent wound breakdown.

The following basic surgical principles should be followed when performing perineal repairs:

- Suture as soon as possible after childbirth to prevent excessive blood loss and to minimise the risk of infection.
- Check equipment and count cotton swabs and sponges prior to commencing the perineal repair and repeat following completion of the procedure.
- Obtain proper lighting to enable the operator to fully visualise the extent of the trauma and to identify the structures involved.
- Transfer the patient to an operating room and have adequate anesthesia regional or general if needed. An indwelling catheter should be

inserted for 24 hours to prevent urinary retention.

- Ask for more experienced assistance if the trauma is beyond the operator's scope of practice.
- Close dead space and ensure haemostasis is achieved to prevent haematoma formation.
- Sutures must not be over-tightened; this might cause tissue hypoxia, which subsequently may delay the healing process.
- Tie sutures securely using a square surgeon's knot.
- Ensure good anatomical alignment of the wound and also give consideration to the cosmetic results.
- Count cotton swabs and sponges to prevent any unwanted packs being left in the vagina.

3.9.2 First Degree Tears and Labial Lacerations

First degree tears must be sutured if there is excessive bleeding or if there is any uncertainty regarding alignment of the traumatised tissue, which may affect the healing process. If the tear is left unsutured, the midwife or doctor must discuss the implications with the woman and obtain her informed consent. Details regarding the discussion and consent must be fully documented in the woman's case notes.

Labial lacerations are usually very superficial but may be very painful. Some practitioners do not recommend suturing, but if the trauma is bilateral the lacerations can sometimes adhere together over the urethra and the woman may present with voiding difficulties. It is important to advise the woman to part the labia daily during bathing to prevent adhesions from occurring.

3.9.3 Repair of Episiotomy and Second Degree Tears

Prior to performing the perineal repair, the practitioner must prepare the equipment according to practice policies and guidelines. Safety glasses and gloves must be worn during all obstetric procedures to protect the operator against HIV and hepatitis infection. The woman should be placed in a comfortable position so that the trauma can easily be visualised and her dignity maintained throughout the procedure. Perineal tears and episiotomies are repaired under aseptic conditions and the area should be cleaned prior to commencing the suturing according to local policy. A rectal examination should be performed routinely when assessing perineal injury to avoid missing trauma to the anal sphincters (internal or external). This should be repeated once the repair is complete to ensure that suture material has not been accidentally inserted through the rectal mucosa.

It is not necessary to use lithotomy poles or stirrups to support the woman's legs during the repair as restraining her legs may bring back repressed memories of sexual abuse, making her feel helpless and out of control.[64] Furthermore, leg restraints (high stirrups or lithotomy poles) as suggested by Borgatta,[21] cause flexion and abduction of the woman's hips, resulting in excessive stretching of the perineum, which may cause the episiotomy or tear to gape. This, apart from being uncomfortable for the woman, may make the trauma difficult for the operator to realign and suture. Furthermore, there is no need to use a tampon, as this may obscure visualisation of the apex of the vaginal trauma. Excessive uterine bleeding should be managed appropriately prior to commencing the perineal suturing.

Ensure that the wound is adequately anaesthetised prior to commencing the repair. It is recommended that 10–20 ml of lignocaine 1% is injected evenly into the perineal wound. If the woman has an epidural, it may be "topped-up" and used to block perineal pain during suturing instead of injecting local anaesthetic. However, Kahn and Lilford[65] recommend that if an epidural is used, the perineal wound should be infiltrated with normal saline or local anaesthetic to mimic tissue oedema and prevent over-tight suturing.

3.9.4 The Continuous Suturing Technique

In can be concluded from current robust research evidence that perineal trauma should be repaired using the continuous non-locking technique to re-approximate all layers (vagina, perineal muscles and skin) with absorbable polyglactin 910 material (Vicryl Rapide).

3.9.4.1   Suturing the Vagina

The first stitch is inserted above the apex of the vaginal trauma to secure any bleeding points that might not be visible. Close the vaginal trauma with a loose, continuous, non-locking technique, making sure that each stitch is inserted not too wide, otherwise the vagina may be narrowed. Continue to suture down to the hymenal remnants and insert the needle through the skin at the fourchette to emerge in the centre of the perineal muscle trauma (Figure 3.4.1).

3.9.4.2   Suturing the Muscle Layer

Check the depth of the trauma and close the perineal muscle (deep and superficial) with continuous non-locking stitches. If the trauma is deep, the perineal muscles can be closed using two layers of continuous stitches. Re-align the muscle so that the skin edges can be re-approximated without tension, ensuring that the stitches are not inserted through the rectum or anal canal (Figure 3.4.2).

3.9.4.3   Suturing the Perineal Skin

At the inferior end of the wound, bring the needle out just under the skin surface, reversing the stitching direction. The skin sutures are placed below the skin surface in the subcutaneous tissue, thus avoiding the profusion of nerve endings. Continue to take bites of tissue from each side of the wound edges until the hymenal remnants are reached. Secure the finished repair with a loop or Aberdeen knot placed in the vagina behind the hymenal remnants (Figure 3.5).

Finally:

- Check that there is no excessive bleeding and that the finished repair is anatomically correct.
- An accurate detailed account of the repair should be documented in the woman's case notes following completion of the procedure, including details of suture method and materials used. It is also useful to include a simple diagram illustrating the structures involved.
- The woman should be informed regarding the use of appropriate analgesia, hygiene and the importance of a good diet and daily pelvic floor exercises.
- It is important that the woman is given a full explanation of the injury sustained and contact details if she has any problems during the postnatal period. Special designated clinics should be available for women with perineal problems to ensure that they receive appropriate, sensitive and effective treatment.

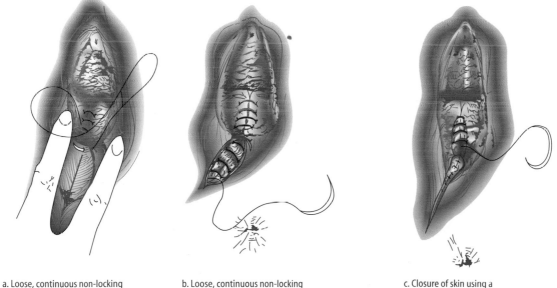

a. Loose, continuous non-locking stitch to vaginal wall

b. Loose, continuous non-locking stitch to perineal muscles

c. Closure of skin using a loose subcutaneous stitch

FIGURE 3.4. Continuous suturing technique for mediolateral episiotomy.

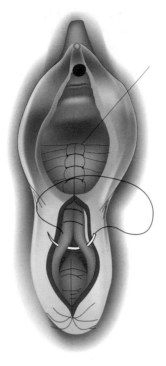

FIGURE 3.5. Continuous suturing technique for midline episiotomy. Once the vaginal mucosa has been closed to the hymenal ring, the needle is passed from the midline to the perineal body and a crown stitch re-approximating the bulbocavernosus muscles is performed. A subcuticular stitch is carried from the inferior perineal margin to the hymen and tied.[66]

3.10 Conclusion

Mismanagement of perineal trauma has a major impact on women's health and significant implications on health service resources. Health professionals must base their practice on current research evidence and be aware of problems associated with perineal trauma and repair. Careful identification and repair of trauma by a skilled practitioner may avoid problems. Furthermore, it is important that prompt sensitive treatment is provided for those women with problems in order to reduce the morbidity associated with perineal injury following childbirth.

References

1. Sleep J. Postnatal perineal care revisited. In: Alexander J, Levy V, Roch S, eds. Aspects of midwifery practice. A research based approach, 1st edn. London: Macmillan Press, 1995, pp 132–53.
2. Sleep J. Perineal care: a series of five randomized controlled trials. In: Robinson S, Thomson A, eds. Midwives, research and childbirth, 1st edn, vol 2. London: Chapman and Hall, 1991, pp 199–251.
3. Kettle C, Hills RK, Jones P, Darby L, Gray R, Johanson R. Continuous versus interrupted perineal repair with standard or rapidly absorbed sutures after spontaneous vaginal birth: a randomised controlled trial. Lancet 2002;359:2217–23.
4. Glazener CMA, Abdalla M, Stroud P, Naji S, Templeton A, Russell IT. Postnatal maternal morbidity: extent, causes, prevention and treatment. Br J Obstet Gynaecol 1995;102:282–7.
5. Sleep J, Grant A. West Berkshire Perineal Management Trial. Three year follow-up. Br Med J 1987; 295(7):749–51.
6. Sultan AH, Kamm MA, Hudson CN, Thomas JM, Bartram CI. Anal-sphincter disruption during vaginal delivery. N Engl J Med 1993;329:1905–11.
7. Sleep J, Grant A, Garcia J, Elbourne D, Spencer J, Chalmers I. West Berkshire perineal management trial. Br Med J 1984;289:587–90.
8. Klein MC, Gauthier RJ, Robbins JM et al. Relationship of episiotomy to perineal trauma and morbidity, sexual function, and pelvic floor relaxation. Am J Obstet Gynecol 1994;171(3):591–8.
9. Department of Health. A first class service – Quality in the new NHS. London: HMSO, 1998.
10. Hurley J. Midwives and research-based practice. Br J Midwifery 1998;6:294–7.
11. McCandlish R, Bowler U, Van Asten H, Berridge G, Winter C, Sames L, Garcia J, Renfrew M, Elbourne D. A randomised controlled trial of care of the perineum during second stage of normal labour. Br J Obstet Gynaecol 1998;105:1262–72.
12. Thacker SB, Banta HD. Benefits and risks of episiotomy: an interpretative review of the English language literature 1860–1980. Obstet Gynecol Survey 1983;38(6):322–34.
13. Kettle C, O'Brien S. Methods and materials used in perineal repair. Guideline no 23. London: Royal College of Obstetricians & Gynaecologists, revised July 2004.
14. Sultan AH, Kamm MA, Bartram CI, Hudson CN. Perineal damage at delivery. Contemp Rev Obstet Gynaecol 1994;6:18–24.
15. UKCC. The midwives' scope of practice. London: UKCC, 1992.
16. Sultan AH, Kamm MA, Hudson CN. Obstetric perineal trauma: an audit of training. J Obstet Gynaecol 1995;15(1):19–23.

17. McClellan MT, Melick CF, Clancy SL, Artel R. Episiotomy and perineal repair. An evaluation of resident education and experience. J Reprod Med 2002;47(12):1025–30.
18. Rix JA. Painful and perineal problem. Daily Telegraph 1992;14.
19. Brimacombe J. Reaping the pain which others have sewn. The Independent (14th March) 1995;21.
20. Lewis L. Are you sitting comfortably? The development of a perineal audit system to enable midwives to follow their perineal management up to 13 months postnatally. Midwives Chronicle 1994; 226–7.
21. Borgatta L, Piening SL, Cohen WR. Association of episiotomy and delivery position with deep perineal laceration during spontaneous delivery in nulliparous women. Am J Obstet Gynecol 1989;160(2): 294–7.
22. Thorp JM, Bowes WA. Episiotomy: can its routine use be defended? Am J Obstet Gynecol 1989; 160:1027–30.
23. Shiono P, Klebanoff MA, Carey JC. Midline episiotomies: more harm than good? Obstet Gynecol 1990;75:765–70.
24. Weaks JD, Kozak LJ. Trends of episiotomy in the United States: 1980–1998. Birth 2001;28(3):152–60.
25. Klein MC. Use of episiotomy in the United States. Birth 2002;29:74.
26. Magdi I. Obstetric injuries of the perineum. J Obstet Gynaecol Br Commonw 1949;49:687–700.
27. McCandlish R, Brocklehurst P, King V, Kettle C. Midwives should offer perineal repair. Pract Midwife 1999;2(7):14–5.
28. Wood T. Not suturing is safe. Pract Midwife 1999; 2(7):15.
29. Gilpin-Blake D, Elliot S. A natural alternative to suturing. Midwifery Today 2001(winter);60:32.
30. Metcalfe A, Tohill S, Williams A, Haldon V, Brown L, Henry L. A pragmatic tool for the measurement of perineal tears. Br J Midwifery 2002;10(7):412–7.
31. Head M. Dropping stitches. Nursing Times 1993; 89(33):64–5.
32. Clement S, Reed B. To stitch or not to stitch? A long-term follow-up study of women with unsutured perineal tears. Pract Midwife 1999;2(4):20–8.
33. Lundquist M, Olsson A, Nissen E, Norman M. Is it necessary to suture all lacerations after a vaginal delivery? Birth 2000;27(2):79–85.
34. Fleming EM, Hagan S, Niven C. Does perineal suturing make a difference? The SUNS trial. Br J Obstet Gynaecol 2003;110:684–9.
35. Lewis P. Poor science makes poor practice. Modern Midwife 1997;7(6):4–5.
36. Kettle C. Perineal repair: a randomised controlled trial of suturing techniques and materials following spontaneous vaginal birth. PhD Thesis, Keele University, UK, 2002.
37. Pretorius GP. Episiotomy. Br Med J 1982;284: 1322.
38. Gordon B, Mackrodt C, Fern E, Truesdale A, Ayers S, Grant A. The Ipswich Childbirth Study: 1. A randomised evaluation of two stage postpartum perineal repair leaving the skin unsutured. Br J Obstet Gynaecol 1998;105(4):435–40.
39. Oboro VO, Tabowei TO, Loto OM, Bosah JO. A multicentre evaluation of the two-layered repair of postpartum perineal trauma. J Obstet Gynaecol 2003;23(1):5–8.
40. Kettle C, Johanson RB. Continuous versus interrupted sutures for perineal repair. The Cochrane Library, Issue 3. Oxford: Update Software, 2003.
41. Banninger U, Buhrig H, Schreiner WE. A comparison between chromic catgut and polyglycolic acid sutures in episiotomy repair (transl.). Geburtshilfe Frauenheilkd 1978;33:30–3.
42. Isager-Sally L, Legarth J, Jacobsen B, Bostofte E. Episiotomy repair – immediate and long-term sequelae. A prospective randomized study of three different methods of repair. Br J Obstet Gynaecol 1986;93:420–5.
43. Mahomed K, Grant A, Ashurst H, James D. The Southmead perineal suture study. A randomized comparison of suture materials and suturing techniques for repair of perineal trauma. Br J Obstet Gynaecol 1989;96:1272–80.
44. Rucker MP. Perineorraphy with longitudinal sutures. Virginia Medical Monthly 1930;July: 238–9.
45. Mandy TE, Christhilf SM, Mandy AJ, Siegel IA. Evaluation of the Rucker method of episiotomy repair as to perineal pain. Am J Surg 1951;82: 251–5.
46. Christhilf SM, Monias MB. Knotless episiorrhaphy as a positive approach towards eliminating postpartum perineal distress. Am J Obstet Gynecol 1962;84(6):812–8.
47. Guilhem P, Pontonnier A, Espagno G. Episiotomie prophylactique. Suture intradermique. Gynécologie et Obstétrique 1960;59(2):261–7.
48. Llewellyn-Jones JD. Commentary. Repair of episiotomies and perineal tears. Br J Obstet Gynaecol 1987;94:92–3.
49. Grant A. The choice of suture materials and techniques for repair of perineal trauma: an overview of the evidence from controlled trials. Br J Obstet Gynaecol 1989;96(11):1281–9.

50. Fleming N. Can the suturing method make a difference in postpartum perineal pain? J Nurse-Midwifery 1990;35(1):19–25.

51. Olah KS. Episiotomy repair – suture material and short term morbidity. J Obstet Gynaecol 1990; 10:503–5.

52. Kettle C, Johanson RB. Absorbable synthetic versus catgut suture material for perineal repair (Cochrane Review). The Cochrane Library, Issue 3. Oxford: Update Software, 2003.

53. Mackenzie D. The history of sutures. History of Medicine 1973;17:158.

54. Cuschieri A, Steele RJC, Moossa AR. Essential surgical practice, 4th edn. Oxford: Butterworth-Heinemann, 2000.

55. Taylor I, Karran SJ. Surgical principles, 1st edn. London: Oxford University Press, 1996.

56. Ethicon. Coated Vicryl polyglactin 910: the gentle approach. Edinburgh: Ethicon Limited, 1992.

57. McCaul LK, Bagg J, Jenkins WMM. Rate of loss of irradiated polyglactin 910 (Vicryl Rapide) from the mouth: a prospective study. Br J Oral Maxillofac Surg 2000;38:328–30.

58. Craig PH, Williams JA, Davis KW, Magoun AD, Levy AJ, Bogdansky S, Jones JP. A biologic comparison of polyglactin 910 and polyglycolic acid synthetic absorbable sutures. Surg Gynecol Obstet 1975;141:1–10.

59. Moy RL, Lee A, Zalka A. Commonly used suture materials in skin surgery. Am Fam Physician 1991; 44(6):2123–38.

60. Mackrodt C, Gordon B, Fern E, Ayers S, Truesdale A, Grant A. The Ipswich childbirth study: 2. A randomised comparison of polyglactin 910 with chromic catgut for postpartum perineal repair. Br J Obstet Gynaecol 1998;105(4):441–5.

61. Ethicon. A unique new product completes the family: VICRYL rapide. Edinburgh: Ethicon Limited, 1991.

62. Gemynthe A, Langhoff-Roos J, Sahl S, Knudsen J. New VICRYL formulation: an improved method of perineal repair? Br J Midwifery 1996;4(5): 230–4.

63. McElhinney BR, Glenn DRJ, Harper MA. Episiotomy repair: vicryl versus vicryl rapide. Ulster Med J 2000;69(1):27–9.

64. Walton I. Sexuality and motherhood. Hale: Books for Midwives Press, 1994, p 125.

65. Kahn GQ, Lilford RJ. Wound pain may be reduced by prior infiltration of the episiotomy site after delivery under spinal epidural anaesthetic. Br J Obstet Gynaecol 1987;94(4):341–4.

66. Hankins GD, Clark SL, Cunningham FG, Gilstrap LC. Operative obstetrics, 1st edn. New York: Appleton and Lange, 1995. Figures 7–10 and 7–11, p 105.

4
Third and Fourth Degree Tears

Abdul H. Sultan and Ranee Thakar

4.1 Historical Perspective

The earliest evidence of severe perineal injury sustained during childbirth is from the mummy of Henhenit, an Egyptian woman approximately 22 years of age from the harem of King Mentuhotep II of Egypt in 2050 BC.[1] Henhenit's pelvis was an abnormal shape, there was a rupture of the vagina into the bladder and the lower bowel was found protruding from the anus. These severe perineal injuries may have been due to cephalo-pelvic disproportion that probably resulted in her early death.[1]

The first mention of the surgical management of severe perineal injury appears in Avicenna's famous Arabic book, *Al Kanoun*. He recommended a form of a crossed or bootlace suture for the repairs of perineal injuries. Celsus offered only bedrest with legs secured together. However, Abroise Pare, Mauriceau and Smellie disagreed with this approach and recommended the use of sutures, although there is no evidence that they actually did use sutures. The first recorded case of perineal suture was by Guillemiau around 1610, when he attempted to repair a fourth degree tear using a suture twisted around a straight needle, but this was unsuccessful.[1] In 1834, Roux described a technique of approximating the torn edges with a quilted suture reinforced by interrupted sutures.[1] Subsequently there have been various reports in which material such as carbolised catgut, silk, silkworm gut and silver wire were used for suturing. However, success rates with primary wound union of perineal wounds reported in the late 1800s were in the region of 50–60%.[2]

In 1930, Royston[3] described a commonly practised technique in which the ends of the torn sphincter were approximated by inserting a deep catgut suture through the inner third of the sphincter muscle and a second set of sutures (mattress or interrupted) through the outer third of the sphincter. As early as 1948, Kaltreider[4] described their series of women since 1935 in whom one mattress or figure-of-eight suture was used to approximate the sphincter ends during primary repair.

Ingraham et al.[5] mentioned the Royston technique as their method of repair, but their description differs in that they indicate that sutures are only inserted in the fascial sheath or capsule of the anal sphincter. Fulsher and Fearl[6] also described this technique and emphasised that no sutures should pass through the sphincter muscle. More specifically, Cunningham and Pilkington[7] described inserting four interrupted sutures in the capsule of the external anal sphincter (EAS) at the anterior, posterior, superior and inferior points. The end-to-end approximation type of repair has been the standard and is still used widely. However, in 1999, Sultan et al.[8] described the overlap technique of primary repair of the EAS (described by Parks previously for secondary sphincter repair). In addition, Sultan et al.[8] highlighted the importance of recognition and separate repair of the freshly torn internal anal sphincter (IAS), which is largely responsible for maintaining the resting tone of the anal sphincter. Damage to the IAS is associated with incontinence to flatus and passive soiling (see Chapter 8).

4.2   Prevalence

The prevalence of third and fourth degree tears, collectively referred to as obstetric anal sphincter injuries (OASIS), appears to be dependent upon the type of episiotomy practised. In centres where mediolateral episiotomies are practised, the rate of OASIS is 1.7% (2.9% in primiparae)[9] compared to 12%[10] (19% in primiparae)[11] in centres practising midline episiotomy.

4.3   Outcome of Primary Repair

A meta-analysis of the literature regarding the outcome of primary repair is difficult to establish due to considerable variability in study design and data collection. There are variations in repair techniques (anaesthesia used, suture material, repair, antibiotics, stool softeners), some studies are multicentre,[12] there is a wide range of follow-up periods and discrepancies exist in subjective and objective assessments. In particular, most studies have used non-validated structured questionnaires, while others[12,13] have used scoring systems, e.g. Pescatori, Wexner. Given these limitations, we have attempted to compile a list of studies in the English literature following a Medline search from January 1980 to December 2005 (Table 4.1).

The extent of the sphincter injury may be related to outcome of repair. However, in some studies, the data were not interpretable,[20] incomplete[28,44] or inclusive of symptoms other than anal incontinence.[37] Nazir et al.[41] evaluated 132 females with OASIS and found that on univariate analysis, the grade of tear correlated with frequency of soiling, but this was no longer statistically significant on multivariate analysis. In Table 4.2 we have included studies that have quantified the degree of sphincter trauma and correlated it with anal incontinence. De Leeuw et al.[26] reported that the odds for the development of faecal incontinence increased more than twofold with each grade (4 > 3b > 3a).

Thirty-five studies were identified over a 20-year period with follow-up ranging from 1 to 30 months. The prevalence of anal incontinence (including flatus as a sole symptom) and faecal incontinence (liquids and solids with or without flatus) following end-to-end repair ranges between 15–61% ($n = 35$; mean = 39%) and 2–29% ($n = 25$; mean = 14%) respectively (Table 4.1). In addition faecal urgency can affect a further 6[30,44]–28%.[46] Despite repair, persistent sonographic anal sphincter defects were identified in 34[21]–91%.[44] Another distressing symptom following OASIS that is not frequently volunteered because of embarrassment is the development of anal incontinence during coitus, affecting about 17% of women.[42] Forceps delivery, first vaginal delivery, large baby, shoulder dystocia and a persistent occipito-posterior position have been identified as the main risk factors for the development of a third/fourth degree tear.[26,29,30,47]

4.4   Repair Techniques

For decades the most popular technique of primary repair following OASIS has been by "end-to-end" approximation with either interrupted or "figure-of-eight" sutures (Figure 4.1).[30] By contrast, when faced with patients with faecal incontinence, colorectal and trained gynaecologic surgeons favour the "overlap technique" of sphincter repair (secondary) as described by Parks and McPartlin.[48] (see Chapter 12A). Jorge and Wexner[49] reviewed the literature and reported on 21 studies using the overlap technique, with good results ranging from 74% to 100%. Unfortunately, as already alluded to above, there are similar limitations in performing a meta-analysis to look at outcomes regarding studies relating to secondary sphincter repair (see Chapter 12A). Engel et al.[50] prospectively studied 55 patients with faecal incontinence undergoing overlap anterior anal sphincter repair and reported a good clinical outcome in 80% at 15 months. A poor result was found to be associated with an EAS defect, while demonstration of an overlap by anal endosonography (Figure 4.2) correlated with a favourable outcome. At 5-years, 46 of the 55 patients were followed up and only 50% remained continent.[51] However, at least one third of these women had more than one attempt at sphincter repair.[51]

Despite scepticism from surgeons that overlapping friable torn muscle as a primary procedure may not be possible, Sultan et al.[8] evaluated the

TABLE 4.1. Prevalence of anal incontinence following primary repair of obstetric anal sphincter rupture (faecal incontinence only, i.e. excluding flatus incontinence, is shown in parentheses).

Author (n = 33)	Year	Country	N	Follow-up (months)	Anal(faecal) incontinence
Sangalli et al.[14]	2000	Switzerland	177	13 years	15% (10%)
Wood et al.[15]	1998	Australia	84	31	17%* (7%)
Walsh et al.[16]	1996	UK	81	3	20% (7%)
Sander et al.[17]	1999	Denmark	48	1	21% (4%)
Pretlove et al.[18]	2004	UK	41	?	22% (22%)
Crawford et al.[19]	1993	USA	35	12	23% (6%)
Sorensen et al.[20]	1993	Denmark	38	3	24% (?)
Mackenzie et al.[21]	2003	UK	53	3	25% (7%)
Nichols et al.[22]	2005	USA	56	3	25% (11%)
Nielsen et al.[23]	1992	Denmark	24	12	29% (?)
Go and Dunselman[24]	1988	Netherlands	20	6	30% (15%)
Fenner et al.[25]	2003	USA	165	6	30% (?)
De Leeuw et al.[26]	2001	Netherlands	125	14 years	31% (?)
Wagenius[27]	2003	Sweden	186	4 years	33% (25%)
Uustal Fornell et al.[28]	1996	Sweden	51	6	40% (16%)
Poen et al.[29]	1998	Netherlands	117	56	40% (?)
Sultan et al.[30]	1994	UK	34	2	41% (9%)
Zetterstrom et al.[31]	1999	Sweden	46	9	41% (2%)
Mellerup Sorensen et al.[32]	1988	Denmark	25	78	42% (?)
Tetzschner et al.[33]	1996	Denmark	72	24–48	42% (17%)
Williams et al.[34]	2003	UK	124	?	42% (?)
Norderval et al.[12]	2004	Norway	156	25	42% (17%)
Garcia et al.[35]	2005	USA	26	3	42% (15%)
Kammerer-Doak et al.[36]	1999	USA	15	4	43% (13%)
Haadem et al.[37]	1988	Sweden	62	3	44% (?)
Rieger et al.[38]	2004	Australia	51	3	45% (25%)
Bek and Laurberg[39]	1992	Denmark	121	?	50% (?)
Davis et al.[40]	2003	UK	52	3.6	50% (?)
Fitzpatrick et al.[13]	2000	Ireland	154	3	53% (6%)
Nazir et al.[41]	2003	Norway	100	18	54% (17%)
Gjessing et al.[42]	1998	Norway	35	12–60	57% (23%)
Savoye-Collet et al.[43]	2003	France	21	4	57% (29%)
Goffeng et al.[44]	1998	Sweden	27	12	59% (11%)
Nyqaard et al.[45]	1997	USA	29	30 years	59% (28%)
Pinta et al.[46]	2004	Finland	52	15	61% (10%)
Mean					39% (14%)

*Includes two with secondary sphincter repair.

TABLE 4.2. Rates of incontinence according to grade of tear.

Author	Year	N	3a	3b	4°	P value
Poen et al.[29]	1998	117		38%	58%	NS
Sangali et al.[14]	2000	177		11.5%	25%	0.049
De Leeuw et al.[26]	2001	125	21%	31%	64%	0.001
Fenner et al.[25]	2003	165		3.6%	31%	0.001
Norderval et al.[12]	2004	156	44%	44%	53%	NS*
Nichols et al.[22]	2005	56		28%	59%	0.03
Mean				22%	48%	

In these studies, 3a = partial thickness, 3b = full thickness, 4° = torn anal sphincter and mucosa. *3a and 3b were combined for the analysis.

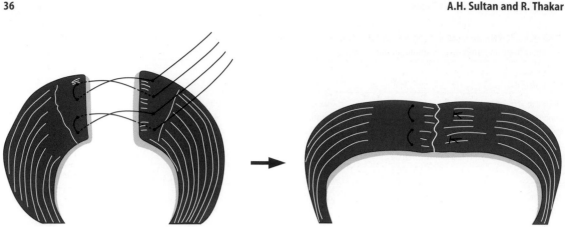

FIGURE 4.1. Diagrammatic representation of an end-to-end repair using "figure-of-eight" sutures.

feasibility of this technique in 27 women and demonstrated that EAS overlap repair as well as identification and end-to-end repair of the IAS was possible following acute OASIS. They observed that compared to matched historical controls[52] who had an end-to-end repair, anal incontinence could be reduced from 41% to 8% using the overlap technique and separate repair of the internal sphincter.[8] Based on this they recommended a randomised trial between end-to-end and overlap repair.

Kairaluoma et al.[53] reported on 31 consecutive women who sustained OASIS (3b and fourth

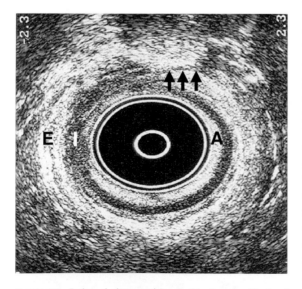

FIGURE 4.2. Endoanal ultrasound image (*E* external sphincter, *I* internal sphincter, *A* anal epithelium) with arrows indicating site of overlap repair of the external anal sphincter.

degree). All had an EAS overlap repair immediately after delivery performed by two colorectal surgeons. In addition to end-to-end repair of the IAS, they also performed a levatorplasty to approximate the levators in the midline with two sutures. At a median follow-up of 2 years, 23% complained of anal incontinence, 23% developed wound infection, 27% complained of dyspareunia and one developed a rectovaginal fistula. Levatorplasty therefore should be avoided during primary anal sphincter repair.

The first randomised trial published was by Fitzpatrick et al.[13] in Dublin, who found no significant difference between the two methods of repair, although there appeared to be trend towards more symptoms in the end-to-end group. There were methodological differences in that the torn IAS was not identified and repaired separately and they used a constipating agent for 3 days after the repair. Unfortunately they included partial EAS tears in their randomised study. A true overlap[8,48] is not possible if the sphincter ends are not completely divided and it would be expected that if an overlap is attempted, the residual intact sphincter muscle would have to curl up and hence there would be undue tension on the remaining torn ends of muscle that would be overlapped. This technique would therefore go against the general principles of surgery of deliberately placing tissue under avoidable tension. Nevertheless as the authors concur, a better outcome would be expected with both techniques as a consequence of focused education and training in anal sphincter repair.

Garcia et al.[35] also performed a randomised trial of the two techniques and took great care to include only complete ruptures of the EAS (full-thickness 3b, 3c and fourth degree tears). There were 23 women in the end-to-end group and 18 in the overlap group. Unfortunately only 15 and 11 women respectively returned for follow-up, which was only at 3 months. No significant difference was found between the groups in terms of symptoms of faecal incontinence or transperineal ultrasound findings. However, the authors acknowledged that the major limitations of their study were that randomisation was inaccurate and that their study was underpowered.

Recently, Williams et al.[54] performed a factorial randomised controlled trial ($n = 112$) in which women were randomised into four groups: overlap with polyglactin (Vicryl; Ethicon, Edinburgh, UK); end-to-end repair with Vicryl; overlap repair with polydiaxanone (PDS; Ethicon, Edinburgh, UK); end-to-end repair with PDS. This trial was specifically designed to test the hypothesis regarding suture-related morbidity (need for suture removal due to pain, suture migration or dyspareunia) using the two techniques. At 6 weeks there were no differences in suture-related morbidity. The authors claim that there were no differences in outcome based on repair technique. Unfortunately, the majority of patients included in this trial had partial tears of the EAS (3a tears) and as mentioned above, a true overlap[8,48] cannot be performed if the EAS is only partially torn. Furthermore, their follow-up rate at 12 months was only 54%. These data therefore need to be interpreted with caution.

Fernando et al.[55] performed a randomised trial of end-to-end vs overlap technique.[8] The study had adequate power ($n = 64$) and the primary outcome was faecal incontinence at 1 year. All repairs were performed by two trained operators and superficial partial tears of the EAS (3a) were excluded. At 12 months (81% follow-up rate), 24% in the end-to-end and none in the overlap group reported faecal incontinence ($P = 0.009$). Faecal urgency at 12 months was reported by 32% in the end-to-end group and 3.7% in the overlap group ($P = 0.02$). There were no significant differences in dyspareunia and quality of life between the groups. At 12 months, 20% reported perineal pain in the end-to-end group and none in the overlap group

($P = 0.04$). During 12 months, 16% in the end-to-end group and none in the overlap group reported deterioration of defaecatory symptoms ($P = 0.01$). Further calculation revealed that four women need to be treated with the overlap technique to prevent one woman with OASIS developing faecal incontinence.

4.5 Principles and Technique of Repair

1. Repair of OASIS should be conducted only by a doctor who has been formally trained (or under supervision) in primary anal sphincter repair.

2. Repair should be conducted in the operating theatre where there is access to good lighting, appropriate equipment and aseptic conditions. In our unit we have a specially prepared instrument tray containing a Weislander self-retaining retractor, four Allis tissue forceps, McIndoe scissors, tooth forceps, four artery forceps, stitch scissors and a needle holder (www.perineum.net). In addition, deep retractors (e.g. Deavers) are useful when there are associated paravaginal tears.

3. A general or regional (spinal, epidural, caudal) anaesthetic provides analgesia as well as muscle relaxation, which is an important pre-requisite to enable proper evaluation of the full extent of the injury. As the inherent tone of the EAS can result in retraction of the torn muscle ends within its capsular sheath, adequate muscle relaxation would allow the torn ends of the EAS to be grasped and retrieved. This would enable repair of the torn muscles without tension, especially if the intention is to overlap the EAS.

4. The full extent of the injury should be evaluated by a careful vaginal and rectal examination in lithotomy and graded according to the recommended classification (see Chapter 2). If there is any ambiguity about the grading of the injury, the next higher grade should be selected, e.g. if there is a discrepancy between grade 3a and 3b, the injury should be classified as 3b.

5. On rare occasions an isolated "buttonhole" type tear (see Chapter 2) can occur in the rectum without disrupting the anal sphincter. This is best repaired transvaginally using interrupted Vicryl sutures. To minimise the risk of a persistent

rectovaginal fistula, a second layer of tissue should be interposed between the rectum and vagina by approximating the rectovaginal fascia. A colostomy is rarely indicated unless there is a large tear extending above the pelvic floor or there is gross faecal contamination of the wound.

6. In the presence of a fourth degree tear, the torn anal epithelium is repaired with interrupted Vicryl 3/0 sutures with the knots tied in the anal lumen. This technique has been widely described[56] and proponents of this technique argue that by tying the knots outside, the quantity of foreign body within the tissue would be reduced, hence reducing the risk of infection. However, this concern probably applies to the use of catgut, which dissolves by proteolysis, as opposed to the newer synthetic materials such as Vicryl or Dexon (polyglycolic acid), which dissolve by hydrolysis. Catgut made from submucosa of sheep gastrointestinal tract has now been withdrawn from the UK and other European countries. A subcuticular repair of the anal epithelium via the transvaginal approach has also been described and could be equally effective provided the terminal knots are secure.[56]

7. The sphincter muscles are repaired with 3/0 PDS dyed sutures (Figure 4.3). Compared to a braided suture material, monofilamentous sutures are believed to lessen the risk of infection.[57] Non-absorbable monofilament sutures such as nylon or Prolene (polypropylene) are preferred by some colorectal surgeons when performing secondary sphincter repair. However, non-absorbable sutures

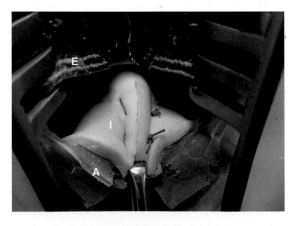

FIGURE 4.3. Internal anal sphincter (*I*) repair using mattress sutures demonstrated on a model (*E* external sphincter, *A* anal epithelium).

can cause stitch abscesses (particularly the knots) and the sharp ends of the suture can cause discomfort, necessitating removal. Complete absorption of PDS takes longer than Vicryl, with 50% tensile strength lasting more than 3 months compared to 3 weeks respectively.[54] To minimise suture migration, care should be taken to cut suture ends short and ensure that they are covered by the overlying superficial perineal muscles. However, a randomised controlled trial revealed no differences in suture-related morbidity between Vicryl and PDS at 6 weeks postpartum.[54]

8. The IAS should be identified and, if torn, repaired separately from the EAS. The IAS lies between the EAS and the anal epithelium. It is thinner and paler than the striated EAS (see Chapter 2). The appearance of the IAS can be described as being analogous to the flesh of raw fish, as opposed to the red meat appearance of the EAS. The ends of the torn muscle are grasped with Allis forceps and an end-to-end repair is performed with interrupted or mattress 3/0 PDS sutures (Figure 4.3). A torn IAS should be approximated with interrupted sutures, as overlapping can be technically difficult. There is some evidence that repair of an isolated IAS defect is beneficial in patients with established anal incontinence.[58] In a recent blinded randomised study of repair after OASIS, all nine women who had a repair of an IAS tear (grade 3c or fourth degree) were found to have an intact IAS at follow-up using anal endosonography.[55]

9. As the EAS is normally under tonic contraction, it tends to retract when torn (Figure 4.4). The torn ends of the EAS therefore need to be identified and grasped with Allis tissue forceps (Figure 4.5). In order to perform an overlap, the muscle may need mobilisation by dissection with a pair of McIndoe scissors separating it from the ischioanal fat laterally. The torn ends of the EAS can then be overlapped in a "double-breasted" fashion (Figure 4.6) using PDS 3/0 (Ethicon) sutures. A proper overlap is possible only when the full length of the torn ends of the EAS is identified (Figure 4.7); overlapping allows for a greater surface area of contact between muscle (Figure 4.6). By contrast, an end-to-end repair can be performed without identifying the full length of the EAS, giving rise to incomplete apposition (Figure 4.8). Consequently, the woman may remain

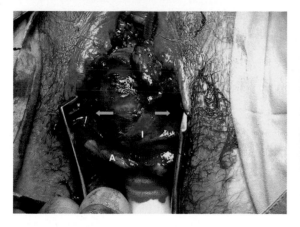

FIGURE 4.4. Third degree tear (grade 3c) with arrows demonstrating retraction of the external sphincter. The internal sphincter (*I*) is also partially torn and the anal epithelium (*A*) is intact.

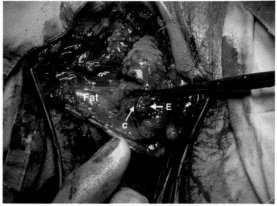

FIGURE 4.5. The external sphincter (*E*) grasped with Allis forceps is surrounded by the capsule (*C*) and lies medial to the ischio-anal fat.

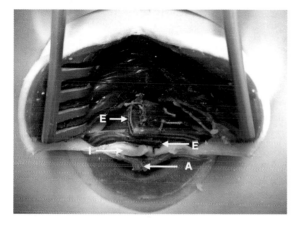

FIGURE 4.6. Repair of a fourth degree tear (demonstrated on a model) using the overlap repair technique of the external sphincter (*E*). The anal epithelium (*A*) and the internal sphincter (*I*) have also been repaired.

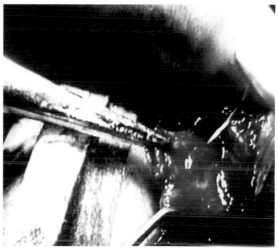

FIGURE 4.7. The full length of the external sphincter should be identified before repair is attempted.

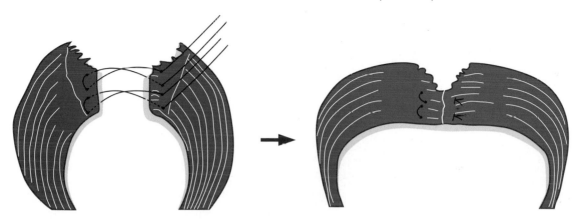

FIGURE 4.8. If the full length of the EAS is not exposed (Figure 4.7), apposition may be incomplete, leading to functional compromise.

continent but would be at an increased risk of developing incontinence later in life. A shorter anal length has been reported following end-to-end primary repair of the EAS.[30] It has also been shown that a shorter anal length is the best predictor of faecal incontinence following secondary sphincter surgery.[59] Unlike end-to-end repair, if further retraction of the overlapped muscle ends were to occur, it is highly probable that muscle continuity would be maintained. However, if the operator is not familiar with the overlap technique or if the EAS is only partially torn (grade 3a/3b), an end-to-end repair should be performed using two or three mattress sutures similar to IAS repair (Figure 4.9) instead of haemostatic "figure-of-eight" sutures (Figure 4.1).

10. After repair of the sphincter, the perineal muscles should be sutured to reconstruct the perineal body to provide support to the repaired anal sphincter. Furthermore, a short deficient perineum would make the anal sphincter more vulnerable to trauma during a subsequent vaginal delivery. Finally, the vaginal skin should be sutured and the perineal skin approximated with a Vicryl 3/0 subcuticular suture.

11. A rectovaginal examination should be performed to confirm complete repair and ensure that all tampons or swabs have been removed.

12. Detailed notes should be made of the findings and repair. Completion of a pre-designed proforma and a pictorial representation of the tears prove very useful when notes are being

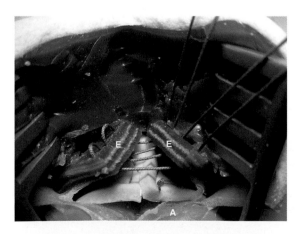

Figure 4.9. End-to-end repair of the external sphincter (*E*) using two mattress sutures (*I* internal sphincter, *A* anal epithelium).

reviewed following complications, audit or litigation (Figure 4.10).

4.6   Postoperative Management

4.6.1   Antibiotics

There are no randomised trials to substantiate the benefits of intraoperative and postoperative antibiotics following repair of OASIS. However, they are now commonly prescribed[60] (especially with fourth degree tears),[56] as infection and wound breakdown could jeopardise the outcome of repair and lead to incontinence or fistula formation. We prescribe intravenous broad-spectrum antibiotics such as cefuroxime 1.5 g and metronidazole 500 mg intraoperatively and continue this orally for 5–7 days.

4.6.2   Bladder Catheterisation

Severe perineal discomfort, particularly following instrumental delivery, is a known cause of urinary retention and following regional anaesthesia it can take up to 12 hours before bladder sensation returns. A Foley catheter should be inserted for about 24 hours unless midwifery staff can ensure that spontaneous voiding occurs at least every 3–4 hours without undue bladder overdistension.

4.6.3   Postoperative Analgesia

The degree of pain following perineal trauma is related to the extent of the injury and OASIS are frequently associated with other more extensive injuries such as paravaginal tears. In one study, 91% of women still complained of severe perineal pain 7 days after OASIS.[61] In a systematic review, Hedayati et al.[62] found that rectal analgesia such as diclofenac is effective in reducing pain from perineal trauma within the first 24 hours after birth and women used less additional analgesia within the first 48 hours after birth (see Chapter 6). Diclofenac is almost completely protein bound and therefore excretion in breast milk is negligible.[63] In women who have had a repair of a fourth degree tear, diclofenac should be administered orally, as insertion of suppositories may be

DETAILS OF PERINEAL TRAUMA REPAIR ___ Mayday University Hospital

Patient Name: ....   Number: .... Date:..................

Tick type of perineal trauma   **First degree** ☐   **Second degree** ☐

Third degree ☐, *if third degree please specify* 3a / 3b /3c   **Fourth degree** ☐
Episiotomy ☐   **If yes, Please state indication..**

Extent of trauma **tick ALL relevant boxes)**   **Unilateral vaginal tear** ☐   **Bilateral vaginal tear** ☐

Labial trauma ☐   **Perineal skin edges down to anal margin**

Anaesthetic for repair   **None** ☐   **Epidural** ☐   **Spinal** ☐   **Lignocaine** ☐_____ **mls**

Repair details
Time of delivery ....**Time repair commenced** ....**Time repair finished** ....

Method of repair
Vagina   **Interrupted / Continuous**   **Suture used Vicryl / Vicryl Rapide**
Perineal muscles   **Interrupted / Continuous**   **Suture used Vicryl / Vicryl Rapide**
Perineal skin   **Interrupted / Continuous**   **Suture used Vicryl / Vicryl Rapide**
Anal mucosa   **Interrupted / Continuous**   **Suture used Vicryl / Vicryl Rapide**
Internal anal sphincter   **Interrupted / Mattress**   **Suture used PDS / Vicryl**
External anal sphincter   **Overlap / End to end**   **Suture used PDS / Vicryl**

Additional information
....

Please complete diagram, mark laccrations and suture repair
Urethra   →→→

Vagina   →→

Anal sphincter   →→→

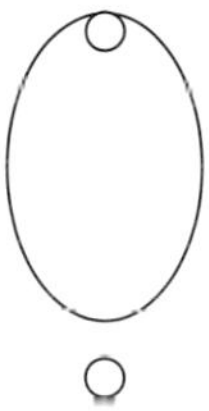

Rectal examination done before repair **Yes / No**   Rectal examination done after repair **Yes / No**
Vaginal examination done **Yes / No** Tampon Removed **Yes /No**
Needle count correct **Yes / No**   Swab count correct **Yes/No**

Estimated blood loss   **After delivery .... mls**   **After suturing ...... mls**   **Total .... mls**

Repaired by
(Print Name) ....   **Midwife / Doctor**
If midwife: **grade** ....   *If* doctor: **Consultant / Staff Grade / SpR / SHO**

FIGURE 4.10. Proforma used at Mayday University Hospital for documentation of perineal trauma.

uncomfortable and there is a theoretical risk of poor healing associated with local anti-inflammatory agents. Codeine-based preparations are best avoided, as they may cause constipation, leading to excessive straining and possible disruption of the repair.

4.6.4 Dietary Advice and Stool Softeners

It is of utmost importance that constipation is avoided, as passage of constipated stool or indeed faecal impaction requiring manual evacuation may disrupt the repair. Although there are conflicting practices described in the literature, the majority consensus is that stool softeners should be prescribed.[56] Mahony et al.[64] performed a randomised trial ($n = 105$) of constipating versus laxative regimens and found that use of laxatives was associated with a significantly earlier and less painful first bowel motion as well as earlier discharge from hospital. Nineteen per cent in the constipated regimen group experienced troublesome constipation (two required hospital admission for faecal impaction) compared to 5% in the laxative regimen group. There were no significant differences in continence scores, anal manometry or endoanal scan findings.

Another prospective, randomised surgeon-blinded study[65] of patients undergoing anorectal reconstructive surgery ($n = 46$) reported a faecal impaction rate of 26% in the group given constipating agents till the third postoperative day compared to 7% in the group allowed a regular diet. We therefore prescribe stool softeners (lactulose 15 ml bd) and a bulking agent (Fybogel [ispaghula husk], one sachet bd) for 10–14 days and we have not encountered any problem with bowel evacuation using this regimen.[8] We prefer not to discharge women from hospital until a bowel action has occurred, unless the community midwife can ensure that constipation is avoided. In the USA, this practice may not be possible since most patients will be discharged within 24 hours following a vaginal delivery. It is recommended that women with OASIS see a healthcare provider 24 or 48 hours after hospital discharge to ensure that bowel evacuation has occurred. If not, early intervention with lactulose, mineral oil, milk of magnesia or other oral bowel stimulant should be given in addition to the stool softeners and bulking agent as described above.

4.6.5 Patient Information

Williams et al.[66] performed a qualitative study of six women who sustained OASIS, and four who had a subsequent pregnancy after OASIS. Some of the themes identified in these women were: apprehension about the consequences of the injury in terms of incontinence, body image and sexual functioning, poor communication and emotional support and unresolved anxieties in partners.

Ideally, these women should be under the care of a specialist team who run the perineal clinic (see Chapter 6). The perineal clinic is viewed as a supportive environment and women feel confident about the information provided by the team.[66] We provide an information booklet to these women to ensure that they understand the implications of sustaining OASIS and secondly provide information as to where and when to seek help if symptoms of infection or incontinence develop. All women complete a validated bowel health and quality-of-life questionnaire relating to issues before the delivery. Following discharge from hospital they should have open access to this clinic until their postnatal appointment, usually between 6 to 8 weeks after delivery. We recommend that pelvic floor and anal sphincter exercises can be initiated when the discomfort resolves and the woman feels comfortable.

If a perineal clinic is not available, women with OASIS should be given clear instructions, preferably in writing before leaving the hospital. In the first 6 weeks following delivery, they should look for signs of infection or wound dehiscence and call with any increase in pain or swelling, rectal bleeding, or purulent discharge. Any incontinence of stool or flatus should also be reported.

4.6.6 Follow-up

We recommend that all women who sustain OASIS should be assessed in hospital by a senior obstetrician 6–8 weeks after delivery. In our practice all women who sustained OASIS are seen usually with their partners in the dedicated perineal clinic (see Chapter 6). They complete the same questionnaires as they did before discharge from hospital. A genital examination is performed, looking specifically for scarring, residual granulation tissue and tenderness. All women then undergo anal manometry and endosonography (see Chapters 9 and10). We ensure that they understand the circumstances surrounding the delivery and provide an explanation if there are concerns. The women are advised to continue pelvic floor exercises while others with minimal sphincter contractility may need electrical stimulation (see Chapter 11).

4.7 Management of Subsequent Pregnancies

Women who sustain anal sphincter injury need careful counselling regarding their management in a subsequent pregnancy. They feel very vulnerable following a previous traumatic delivery and often find the advice inconsistent and biased towards caesarean section (CS).[66] In one survey,[60] 71% of colorectal surgeons recommended CS (a further 19% admitted they were uncertain) compared to fewer than 22% of obstetricians who recommended CS. Unfortunately, the data currently available to develop evidence-based guidelines are limited and therefore we have to rely largely on recommended practice. There are two major issues that concern most women following OASIS when contemplating delivery in a subsequent pregnancy: namely, the risk of recurrence and the risk of developing anal incontinence.

4.7.1 What Is the Risk of Recurrence of OASIS?

The risk of recurrence is dependent upon the type of episiotomy practised in any unit. Most of the published studies are in centres practising midline episiotomy.[11,67]

Peleg et al.[11] studied 4,015 consecutive primiparae who had a singleton, cephalic presentation at term and found 704 sustained OASIS (19%). The risk of recurrence of OASIS in these women was 2.1% when no episiotomy was performed, 11% when a midline episiotomy was performed and 21% when a midline episiotomy was accompanied by instrumental delivery. In another study where midline episiotomies were practised, the recurrence rate of OASIS was reported to be 11%.[67] Harkin et al.[9] studied 20,111 consecutive vaginal deliveries in a unit that practises only mediolateral episiotomies and OASIS occurred in 342 women (2.9% in primiparae and 0.8% in multiparae). Obstetric anal sphincter injuries recurred in two (4.4%) of the 45 women who had sustained OASIS previously. Although risk of OASIS was increased fivefold in a subsequent pregnancy, 95% of women who had sustained previous sphincter injury did not sustain a recurrence.

4.7.2 What Is the Risk of Anal Incontinence after Another Vaginal Delivery?

Poen et al.[29] identified 43 women (out of original cohort of 117) who had subsequent vaginal deliveries following previous OASIS. The rate of anal incontinence was 56% compared to 34% in those who did not subsequently deliver (relative risk 1.6; 95% confidence interval 1.1–2.5). There was no comparable CS group.

Sangalli et al.[14] studied 177 women some 13 years after OASIS (48 fourth degree tears). Anal incontinence was significantly more common in women who had sustained fourth degree tears compared with those with third degree tears (25 vs 11.5%; $P = 0.049$). Unlike women with previous fourth degree tears, those who had sustained a previous third degree tear did not demonstrate an increase in anal incontinence symptoms after a subsequent vaginal delivery. This is in keeping with the findings of Fenner et al.,[25] who found that the symptom of worse bowel control was 10 times higher in women who sustained fourth as opposed to third degree tears. This could be attributed to persistent injury of the IAS.

Overall, the answer to this question remains inconclusive as the data available are retrospective and very limited.

4.7.3 What Is Recommended Practice?

If there are no facilities for anal manometry and endosonography (Figure 4.11), the management of a subsequent pregnancy will depend on symptomatic and clinical evaluation. Asymptomatic women without any clinical evidence of sphincter compromise ascertained by assessment of anal tone could be allowed to have a vaginal delivery. All women who are symptomatic should be referred to a centre with facilities for anorectal assessment and should be counselled for CS.

4.7.3.1 Asymptomatic Women

Asymptomatic women who have minimal compromise of their anal sphincter function (satisfactory pressure measurements and ultrasound images) should be allowed to have a vaginal delivery. These women should be counselled that they

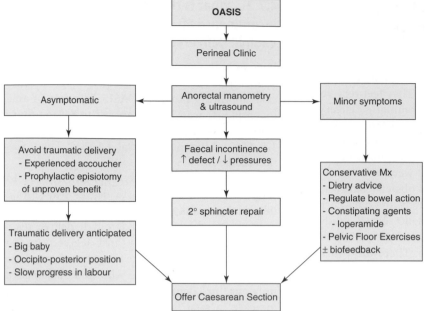

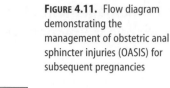

Figure 4.11. Flow diagram demonstrating the management of obstetric anal sphincter injuries (OASIS) for subsequent pregnancies

have a 95% chance of not sustaining recurrent OASIS[9] or developing de novo anal incontinence following delivery.[68] However, the delivery should be conducted by an experienced doctor or midwife. If an episiotomy is considered necessary, e.g. because of a thick inelastic or scarred perineum, a mediolateral episiotomy should be performed. There is no evidence that routine episiotomies prevent recurrence of OASIS. The threshold at which these women may be considered for a CS may be lowered if a traumatic delivery is anticipated, e.g. in the presence of one or more additional relative risk factors such as a big baby, shoulder dystocia, prolonged labour, difficult instrumental delivery. However, in deciding the mode of delivery, counselling (and its clear documentation) is extremely important. Some of these women who have sustained OASIS may be scarred both physically and emotionally and may find it difficult to cope with the thought of another vaginal delivery. These women will require sympathy, psychological support and consideration to their request for CS.

4.7.3.2 Symptomatic Women

All symptomatic women are first treated conservatively (see Chapter 11) depending on their main symptoms and findings at investigation.

Women who suffer from varying degrees of irritable bowel syndrome will need evaluation and appropriate dietary advice depending on whether their bowel pattern is diarrhoea or constipation predominant. It has been shown that in women who have pre-existing irritable bowel syndrome, symptoms of defaecatory urgency and/or flatus incontinence deteriorate significantly following vaginal delivery independent of anal sphincter injury.[69]

Conservative management of anal incontinence is described in detail in Chapter 11 and is summarised as follows:

- All women are included in the biofeedback programme (Chapter 11).
- If muscle contractility is weak or absent, electrical muscle stimulation is commenced.
- Women with flatus incontinence are given dietary advice, especially the avoidance of gas-producing foods such as legumes.
- Women with faecal incontinence are commenced on a low residue diet and constipating agents such as loperamide can be used.

Women whose symptoms are adequately controlled by conservative measures are offered CS in any subsequent delivery so as to minimise the risk of further compromise to anal sphincter function.

Women with faecal incontinence in whom conservative measures have failed should be offered anal sphincter surgery (Chapter 12A), while others may need advanced surgical techniques as described in Chapter 12B. All women who have undergone successful incontinence surgery should be delivered by CS.

A management dilemma arises in women who suffer from faecal incontinence but who wish further pregnancies. These women could avoid a CS and undergo a vaginal delivery followed by a secondary sphincter repair at a later date. The only rationale behind this is that most of the damage that occurs during childbirth occurs with the first vaginal delivery[68,70] and therefore the risk of further damage during a subsequent vaginal delivery is relatively small. However, there is a potentially unquantified risk of deteriorating pudendal neuropathy. By contrast, CS is not without major morbidity and mortality.[71] Therefore counselling plays an important role in the decision-making process.

4.7.4   How Safe Is Caesarean Section?

The greatest fear of women who have sustained OASIS is a recurrence of the injury and associated risk of faecal incontinence. Clearly CS alleviates these fears but it has a greater impact on morbidity and mortality (see Chapter 5). In particular, CS is associated with an increased risk of maternal mortality, peripartum hysterectomy, urinary tract injury, thromboembolic disease, etc.[72] Furthermore, there are implications for future pregnancies, as there is an increased risk of placenta praevia, uterine rupture, antepartum stillbirth and infertility.[72] In an analytical model looking at elective CS for women with previous OASIS,[73] McKenna reported that a woman who chooses a CS has an 11.3% risk of morbidity compared to 4.2% following vaginal delivery (relative risk 2.7) and the relative risk of maternal death was 2.6 following CS. It is therefore important that women who request CS on demand are made fully aware of the associated risks. In the UK, an obstetrician can refuse to perform a CS on request without a medical indication, although the woman has the right to seek a second opinion. In the USA, an obstetrician can also refuse to perform a CS on request. However, the woman has the right to seek a second opinion and to change doctors. In many cases, the third-party payer will not pay for a CS on request without a medical indication.

4.7.5   Can Objective Assessments Predict Who Will Develop Incontinence?

There are limited prospective studies to address this issue. Fynes et al.[68] performed a prospective study of 59 women at three time points: 34 weeks gestation of their first pregnancy and 6–12 weeks after two consecutive vaginal deliveries. They found that out of all the asymptomatic women after the first vaginal delivery who were found to have a large "occult" sonographic anal sphincter defect (>one quadrant) or anal squeeze pressures of less than 20 mmHg, 75% (six of eight) became symptomatic after the second vaginal delivery. By contrast, only 5% (two of the 43) with less extensive defects became symptomatic ($P < 0.0001$). There is an increasing awareness of the role of the IAS in maintaining continence. Nichols et al.[22] followed up 56 women who sustained OASIS and found that combined defects of the IAS and EAS were associated with the highest risk of bowel symptoms compared to an intact sphincter (odds ratio 18.7; CI 3–101, $P < 0.001$) and isolated defects of the EAS (odds ratio 15.7; 95% CI 3–76; $P = 0.003$).

4.8   Who Should Be Performing Acute Primary Obstetric Sphincter Repairs?

In view of the observed suboptimal outcome associated with primary anal sphincter repair when performed by obstetricians with varying degrees of experience (Table 4.1), it has been suggested that perhaps a repair performed by colorectal surgeons may be associated with a better outcome.[16,74,75] However, in a study (described above)[53] the outcome was no better. Furthermore, in a survey of colorectal practice in the UK,[60] only 6.7% of colorectal surgeons reported that they performed more than ten acute repairs per year, 60% had never performed an acute sphincter repair and 30% performed fewer than five per year. It is

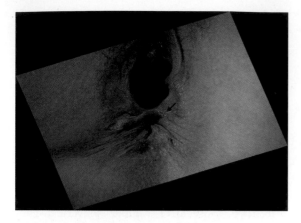

FIGURE 4.12. Demonstration of a cloacal defect following a missed third degree tear. The perineal body is absent and the external sphincter is deficient between 10 and 2 o'clock (between arrows) as noted by the absence of the corrugator cutis ani.

therefore not surprising that only 19% of colorectal surgeons believed that they should be involved in the acute management of OASIS. We believe that the most experienced clinician should perform the repair as soon as possible after the injury. Ideally, the most appropriate trained clinician should be an obstetrician who would be easily accessible at any time. It has been suggested that perhaps it may be prudent to leave women with OASIS overnight, particularly those who have delivered at night, until a colorectal surgeon becomes available to perform the repair.[76] We believe that it would be unkind to leave a woman who had just delivered until the morning. She may be actively bleeding, the tissues may become oedematous and there is an added risk of infection. This delay would create unnecessary anxiety at a time when the parents should be celebrating the birth of their child. However, a delay in repair may be justified in exceptional circumstances when an experienced obstetrician may not be available. Furthermore, women who sustain OASIS often have concomitant vaginal lacerations (some multiple and deep) that will need to be repaired by an obstetrician (as well as reconstruction of the perineal body). It was concerning to note that 30% of colorectal surgeons recommended a covering colostomy for OASIS, confirming that while they may have expertise in dealing with women presenting with faecal incontinence (Figure 4.12),

(see Chapters 12a and 12b) very few have any experience with acute OASIS.[60]

4.9   Education and Training

Deficiencies in training programmes of doctors and midwives have already been alluded to in Chapters 2 and 3. Doctors and midwives have indicated that their training in perineal anatomy and ability to recognise OASIS are suboptimal.[77] There are also inconsistencies in classification of perineal trauma, as one third of doctors were classifying third degree tears as second degree (see Chapter 2). Most trainee doctors admitted that their training in recognising (84%) and repairing (94%) OASIS was poor[77] and 64% of consultants reported unsatisfactory or no training in the management of OASIS.[60]

In view of this, we initiated an international hands-on workshop on the management of OASIS in February 2000 (www.perineum.net). The OASIS workshop is structured to include lectures and demonstrations of anatomy and repair using a specifically designed latex anal sphincter model (Figure 4.13), video demonstrations and pig anal sphincters (Figure 4.14). By February 2006, we had conducted 30 such hands-on workshops in the UK and in order to establish the usefulness of such a course we conducted an audit of the first 80 delegates. The delegates completed a questionnaire before and 3 months after attending the workshop. Only 33% admitted to any prior formal

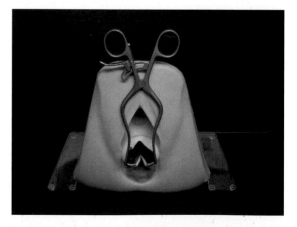

FIGURE 4.13. The Sultan anal sphincter trainer with a central replaceable block has been designed for hands-on teaching (www.perineum.net).

training in repair of OASIS. At 3 months, 78% admitted to a change in clinical practice in terms of repairing the IAS, 29% introduced a protocol for repair of OASIS and 34% changed their management of subsequent pregnancies.[78] The feedback from attendees was that this programme should become an essential part of the modular training for career trainees. A number of similar courses have now been established nationally and internationally.

Since October 2002, we have introduced a second international hands-on workshop specifically for midwives and trainee doctors, in which we teach anatomy and emphasise the need for rectal examinations to ensure that OASIS do not remain undiagnosed.[79] The delegates are also taught repair of episiotomy and spontaneous first and secondary tears. A prospective audit of knowledge and practice was conducted by completion of a questionnaire before and 2 months after the course ($n = 147$). This revealed a significant improvement in accurate classification of perineal trauma as well as in repair technique. All doctors and most midwives changed their practice in that they routinely performed a rectal examination to evaluate the full extent of perineal trauma (and to exclude OASIS) prior to suturing.[80]

Concern about training has also been raised by McLennan et al.,[81] who surveyed 1,177 fourth-year residents and had a 25% response rate. They found that the majority of residents had received no formal training in pelvic floor anatomy, episi-

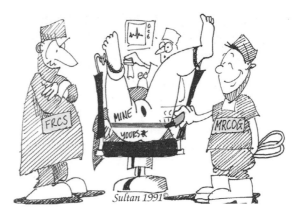

FIGURE 4.15. Political interaction between the obstetrician (MRCOG) and the surgeon (FRCS) regarding the "bottom line".

otomy or perineal repair, and supervision during perineal repair was limited. Similar to the findings of our survey of popular textbooks in the UK,[56] Stepp et al.[82] found that textbooks used in American practice offered little in terms of prevention and repair of perineal trauma. Strategies for prevention of OASIS are discussed in Chapter 5. One explanation for the inadequate training in anatomy and pathophysiology can be attributed to the compartmentalisation of the pelvic floor such that many specialities (obstetricians, colorectal surgeons, urologists, gastroenterologists, etc.) deal with conditions that are in close proximity to each other. The territorial effects have been well illustrated by Wall and DeLancey[83] in an excellent article on the "politics of the pelvic floor". Unfortunately, the "bottom line" is that politics also exist on the perineum, where an arbitrary dividing line has been drawn separating the territory of the obstetrician from that of the surgeon (Figure 4.15). The problem to hand is that no one can identify the exact location of this line. Consequently there is a large grey zone on either side of this line that each speciality believes belongs to the other . . . leaving a chasm in education and training that this book endeavours to fill.

4.10 Conclusion

Obstetric anal sphincter injuries occur in about 20% of women undergoing their first vaginal delivery (in centres that practise midline episiotomy).

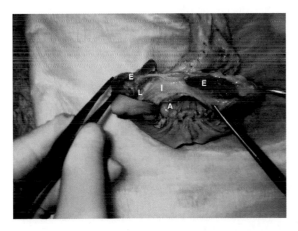

FIGURE 4.14. The pig anal sphincter demonstrating the external sphincter (*E*), longitudinal muscle coat (*L*), internal sphincter (*I*) and anal epithelium (*A*).

Overall, although there has been a notable increase in the prevalence of OASIS, it could be largely attributed to improvements in detection of such injuries. When such injuries are identified, it is imperative that they are repaired by a skilled clinician under optimal conditions. A good understanding of perineal and anal sphincter anatomy and adherence to sound principles (described above) are essential. Although the technique of overlap repair of the external sphincter may be associated with a better outcome, it remains to be established whether this could be achieved universally. Until then, depending on the expertise of the operator, either the overlap or end-to-end repair technique can be used for repair. There is an obvious demand for focused education and training in perineal anatomy, recognition of OASIS and training in repair techniques. Hands-on workshops with video recordings, models and pig anal sphincters are now very popular and have proved to be very successful.

References

1. Magdi I. Obstetric injuries of the perineum. J Obstet Gynaecol Br Commonw 1949;49:687–700.
2. Garrigues HJ. The obstetric treatment of the perineum. Am J Obstet Gynecol 1880;13(2): 231–64.
3. Royston GD. Repair of complete perineal laceration. Am J Obstet Gynecol 1930;19:185–95.
4. Kaltreider DF. A study of 710 complete lacerations following central episiotomy. South Med J 1948;41: 814–20.
5. Ingraham HA. A report on 159 third degree tears. Am J Obstet Gynecol 1949;57:730–5.
6. Fulsher RW, Fearl CL. The third-degree laceration in modern obstetrics. Am J Obstet Gynecol 1955; 69:786–93.
7. Cunningham CB, Pilkington JW. Complete perineotomy. Am J Obstet Gynecol 1955;70:1225–31.
8. Sultan AH, Monga AK, Kumar D, Stanton SL. Primary repair of obstetric anal sphincter rupture using the overlap technique. Br J Obstet Gynaecol 1999;106:318–23.
9. Harkin R, Fitzpatrick M, O'Connell PR, O'Herlihy C. Anal sphincter disruption at vaginal delivery: is recurrence predictable? Eur J Obstet Gynecol Reprod Biol 2003;109(2):149–52.
10. Coats PM, Chan KK, Wilkins M, Beard RJ. A comparison between midline and mediolateral episiotomies. Br J Obstet Gynaecol 1980;87:408–12.
11. Peleg D, Kennedy CM, Merrill D, Zlatnik FJ. Risk of repetition of a severe perineal laceration. Obstet Gynecol 1999;93(6):1021–4.
12. Norderval S, Nsubuga D, Bjelke C, Frasunek J, Myklebust I, Vonen B. Anal incontinence after obstetric sphincter tears: incidence in a Norwegian county. Acta Obstet Gynecol Scand 2004;83(10): 989–94.
13. Fitzpatrick M, Behan M, O'Connell R, O'Herlihy C. A randomized clinical trial comparing primary overlap with approximation repair of third-degree obstetric tears. Am J Obstet Gynecol 2000;183: 1220–4.
14. Sangalli MR, Floris L, Faltin D, Weil A. Anal incontinence in women with third or fourth degree perineal tears and subsequent vaginal deliveries. Aust N Z J Obstet Gynaecol 2000;40(3):244–8.
15. Wood J, Amos L, Rieger N. Third degree anal sphincter tears: risk factors and outcome. Aust N Z J Obstet Gynaecol 1998;38(4):414–17.
16. Walsh CJ, Mooney EF, Upton GJ, Motson RW. Incidence of third-degree perineal tears in labour and outcome after primary repair. Br J Surg 1996;83(2): 218–21.
17. Sander P, Bjarnesen J, Mouritsen L, Fuglsang-Frederiksen A. Anal incontinence after obstetric third-/fourth-degree laceration. One-year follow-up after pelvic floor exercises. Int Urogynecol J Pelvic Floor Dysfunct 1999;10(3):177–81.
18. Pretlove SJ, Thompson PJ, Guest P, Toozs-Hobson P, Radley S. Detecting anal sphincter injury: acceptability and feasibility of endoanal ultrasound immediately postpartum. Ultrasound Obstet Gynecol 2003;22(2):215–17.
19. Crawford LA, Quint EH, Pearl ML, DeLancey JO. Incontinence following rupture of the anal sphincter during delivery. Obstet Gynecol 1993;82(4 Pt 1):527–31.
20. Sorensen M, Tetzschner T, Rasmussen OO, Bjarnesen J, Christiansen J. Sphincter rupture in childbirth. Br J Surg 1993;80(3):392–4.
21. Mackenzie N, Parry L, Tasker M, Gowland MR, Michie HR, Hobbiss JH. Anal function following third degree tears. Colorectal Dis 2004;6(2):92–6.
22. Nichols CM, Lamb EH, Ramakrishnan V. Differences in outcomes after third- versus fourth-degree perineal laceration repair: a prospective study. Am J Obstet Gynecol 2005;193(2):530–4.
23. Nielsen MB, Hauge C, Rasmussen OO, Pedersen JF, Christiansen J. Anal endosonographic findings in the follow-up of primarily sutured sphincteric ruptures. Br J Surg 1992;79(2):104–6.
24. Go PM, Dunselman GA. Anatomic and functional results of surgical repair after total perineal rupture

at delivery. Surg Gynecol Obstet 1988;166(2): 121–4.

25. Fenner DE, Genberg B, Brahma P, Marek L, DeLancey JOL. Fecal and urinay incontinence after vaginal delivery with anal sphincter disruption in an obstetrics unit in the United States. Am J Obstet Gynecol 2003;189:1543–50.

26. De Leeuw JW, Vierhout ME, Struijk PC, Hop WC, Wallenburg HC. Anal sphincter damage after vaginal delivery: functional outcome and risk factors for fecal incontinence. Acta Obstet Gynecol Scand 2001;80:830–4.

27. Wagenius J, Laurin J. Clinical symptoms after anal sphincter rupture: a retrospective study. Acta Obstet Gynecol Scand 2003;82(3):246–50.

28. Uustal Fornell, Berg G, Hallbook O, Matthiesen LS, Sjodahl R. Clinical consequences of anal sphincter rupture during vaginal delivery. J Am Coll Surg 1996;183(6):553–8.

29. Poen AC, Felt-Bersma RJ, Strijers RL, Dekker GA, Cuesta MA, Meuwissen SG. Third-degree obstetric perineal tear: long-term clinical and functional results after primary repair. Br J Surg 1998;85(10): 1433–8.

30. Sultan AH, Kamm MA, Hudson CN, Bartram CI. Third degree obstetric anal sphincter tears: risk factors and outcome of primary repair. Br Med J 1994;308:887–91.

31. Zetterstrom J, Lopez A, Anzen B, Norman M, Holmstrom B, Mellgren A. Anal sphincter tears at vaginal delivery: risk factors and clinical outcome of primary repair. Obstet Gynecol 1999;94(1): 21–8.

32. Mellerup Sorensen S, Bondesen H, Istre O, Vilmann P. Perineal rupture following vaginal delivery. Long term consequences. Acta Obstet Gynecol Scand 1988;67(4):315–18.

33. Tetzschner T, Sorensen M, Lose G, Christiansen J. Anal and urinary incontinence in women with obstetric anal sphincter rupture. Br J Obstet Gyn aecol 1996;103(10):1034–40.

34. Williams A, Adams EJ, Bolderson J, Tincello DG, Richmond DH. Effect of a new guideline on outcome following third-degree perineal tears: results of a 3-year audit. Int Urogynecol J Pelvic Floor Dysfunct 2003;14(6):385–9.

35. Garcia V, Rogers RG, Kim SS, Hall RJ, Kammerer-Doak DN. Primary repair of obstetric anal sphincter laceration: a randomized trial of two surgical techniques. Am J Obstet Gynecol 2005;192(5): 1697–701.

36. Kammerer-Doak DN, Wesol AB, Rogers RG, Dominguez CE, Dorin MH. A prospective cohort study of women after primary repair of obstetric

anal sphincter laceration. Am J Obstet Gynecol 1999;181(6):1317–22.

37. Haadem K, Ohrlander S, Lingman G. Long-term ailments due to anal sphincter rupture caused by delivery–a hidden problem. Eur J Obstet Gynecol Reprod Biol 1988;27(1):27–32.

38. Rieger N, Perera S, Stephens J, Coates D, Po D. Anal sphincter function and integrity after primary repair of third-degree tear: uncontrolled prospective analysis. ANZ J Surg 2004;74(3): 122–4.

39. Bek KM, Laurberg S. Risks of anal incontinence from subsequent vaginal delivery after a complete obstetric anal sphincter tear. Br J Obstet Gynaecol 1992;99(9):724–6.

40. Davis K, Kumar D, Stanton SL, Thakar R, Fynes M, Bland J. Symptoms and anal sphincter morphology following primary repair of third-degree tears. Br J Surg 2003;90(12):1573–9.

41. Nazir M, Stien R, Carlsen E, Jacobsen AF, Nesheim BI. Early evaluation of bowel symptoms after primary repair of obstetric perineal rupture is misleading: an observational cohort study. Dis Colon Rectum 2003;46(9):1245–50.

42. Gjessing H, Backe B, Sahlin Y. Third degree obstetric tears; outcome after primary repair. Acta Obstet Gynecol Scand 1998;77(7):736–40.

43. Savoye-Collet C, Savoye G, Koning E, Sassi A, Leroi AM, Dacher JN. Endosonography in the evaluation of anal function after primary repair of a third-degree obstetric tear. Scand J Gastroenterol 2003; 38(11):1149–53.

44. Goffeng AR, Andersch B, Andersson M, Berndtsson I, Hulten L, Oresland T. Objective methods cannot predict anal incontinence after primary repair of extensive anal tears. Acta Obstet Gynecol Scand 1998;77(4):439–43.

45. Nygaard IE, Rao SS, Dawson JD. Anal incontinence after anal sphincter disruption: a 30-year retrospective cohort study. Obstet Gynecol 1997;89(6): 896–901.

46. Pinta TM, Kylanpaa ML, Salmi TK, Teramo KA, Luukkonen PS. Primary sphincter repair: are the results of the operation good enough? Dis Colon Rectum 2004;47(1):18–23.

47. Abramowitz L, Sobhani I, Ganansia R, Vuagnat A, Benifla JL, Darai E, et al. Are sphincter defects the cause of anal incontinence after vaginal delivery? Results of a prospective study. Dis Colon Rectum 2000;43(5):590–6.

48. Parks AG, McPartlin JF. Late repair of injuries of the anal sphincter. Proc R Soc Med 1971;64(12): 1187–9.

49. Jorge JM, Wexner SD. Etiology and management of fecal incontinence. Dis Colon Rectum 1993;36(1): 77–97.

50. Engel AF, Kamm MA, Sultan AH, Bartram CI, Nicholls RJ. Anterior anal sphincter repair in patients with obstetric trauma. Br J Surg 1994;81(8): 1231–4.

51. Malouf AJ, Norton CS, Engel AF, Nicholls RJ, Kamm MA. Long-term results of overlapping anterior anal-sphincter repair for obstetric trauma. Lancet 2000;355(9200):260–5.

52. Sultan AH. Third degree tear repair. In: MacClean AB, Cardozo L, eds. Incontinence in women. London: RCOG Press, 2002, pp 379–90.

53. Kairaluoma MV, Raivio P, Aarnio MT, Kellokumpu IH. Immediate repair of obstetric anal sphincter rupture: medium-term outcome of the overlap technique. Dis Colon Rectum 2004;47(8):1358–63.

54. Williams A, Adams EJ, Tincello DG, Alfirevic Z, Walkinshaw SA, Richmond DH. How to repair an anal sphincter injury after vaginal delivery: results of a randomised controlled trial. BJOG 2006;113(2): 201–7.

55. Fernando R, Sultan AH, Kettle C, Radley S, Jones P, O'Brien S. Repair techniques for obstetric anal sphincter injuries: a randomized trial. Obstet Gynecol 2006;107:1261–8.

56. Sultan AH, Thakar R. Lower genital tract and anal sphincter trauma. Best Pract & Res – Clin Obstet Gynaecol 2002;16:99–116.

57. Katz S, Izhar M, Mirelman D. Bacterial adherence to surgical sutures. A possible factor in sutures induced infection. Annals Surg 1981;194(1):35–41.

58. Meyenberger C, Bertschinger P, Zala GF, Buchmann P. Anal sphincter defects in fecal incontinence: correlation between endosonography and surgery. Endoscopy 1996;28(2):217–24.

59. Hool GR, Lieber ML, Church JM. Postoperative anal canal length predicts outcome in patients having sphincter repair for fecal incontinence. Dis Colon Rectum 1999;42(3):313–18.

60. Fernando RJ, Sultan AH, Radley S, Jones PW, Johanson RB. Management of obstetric anal sphincter injury: a systematic review and national practice survey. BMC Health Serv Res 2002;2(1):9.

61. MacArthur AJ, MacArthur C. Incidence, severity, and determinants of perineal pain after vaginal delivery: a prospective cohort study. Am J Obstet Gynecol 2004;191(4):1199–204.

62. Hedayati H, Parsons J, Crowther CA. Rectal analgesia for pain from perineal trauma following childbirth. Cochrane Database Syst Rev 2003(3): CD003931.

63. Kettle C, Hills RK, Jones P, Darby L, Gray R, Johanson R. Continuous versus interrupted perineal repair with standard or rapidly absorbed sutures after spontaneous vaginal birth: a randomised controlled trial. Lancet 2002;359(9325):2217–23.

64. Mahony R, Behan M, O'Herlihy C, O'Connell PR. Randomized, clinical trial of bowel confinement vs. laxative use after primary repair of a third-degree obstetric anal sphincter tear. Dis Colon Rectum 2004;47(1):12–17.

65. Nessim A, Wexner SD, Agachan F, Alabaz O, Weiss EG, Nogueras JJ, et al. Is bowel confinement necessary after anorectal reconstructive surgery? A prospective, randomized, surgeon-blinded trial. Dis Colon Rectum 1999;42(1):16–23.

66. Williams A, Lavender T, Richmond DH, Tincello DG. Women's experiences after a third-degree obstetric anal sphincter tear: a qualitative study. Birth 2005;32(2):129–36.

67. Payne TN, Carey JC, Rayburn WF. Prior third- or fourth-degree perineal tears and recurrence risks. Int J Gynecol Obstet 1999;64:55–7.

68. Fynes M, Donnelly V, Behan M, O'Connell PR, O'Herlihy C. Effect of second vaginal delivery on anorectal physiology and faecal continence: a prospective study [see comments]. Lancet 1999; 354(9183):983–6.

69. Donnelly V, Fynes M, Campbell D, Johnson H, O'Connell PR, O'Herlihy C. Obstetric events leading to anal sphincter damage. Obstet Gynecol 1998; 92(6):955–61.

70. Sultan AH, Kamm MA, Hudson CN, Thomas JM, Bartram CI. Anal sphincter disruption during vaginal delivery. New Engl J Med 1993;329: 1905–11.

71. Sultan AH, Stanton SL. Preserving the pelvic floor and perineum during childbirth – elective caesarean section? Br J Obstet Gynaecol 1996;103(8): 731–4.

72. National Institute for Health and Clinical Excellence. Caesarean section: clinical guideline. London: NICE, 2004.

73. McKenna DS, Ester JB, Fischer JR. Elective cesarean delivery for women with a previous anal sphincter rupture. Am J Obstet Gynecol 2003;189(5):1251–6.

74. Sultan AH, Kamm MA. Faecal incontinence after childbirth. Br J Obstet Gynaecol 1997;104(9): 979–82.

75. Cook TA, Mortensen NJ. Management of faecal incontinence following obstetric injury. Br J Surg 1998;85(3):293–9.

76. Sultan AH. Third degree tear repair. In: MacClean AB, Cardozo L, eds. Incontinence in women. London: RCOG Press, 2002, pp 420–30.

77. Sultan AH, Kamm MA, Hudson CN. Obstetric perineal tears: an audit of training. J Obstet Gynaecol 1995;15:19–23.

78. Thakar R, Sultan AH, Fernando R, Monga A, Stanton S. Can workshops on obstetric anal sphincter rupture change practice? Int Urogynecol J 2001; 12:S5.

79. Andrews V, Thakar R, Sultan AH, Kettle C. Can hands-on perineal repair courses affect clinical practice? Br J Midwifery 2005;13(9).

80. Andrews V, Sultan AH, Thakar R, Jones PW. Occult anal sphincter injuries–myth or reality? BJOG 2006; 113(2):195–200.

81. McLennan MT, Melick CF, Clancy SL, Artal R. Episiotomy and perineal repair. An evaluation of resident education and experience. J Reprod Med 2002;47(12):1025–30.

82. Stepp KJ, Siddiqui NY, Emery SP, Barber MD. Textbook recommendations for preventing and treating perineal injury at vaginal delivery. Obstet Gynecol 2006;107(2):361–6.

83. Wall LL, DeLancey JO. The politics of prolapse: a revisionist approach to disorders of the pelvic floor in women. Perspect Biol Med 1991;34(4): 486–96.

5
Prevention of Perineal Trauma

Ranee Thakar and Erica Eason

Perineal trauma can be associated with considerable short- and long-term morbidity. Perineal laceration and episiotomy are painful, incur blood loss, and may become infected; fistulae occasionally follow. Long-term, other complications of obstetrical trauma to the pelvic floor may affect women's lives even more than the immediately apparent laceration. Dyspareunia related to the tear and its repair may last for months or even years. Pelvic floor muscles and nerves may be stretched, torn or sheared from their attachments, as shown in magnetic resonance imaging studies,[1] resulting in urine leakage, urgency or incontinence of faeces or flatus, or pelvic organ prolapse. Apart from the physical and hormonal aspects of pregnancy, the specific effects of childbirth have not yet been clearly distinguished, although some light has been shed by prospective studies, especially by the Term Breech Trial, in which planned vaginal or caesarean birth was randomly assigned.[2] On the other hand, some symptoms present at 3 months postpartum (a time frequently chosen by researchers for postpartum assessment) may be caused in part by the very low oestrogen levels, which are due to breast feeding but resolve after weaning the infant. For instance, dyspareunia may be due to atrophic vaginitis, and urinary urgency to thinned uroepithelium of the urethra and bladder base. While a good deal of research into the sequelae of obstetric perineal trauma has focussed on urodynamics, pudendal nerve function, or imaging of the muscles of the pelvic floor and anal canal, one must keep in mind that these, and even observed anal sphincter lacerations, are proxy measures for the outcomes of importance to women: continence and comfort.

On a population health basis, preventing perineal trauma in even a modest proportion of childbearing women would benefit large numbers of women. It would also reduce both the cost of childbirth (with fewer sutures and less suturing time required[3]) and the need of medical care for sequelae such as urinary and faecal incontinence.

5.1 Interventions to Prevent Obstetrical Perineal Trauma

The case for perineal trauma prevention during childbirth is compelling, and the low trauma rates achieved by some practitioners attest that there are effective ways to do so. In the past few decades, great strides have been made toward subjecting traditional care practices in care during pregnancy and childbirth to randomised controlled trial (RCT) and systematic review. Regrettably, these studies have had flaws assessing a limited range of perineal outcomes and following participants for a few months at best. Many aspects of pregnancy, labour and delivery care thought to affect perineal trauma have yet to be subjected to rigorous assessment. Birthing methods used by practitioners with low rates of perineal trauma need to be identified and evaluated. Therefore we will summarise the evidence for interventions potentially affecting the rate of perineal trauma, focusing primarily on the evidence from RCTs.

We first discuss interventions with evidence from RCTs, in the order in which a decision about whether an intervention might have to be made in the course of patient care. We then mention other interventions for which evidence is weaker or lacking, in like order. Outcomes presented include perineal and anal sphincter trauma, and when available, various perineal functions such as continence, pelvic organ support and sexual comfort. Table 5.1 lists the interventions discussed. For each effective intervention, we present the risk difference along with the "number needed to treat" (NNT): the number of women who need to receive or avoid an intervention to prevent one case of sutured perineal trauma or anal sphincter trauma (Table 5.2). Possible risks factors not amenable to intervention are discussed last.

TABLE 5.1. Interventions to prevent obstetrical perineal trauma.

Interventions about which sound evidence is available
Planned caesarean vs planned vaginal birth
Antenatal perineal massage
Exercise in pregnancy
Water labour/birth
Position during labour
Position during giving birth
Epidural vs narcotic pain relief
Early or delayed pushing with epidural
Coaching: pushing vs no instruction
Spontaneous vs forceps birth
Episiotomy or not, type of episiotomy
Second stage stretching massage of the perineum
Hands on vs hands poised: perineal support
Vacuum vs forceps

Interventions lacking sound evidence
Head flexion
Head restraint (physical) to slow the delivery
Head restraint (verbal): preventing pushing when the perineum is tense
Perineal analgesia
Delivery with or between contractions
Delivering the posterior shoulder – firstly or secondly, inferiorly or anteriorly
Operative vaginal delivery vs caesarean section
Interventions for occiput posterior malposition

TABLE 5.2. Summary of RCT-proven effects on perineal trauma.

Intervention	Outcome	Risk difference	NNT*
Avoiding episiotomy	Perineal trauma	−20%	5
Mediolateral vs midline episiotomy	Anal trauma	−15%	6.7
Spontaneous birth vs forceps	Anal trauma	−11%	9
Narcotic vs epidural analgesia	Operative delivery	−10%	10
Antenatal massage in nulliparae	Perineal trauma	−7%	13
Antenatal pelvic floor exercise	Urinary incontinence	−6%	17
Vacuum vs forceps	Anal trauma	−6%	18
Planned caesarean section	Urinary incontinence	−2.8%	36
	Anal incontinence	n.s.	
Water labour/birth	Perineal trauma	n.s.	
Recumbent vs upright position	Perineal trauma	n.s.	
Delayed vs early pushing with epidural	Perineal trauma	n.s.	
Directed vs spontaneous pushing	Perineal trauma	n.s.	
Hands on vs poised	Perineal trauma	n.s.	
Second stage perineal stretching	Perineal trauma	n.s.	

*Number of women needing to receive intervention for one to benefit.

5.2 Interventions with RCT Evidence Regarding Effectiveness

5.2.1 Planned Caesarean vs Planned Vaginal Birth

The Term Breech Trial was a pioneering RCT of planned caesarean section versus planned vaginal birth for the term fetus in breech position.[2] Mindful of the unique and rare opportunity this trial presented, it was designed with careful assessment of the impact of the planned delivery route on maternal outcomes including perineal functions. Because the primary goal of the trial was to assess the safest route of delivery for the baby, the proportion of women not delivering by the route to which they were randomised was substantial, so analysis by intention-to-treat may underestimate the true effects of route of delivery. Table 5.3 shows 1,592 women's responses to a 3-month postpartum questionnaire regarding pelvic floor and perineal outcomes. The only significant difference between the groups in these outcomes was a lower risk of urinary incontinence after planned

TABLE 5.3. Perineal outcomes from the Term Breech Trial.[2,66]

Outcome at 3 months (except tears)	Planned caesarean (n = 798)	Planned vaginal (n = 797)
Perineal tear	Not reported	72.8%
Anal sphincter tear	0.1%	1.3%
Urinary incontinence in previous week	4.5%*	7.3%
Faecal incontinence	0.8%	1.5%
Flatal incontinence	10.7%	9.7%
Pain of any kind	27.3%	25.0%
Dyspareunia	17.0%	18.7%

*$P < 0.05$.

caesarean section: absolute risk difference was −2.8% with a 95% confidence interval (CI) (−5.1%, −0.5%). Thirty-six elective caesarean sections will need to be performed to prevent one woman developing urinary incontinence at 3 months.[2] There was no significant difference in faecal or flatal incontinence. At 2-year follow-up of a subset of 917 of these women, the risk difference was −4% (n.s.).[4] While planned caesarean section decreases perineal trauma and urinary incontinence compared to planned vaginal delivery, a Cochrane meta-analysis of RCTs of planned caesarean vs vaginal birth found a greater risk of short-term maternal morbidity with planned caesarean (risk difference 2%, 95% CI 0%, 4%.).[5] Since the relative risks of maternal mortality and disastrous morbidity cannot be assessed with the small numbers of participants in RCTs, cohort data must be used. In the mid-1990s, elective caesarean section in the UK was associated with an excess of 3.8 maternal deaths per 100,000.[6] Caesar-

ean section increases the risk of a emergency hysterectomy more than tenfold.[7] Caesarean section to prevent perineal trauma is a recurrent indication in subsequent pregnancies, so cumulative mortality and morbidity must be considered. Clarke et al.'s review of 100,000 deliveries found that the risk of placenta praevia increased linearly with the number of previous caesarean sections, rising to 10% in women with four or more caesarean sections. The risk of placenta accreta also increased to 67% after four caesarean sections.[8]

5.2.2 Antenatal Perineal Massage

Can women planning a vaginal birth do any preparation during pregnancy to decrease their risk of perineal damage? There is good evidence of a modest protective effect of third trimester perineal stretching massage in nulliparous women. Three published RCTs have evaluated the effectiveness of prenatal perineal massage with sweet almond oil by the pregnant woman or her partner.[9-11] Shipman's trial in nulliparous women found an absolute increase of 6.2% intact perineum in the massage group compared to a control group, and Labrecque's RCT found an absolute increase of 9.2% in women having a first vaginal birth. Labrecque found no significant benefit of perineal massage in women having a second or subsequent vaginal birth, even if they had a previous episiotomy scar.[10] The weighted risk difference in sutured perineal trauma in nulliparous women obtained by combining the results of these trials is −7% (95% CI −12%, −3% (Figure 5.1). One

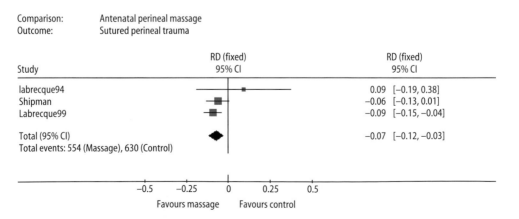

FIGURE 5.1. Forest plot of the risk difference in sutured perineal trauma in RCTs of antenatal perineal massage.

case of perineal trauma requiring suturing would be avoided for every 13 nulliparous women doing prenatal perineal massage. There was no significant risk difference in anal sphincter trauma. At 3 months postpartum, there was no difference in urinary incontinence, anal incontinence or sexual function between women in the massage and control groups.[12] Study participants found perineal massage acceptable.[13] It is encouraging that this simple, woman-controlled intervention to maintain perineal integrity is effective.

5.2.3 Exercise in Pregnancy

Harvey reviewed RCTs of antepartum pelvic floor exercises in primiparous women to prevent long-term urinary incontinence and pelvic floor weakness caused by pregnancy and childbirth.[14] Her quantitative summary of three high-quality RCTs showed a modest effect (risk difference −6%, 95% CI −11%, −2%): she calculated that 17 women would have to do pelvic floor exercises to prevent one case of urinary incontinence (Figure 5.2). A Cochrane review of all sorts of physical therapies for urinary and anal incontinence concluded that there is insufficient evidence at present to determine whether any physical therapy is effective in preventing urinary or faecal incontinence in childbearing women.[15]

5.2.4 Water Birth

Once labour begins, what interventions may be useful to decrease perineal trauma? A recent Cochrane review of seven RCTs of labouring in water baths (one during the second stage) showed no significant difference in second degree (risk difference −2%, 95% CI −6%, 3%) or third and fourth degree (risk difference +1%, 95% CI 0%, 2%) tears. There was no significant difference in vaginal operative delivery (risk difference −2%, 95% CI −5%, 1%) or caesarean section (risk difference +1%, 95% CI 0%, 3%). The use of any analgesia (regional block or narcotic injection) also did not differ: risk difference 0%, 95% CI −8%, 7%.[16]

5.2.5 Position During Labour and Birth

There have been many randomised trials of birth position for the second stage of labour, but the maternal position when the baby is actually born over the perineum is usually unclear. This is unfortunate because the optimal position to assist fetal descent during second stage may not be the best position to prevent perineal trauma as the baby delivers over the perineum. The current evidence on the effectiveness of various delivery positions in the prevention of perineal trauma remains inconclusive.

In Eason et al.'s review of studies meeting inclusion criteria, seven RCTs compared upright birth position using supporting furniture (birthing chair, low stool, or cushion) to recumbent positions (supine or lateral, propped up to 20° or 30° from horizontal.[17] While women assigned to upright positions were less likely to have an episiotomy, they had more lacerations; overall,

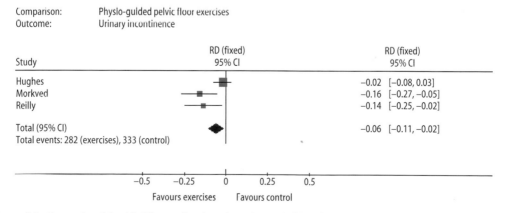

FIGURE 5.2. Forest plot of the risk difference in urinary incontinence in RCTs of physiotherapist-guided pelvic floor exercises.

perineal trauma requiring suturing occurred in slightly more women in upright than in recumbent groups: the weighted risk difference was 2% (95% CI −2%, 5%).

Two studies assessed unsupported upright compared to recumbent positions for the second stage of labour. In one, squatting women were moved to a semi-recumbent position for the actual birth "to avoid perineal trauma".[18] Gardosi compared squatting or other upright positions to a semi-recumbent second stage, but only 36% of women randomised to be upright actually were upright for the birth, since squatting was too strenuous to maintain. There was no significant difference in perineal trauma between groups.[19] Gupta's Cochrane review of position for birth concluded "Overall the quality of the studies was poor and, therefore, the conclusions must be regarded as tentative" but the one finding of note was that upright positions increased blood loss with delivery.[20] Genital prolapse and incontinence have not been assessed in studies of position for birth.

Downe's small RCT in women with epidural analgesia of lateral vs supported sitting in second stage[21] suggested that operative delivery and perineal trauma may be decreased; larger trials are in order.

5.2.6 Epidural vs Narcotic Pain Relief

Howell's review of several RCTs of epidural vs narcotic pain relief[22] documented that 10% more women with epidurals have operative vaginal deliveries (95% CI 6%, 14%) (number needed to cause = 10) and fetal malposition. There was a trend towards more caesarean sections. No summary data on perineal trauma or perineal functions in the longer term were presented, but operative vaginal births are known to increase perineal trauma. Overall it is likely that increased perineal trauma with epidural is due to the associated increase in instrumental delivery.[23,24]

5.2.7 Early vs Delayed Pushing with Epidural

Once the second stage is reached and the fetal head descends, women without epidural generally feel a strong urge to push. In women with epidural, the urge to push is often absent, and different strategies have been taken to second stage management.

In a RCT of 1,862 nulliparous women with epidurals (People Study), Fraser et al. advised women at full dilatation to push early (as soon as randomised) or delay pushing (wait at least 2 hours before pushing) unless the urge was strong or the baby visible. The principal hypothesis, that delayed pushing would reduce the risk of difficult operative delivery defined as caesarean section, mid-pelvic delivery or low pelvic procedure with rotation greater than 45 degrees, was confirmed. Delayed pushing was associated with a reduction in difficult operative deliveries compared with early pushing (NNT = 20) but also with an increase in umbilical cord pH < 7.10 (NNT = 43). There was no difference in episiotomy and third and fourth degree tears.[25] Fitzpatrick et al.[26] and others have conducted RCTs of early vs delayed pushing and also found no difference in perineal or anal sphincter trauma; Fitzpatrick in addition found that instrumental delivery rates, anal incontinence, anal manometry and ultrasound neurophysiology studies did not differ between the two groups.

5.2.8 Second Stage Pushing Advice

Coaching women to hold their breath and push throughout each contraction ("purple pushing") during the second stage or once the head is on the pelvic floor is commonplace. Some have questioned whether these prolonged Valsalva manoeuvres increase pressure on the pelvic floor, secondarily increasing prolapse and urinary incontinence. Two RCTs of directed pushing versus spontaneous pushing in the second stage found no difference in perineal trauma, which was very high in both studies.[27,28]

5.2.9 Spontaneous vs Forceps Birth

In the early decades of the twentieth century, forceps delivery (usually in association with generous episiotomy) was promoted to protect the maternal pelvic floor and the fetal head.[29] Yancey compared spontaneous delivery to elective outlet forceps in a RCT and showed that forceps did not improve neonatal outcomes but did increase maternal trauma:[30] third degree tears were observed in 12 of 168 women who delivered spontaneously compared to 30 of 165 women delivered with forceps. This risk difference of −11% (95% CI −18%, −4%) means that for every nine women giving birth spontaneously instead of by forceps, a third degree tear is avoided.

5.2.10   Routine Episiotomy or Episiotomy "to Prevent a Tear"

Episiotomy has been promoted to prevent more serious tears, allow better healing than tears, and prevent pelvic floor relaxation.[29,31] A Cochrane review of six RCTs of episiotomy showed definitively that restrictive rather than routine episiotomy caused less posterior perineal trauma and less severe vaginal or perineal trauma, as well as less suturing and fewer healing complications.[32] Eason's review of RCTs,[17] updated to include Dannecker's trial, shows a weighted risk difference in sutured perineal trauma between the restrictive and liberal episiotomy policies of −20% (95% CI −22%, −18%) (Figure 5.3). Avoiding routine episiotomy in five women would prevent one case of perineal trauma requiring suturing. The weighted risk difference in anal sphincter tears was −1% (95% CI −1%, 0%): liberal use of midline or mediolateral episiotomy does not prevent anal sphincter tears at spontaneous delivery.[17] The only trial in which episiotomy was midline rather than mediolateral reported no difference in anal sphincter tears between groups randomised to liberal or restrictive episiotomy[33] but 52 of the 53 anal sphincter tears were extensions of episiotomies. This markedly increased relative risk of anal sphincter tear with midline episiotomy has been repeatedly documented.[17] Performing an episiotomy to prevent a tear at spontaneous delivery has no place in modern obstetrics.

What about other effects of episiotomy? There is good RCT evidence that liberal episiotomy increases pain and likely dyspareunia.[32] Routine episiotomy does not prevent urinary incontinence, assessed at 3 months postpartum[33] and at 3 months and 3 years.[34] One trial showed no significant difference in symptoms of perineal bulging and measurements of pelvic muscle strength 3 months postpartum.[33]

There are some cohort data but no RCT data about whether mediolateral episiotomy is protective against anal sphincter laceration compared to no episiotomy in the context of operative vaginal delivery. There is an urgent need for such a RCT, given the high rate of serious lacerations in this situation.

5.2.11   If Episiotomy Is Needed, What Type of Episiotomy Is Safest?

Whether midline episiotomy results in better outcome than mediolateral episiotomy has not

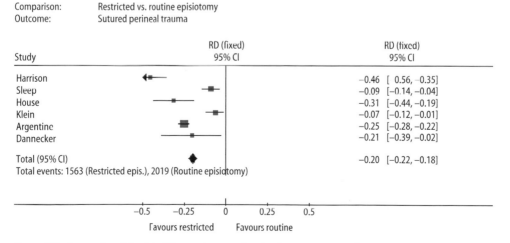

FIGURE 5.3. Forest plot of the risk difference in sutured perineal trauma in RCTs of restricted vs routine episiotomy.

been answered definitely.[32] Midline episiotomies are more popular in North America as it is believed that they are more comfortable. However, a quasi-randomised study by Coats[35] in 407 nulliparous women of mediolateral vs midline episiotomy when episiotomy was needed found that tears into or through the anal sphincter occurred with 12% of midline and 2% of mediolateral episiotomies. In this study subjects not receiving their assigned treatment were excluded from analysis. Since the number of women in the midline episiotomy group is rather smaller, there seems to have been a bias against midline episiotomy, presumably due to concern that it might extend into the anal sphincter. This selection bias would lead to a lower anal sphincter trauma rate in the remaining women in the midline episiotomy group, so their higher trauma rate suggests that midline episiotomy does increase anal sphincter tears. In this trial, pain and dyspareunia were similar in both groups, and more women resumed sexual intercourse in the first month in the midline episiotomy group. In Klein's RCT of midline episiotomy, 7.6% of women had anal sphincter tears, compared to 1.1% in trials of mediolateral episiotomy.[3,36–38]

5.2.12 Second Stage Perineal Stretching Massage

Since episiotomy is not helpful, is there any other action that can protect the perineum during childbirth? A remarkable variety of techniques either to support the perineum or to stretch the perineal borders back over the advancing head have been championed. Recently, RCTs assessing their effectiveness have begun to appear. One popular technique is a stretching massage or "stripping" of the perineum in the second stage to ease the perineum back over the head as it crowns. Stamp et al. did an RCT of perineal sweeping massage with two lubricated fingers in the vagina during each uterine contraction in the second stage of labour.[39] While there were clearly problems with randomisation in this trial (708 in massage group vs 632 in control group), massage did not decrease perineal trauma, postpartum pain, or change perineal functions assessed 3 months later.

5.2.13 Perineal Support: Hands on vs Hands Poised at Delivery

Other practitioners have strongly advocated "support" to the perineum instead of stretching massage during delivery to reduce perineal trauma. In a large ($n = 5,471$) RCT of "hands on or poised" methods of delivery, McCandlish et al. allocated women at the end of second stage of labour to either "hands on" (the midwife's hands put pressure on the baby's head and support the perineum; lateral flexion used to facilitate the delivery of the shoulders) or "hands poised" (the midwife keeps her hands poised, not touching the head or perineum except if light pressure on the head is needed to prevent rapid expulsion, and allowing spontaneous delivery of the shoulders).[40] Unfortunately, assessing whether or not delivery of the baby's head should be restrained was a simultaneous rather than a separately randomised intervention (the study design was not factorial) so we cannot assess the effects of controlling delivery of the head separately from perineal support. The technique for perineal support was not specified in sufficient detail in the protocol to replicate it or to know if all midwives in this trial used the same technique; techniques proposed to support the perineum abound.[41] About 30% of the "hands poised" group were actually delivered "hands on" because the midwife feared impending perineal trauma. There was less pain at 10 days after giving birth in the "hands on" group (31.1% vs 34.1%, $P = 0.02$) but no difference in sutured perineal trauma (58.8% "hands on" vs 59.7% "hands poised": risk difference −1%, 95% CI −4%, 2%). No differences in anal sphincter tears, dyspareunia or urinary or bowel problems were found 3 months postpartum.

5.2.14 Vacuum vs Forceps for Operative Delivery

If operative vaginal delivery is required, should it be accomplished by vacuum extraction or forceps? Perineal trauma after forceps vs vacuum-assisted delivery has been compared in eight RCTs summarised by Eason et al.[17] and in two more recent RCTs.[42,43] The results are consistent and clear: fewer women have anal sphincter trauma with vacuum delivery than with forceps (weighted risk

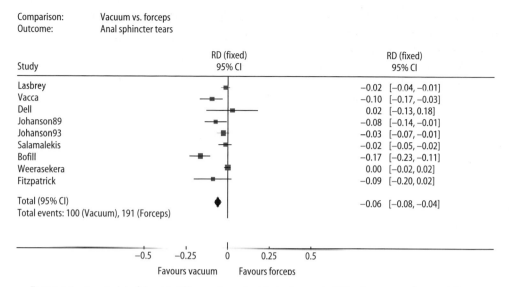

Comparison: Vacuum vs. forceps
Outcome: Anal sphincter tears

Study	RD (fixed) 95% CI	RD (fixed) 95% CI
Lasbrey		−0.02 [−0.04, −0.01]
Vacca		−0.10 [−0.17, −0.03]
Dell		0.02 [−0.13, 0.18]
Johanson89		−0.08 [−0.14, −0.01]
Johanson93		−0.03 [−0.07, −0.01]
Salamalekis		−0.02 [−0.05, −0.02]
Bofill		−0.17 [−0.23, −0.11]
Weerasekera		0.00 [−0.02, 0.02]
Fitzpatrick		−0.09 [−0.20, 0.02]
Total (95% CI)		−0.06 [−0.08, −0.04]
Total events: 100 (Vacuum), 191 (Forceps)		

−0.5 −0.25 0 0.25 0.5

Favours vacuum   Favours forceps

FIGURE 5.4. Forest plot of the risk difference in anal sphincter trauma in RCTs of vacuum vs forceps delivery.

difference −6%, 95% CI −8%, −4%) (Figure 5.4). One anal sphincter tear is avoided for every 18 women delivered by vacuum extraction instead of forceps. Rates of anal sphincter trauma with operative delivery and episiotomy are appalling: a UK RCT[44] where mediolateral episiotomy was practised reported severe vaginal lacerations in 17% of forceps compared to 11% of vacuum deliveries and a Canadian RCT[45] where midline episiotomy was practised reported third/fourth degree tears in 29% of forceps compared to 12% of vacuum deliveries. Occult trauma to the anal sphincter has been detected by anal endosonography in 56%[42]–80%[46] of women delivered by forceps. Compared to vacuum extraction, forceps delivery was associated with almost twice the risk of developing faecal incontinence.[42] These studies support the recommendation by the Royal College of Obstetricians and Gynaecologists that the vacuum extractor should be the instrument of choice for operative vaginal birth.[47] A Cochrane review of forceps vs vacuum-assisted delivery[48] also noted that the vacuum extractor was associated with more vaginal births and less general and regional anaesthesia. What about the neonatal risks? RCTs usually lack the power to address rare adverse outcomes. A population-based study of US singleton live births showed that while neonatal mortal-

ity was similar with both instruments, vacuum delivery was associated with fewer birth injuries (odds ratio 0.69, 95% CI 0.66, 0.72), seizures (0.78, 95% CI 0.68, 0.90) and assisted ventilation (0.94, 95% CI 0.92, 0.97).[49] A 5-year follow-up of infants who participated in a randomised study of forceps and vacuum delivery has confirmed that there is no difference in terms of neurological development and visual acuity with use of either instrument.[50]

5.3 Techniques Proposed but Not Proven to Decrease Perineal Trauma

5.3.1 Head Flexion

The smallest diameters present when the fetal head is in occiput anterior position and well flexed. Various techniques recommended to maintain head flexion during birth include pressing the baby's chin towards its chest through the posterior perineum,[1] restraint of the sinciput just anterior to the perineum, and downwards (posterior) pressure on the occiput between contractions when the perineum is less tense. Many practitioners value maintaining head flexion to minimise perineal trauma. While the "hands on or poised" trials included one hand on the fetal head, the purpose (slowing delivery or flexion or both) and technique was not specified, so conclusions about head flexion cannot be drawn from these studies.

5.3.2 Active Restraint of Delivery of the Head

If it seems obvious that a tense perineum will tear due to rapid egress of the fetal head, should the head be gently restrained, either verbally or manually? Uterine contractions alone may advance the baby as fast or faster than the perineum can stretch. Ritgen recommended slowing egress of the head[51] and his exemplary intact perineum rate (96%) suggests that we should evaluate this. Myles' *Textbook for midwives*[52] recommended that active pushing be discouraged once the perineum is tense. In the "hands on or poised" trials,[40] preventing rapid delivery of the head was considered sufficient justification to abandon the "hands poised" approach. Yet a prevalent approach to delivery in North America is to encourage the mother to push vigorously while the head delivers. Although practice varies diametrically, no controlled trials have addressed either verbal instructions to "breathe the head out" rather than pushing, or manual slowing of the head's delivery.

5.3.3 Perineal Analgesia

Resisting pushing despite the tremendous urge to push and the "ring of fire" sensation of perineal stretching is virtually impossible for many women. Older texts emphasise the importance of allowing time for the perineum to stretch, and chloroform was used a century ago for precisely this purpose.[53] If slowing delivery over the perineum to allow stretching is important, as many believe, is this more feasible with effective perineal analgesia? Although there have been RCTs of epidural analgesia, achieving perineal integrity was not the focus of these trials and co-interventions (such as operative delivery and episiotomy) made possible by epidural analgesia were often used more liberally. The question is unanswered.

5.3.4 Delivery with or Between Contractions

Some practitioners feel that better control over the delivery of the head is obtained by delivering between contractions; this was once part of the British Central Midwives Board instruction.[54] Others feel that by thus hastening delivery, less time is given for the perineum to distend than waiting until delivery is effected by the contraction. Which approach best prevents perineal trauma is unknown.

5.3.5 Delivery of the Shoulders

Perineal trauma is often minimal during delivery of the head, but becomes severe with delivery of the shoulders. There has been no rigorous study of whether the anterior or posterior shoulder should be delivered first. Perhaps more importantly, the optimal technique for delivering the posterior shoulder, in terms of direction and support, has not been studied. It is clear from the "hands on or poised" trials that there was minimal difference between allowing the shoulders to deliver spontaneously and "lateral flexion to facilitate delivery of the shoulders".[40]

5.3.6 Interventions to Correct or Deliver with Occiput Posterior Position

Persistent occipito-posterior (OP) position of the fetal head is a risk factor for prolonged labour, instrumental delivery and perineal trauma in primiparous and multiparous women, likely due to the greater presenting cephalic diameters.[55] Fitzpatrick et al. compared 246 cases with persistent OP position in labour to 13,543 controls delivered with occipito-anterior (OA) position. Although (mediolateral) episiotomy rates were similarly high, anal sphincter trauma was significantly more common in the OP group (7% vs 1%) irrespective of parity.[56] Various methods of preventing OP position during labour and delivery have been proposed, including positioning the labouring woman on hands and knees, oxytocin stimulation of labour, and manual or instrumental rotation of the head to OA. None have been demonstrated by RCT to be effective in decreasing perineal trauma or injury to the pelvic floor.

5.3.7 Operative Vaginal vs Caesarean Birth

If operative delivery is required, is it best accomplished by the vaginal or abdominal route? Since perineal trauma is greater in planned vaginal than caesarean birth, it can be reasonably assumed that perineal and pelvic floor outcomes are better with caesarean compared to vacuum-assisted vaginal birth. However, the balance of risk and benefit with respect to overall maternal morbidity and neonatal outcomes with operative vaginal compared to caesarean delivery when operative delivery is deemed necessary, has not yet been directly subjected to RCT. In the present context of consumer pressures for elective caesarean section, physician concerns with long-term continence and pelvic floor damage, and malpractice liabilities related to neonatal outcomes, the time is ripe for such a trial.

5.3.8 Subsequent Delivery after Anal Sphincter Tear

The risk of recurrence of an anal sphincter tear at a subsequent delivery is 4.4%.[57] There are no RCTs in women with a previous third/fourth degree tear to assess the risks and benefits of planned caesarean section or protective mediolateral episiotomy compared to planned vaginal birth without episiotomy. Experts recommend that women who have needed secondary anal sphincter repairs (remote from childbirth) or who have poor anal sphincter function after primary repair have a better benefit to risk ratio from planned caesarean section to protect the anal sphincter.[7,58]

5.4 Potential Risk Factors for Perineal Trauma

5.4.1 Duration of Second Stage of Labour

In a cohort study of 949 women, Eason et al. found that after controlling for the effects of primiparity, operative delivery and episiotomy, length of second stage was not predictive of anal sphincter trauma.[59] Similarly, in MacArthur's cohort study of 906 women, a prolonged second stage was not predictive of new faecal incontinence after con-

trolling for operative delivery.[60] Farrell also found no relation between active, passive or total second stage length and flatal or faecal incontinence.[61]

5.4.2 Perineal Trauma at a Previous Birth

More women have perineal trauma during a first vaginal birth than during later ones. In a retrospective study of 1,895 women, Martin et al. found that having perineal trauma at the first delivery more than tripled the risk of spontaneous tears at the second delivery.[62] The risk of spontaneous tears at the second delivery increased with the severity of the perineal trauma at the first delivery. A previous anal sphincter laceration is a risk factor for a repeat sphincter tear in centres practising midline episiotomy,[63,64] but does not appear to be a risk factor in centres practising mediolateral episiotomy.[57]

5.4.3 Birth Weight

Increasing size of the newborn is associated with greater anal sphincter trauma, primarily through its association with episiotomy and operative delivery.[59–61] It was not an independent predictor of anal incontinence in any of these studies, although this finding is not universal.

5.4.4 Perineal Length

Women with a perineal body length of less than 2.5 cm have a higher risk of anal sphincter tears.[65]

5.5 Summary

Every attempt should be made to prevent perineal trauma with its attendant pain, dyspareunia and longer-term damage such as prolapse and incontinence. Factors in pregnancy and delivery care whose effects on perineal trauma have been rigorously studied are summarised in Table 5.2, along with the difference in absolute risk of perineal trauma obtainable by applying these interventions and the NNT for each. While certain interventions may reduce perineal trauma, their global impact on maternal and fetal well-being must always be assessed in research studies and kept in mind when caring for pregnant women.

References

1. DeLancey JO, Kearney R, Chou Q, Speights S, Binno S. The appearance of levator ani muscle abnormalities in magnetic resonance images after vaginal delivery. Obstet Gynecol 2003;101(1):46–53.

2. Hannah ME, Hannah WJ, Hewson SA, Hodnett ED, Saigal S, Willan AR. Planned caesarean section versus planned vaginal birth for breech presentation at term: a randomised multicentre trial. Term Breech Trial Collaborative Group. Lancet 2000; 356(9239):1375–83.

3. Sleep J, Grant A, Garcia J, Elbourne D, Spencer J, Chalmers I. West Berkshire perineal management trial. BMJ 1984;289:587–90.

4. Hannah ME, Whyte H, Hannah WJ et al. Maternal outcomes at 2 years after planned cesarean section versus planned vaginal birth for breech presentation at term: the international randomized Term Breech Trial. Am J Obstet Gynecol 2004;191(3): 917–27.

5. Hofmeyr GJ, Hannah ME. Planned caesarean section for term breech delivery (Cochrane Review). The Cochrane Library, Issue 3, 2004. Chichester, UK: John Wiley & Sons, Ltd.

6. Hall MH, Bewley S. Maternal mortality and mode of delivery. Lancet 1999;354:776.

7. Sultan AH, Stanton SL. Preserving the pelvic floor and perineum during childbirth – elective caesarean section? Br J Obstet Gynaecol 1996;103(8): 731–4.

8. Clarke SL, Koongins PP, Phelan JP. Placenta praevia, accreta and prior cesarean section. Obstet Gynecol 1985;89:89–92.

9. Labrecque M, Marcoux S, Pinault JJ, Laroche C, Martin S. Prevention of perineal trauma by perineal massage during pregnancy: a pilot study. Birth 1994;21(1):20–5.

10. Labrecque M, Eason E, Marcoux S et al. Randomized controlled trial of prevention of perineal trauma by perineal massage during pregnancy. Am J Obstet Gynecol 1999;180(3 Pt 1):593–600.

11. Shipman MK, Boniface DR, Tefft ME, McGlohry F. Antenatal perineal massage and subsequent perineal outcomes: a randomised controlled trial. Br J Obstet Gynaecol 1997;104:787–91.

12. Labrecque M, Eason E, Marcoux S. Randomized trial of perineal massage during pregnancy: perineal symptoms three months after delivery. Am J Obstet Gynecol 2000;182(1 Pt 1):76–80.

13. Labrecque M, Eason E, Marcoux S. Women's views on the practice of prenatal perineal massage. Br J Obstet Gynaecol 2001;108(5):499–504.

14. Harvey MA. Pelvic floor exercises during and after pregnancy: a systematic review of their role in preventing pelvic floor dysfunction. J Obstet Gynaecol Can 2003;25:487–98.

15. Hay-Smith J, Herbison P, Morkved S. Physical therapies for prevention of urinary and faecal incontinence in adults (Cochrane Review). The Cochrane Library, Issue 3, 2004. Chichester, UK: John Wiley & Sons, Ltd.

16. Cluett ER, Nikodem VC, McCandlish RE, Burns EE. Immersion in water in pregnancy, labour and birth (Cochrane Review). The Cochrane Library, Issue 2, 2004. Chichester, UK: John Wiley & Sons, Ltd.

17. Eason E, Labrecque M, Wells G, Feldman P. Preventing perineal trauma during childbirth: a systematic review. Obstet Gynecol 2000;95(3):464–71.

18. Gupta JK, Brayshaw EM, Lilford RJ. An experiment of squatting birth. Eur J Obstet Gynecol Reprod Biol 1989;30:217–20.

19. Gardosi J, Sylvester S, B-Lynch C. Alternative positions in the second stage of labour: a randomised controlled trial. Br J Obstet Gynaecol 1989;96: 1290–6.

20. Gupta JK, Hofmeyr GJ. Position for women during second stage of labour (Cochrane Review). The Cochrane Library, Issue 3, 2004. Chichester, UK: John Wiley & Sons, Ltd.

21. Downe S, Gerrett D, Renfrew MJ. A prospective randomised trial on the effect of position in the passive second stage of labour on birth outcome in nulliparous women using epidural analgesia. Midwifery 2004;20:157–68.

22. Howell CJ. Epidural versus non-epidural analgesia for pain relief in labour (Cochrane Review). The Cochrane Library, Issue 3, 2004. Chichester, UK: John Wiley & Sons, Ltd.

23. Robinson JN, Norwitz ER, Cohen AP, Mcelrath TF, Leiberman ES. Epidural analgesia and third- or fourth-degree lacerations in nulliparas. Obstet Gynecol 1999;94(259):262.

24. Lieberman E, O'Donoghue C. Unintended effects of epidural analgesia during labor: a systematic review. Am J Obstet Gynecol 2002;186:S31–S68.

25. Fraser WD, Marcoux S, Krauss I, Douglas J, Goulet C, Boulvain M. Multicenter, randomised trial, controlled trial of delayed pushing for nulliparous women in second stage of labor with continuous epidural. Am J Obstet Gynecol 2000; 182:1165–72.

26. Fitzpatrick M, Harkin R, Mcquillan K, O'Brien C, O'Connell PR, O'Herlihy C. A randomised clinical

trial comparing the effects of delayed versus immediate pushing with epidural analgesia on mode of delivery and faecal incontinence. Br J Obstet Gynaecol 2002;109:1359–65.

27. Parnell C, Langhoff-Roos J, Iversen R, Damgaard P. Pushing method in the expulsive phase of labor. Acta Obstet Gynecol Scand 1993;72:31–5.

28. Thomson AM. Pushing techniques in the second stage of labour. J Adv Nursing 1993;18:171–7.

29. DeLee JB. The prophylactic forceps operation. Am J Obstet Gynecol 1920;1:34–44.

30. Yancey MK, Herpolsheimer A, Jordan GD, Benson WL, Brady K. Maternal and neonatal effects of outlet forceps delivery compared with spontaneous vaginal delivery in term pregnancies. Obstet Gynecol 1991;78:646–50.

31. Pomeroy RH. Shall we cut and reconstruct the perineum for every primipara? Am J Obstet 1918; 78:211–19.

32. Carroli G, Belizan J. Episiotomy for vaginal birth (Cochrane Review). The Cochrane Library, Issue 3, 2004. Chichester, UK: John Wiley & Sons, Ltd.

33. Klein MC, Gauthier RJ, Jorgensen SH et al. Does episiotomy prevent perineal trauma and pelvic floor relaxation? Online J Curr Clin Trials 1992;1: Doc No 10.

34. Sleep J, Grant A. West Berkshire management trial: three year follow-up. BMJ 1987;295:749–51.

35. Coats PM, Chan KK, Wilkins M, Beard RJ. A comparison between midline and mediolateral episiotomies. Br J Obstet Gynaecol 1980;87:408–12.

36. Harrison RF, Brennan M, North PM, Reed JV, Wickham EA. Is routine episiotomy necessary? BMJ 1984;288:1971–5.

37. House MJ, Cario G, Jones MH. Episiotomy and the perineum: a random controlled trial. J Obstet Gynaecol 1986;7:107–10.

38. Argentine Episiotomy Trial Collaborative Group. Routine vs selective episiotomy: a randomised controlled trial. Lancet 1993;42:1517–18.

39. Stamp G, Kruzins G, Crowther C. Perineal massage in labour and prevention of perineal trauma: randomised controlled trial. BMJ 2001;322:1277–80.

40. McCandlish R, Bowler U, van Asten H et al. A randomised controlled trial of care of the perineum during second stage of normal labour. Br J Obstet Gynaecol 1998;105:1262–72.

41. Goodell W. Management of the perineum during labour. Am J Med Sciences 1871;61:53–79.

42. Fitzpatrick M, Behan M, O'Connell PR, O'Herlihy C. Randomised clinical trial to assess anal sphincter function following forceps or vacuum assisted vaginal delivery. Br J Obstet Gynaecol 2003;110: 424–9.

43. Weerasekera DS, Premaratne S. A randomised prospective trial of the obstetric forceps versus vacuum extraction using defined criteria. J Obstet Gynaecol 2002;22(4):344–5.

44. Johanson RB, Rice C, Doyle M. A randomised prospective study comparing the new vacuum extractor policy with forceps delivery. Br J Obstet Gynaecol 1993;100:524–30.

45. Bofill JA, Rust OA, Schorr SJ et al. A randomized prospective trial of the obstetric forceps versus the M-cup vacuum extractor. Am J Obstet Gynecol 1996;175(5):1325–30.

46. Sultan AH, Johanson RB, Carter JE. Occult anal sphincter trauma following randomized forceps and vacuum delivery. Int J Gynecol Obstet 1998;61: 113–19.

47. RCOG Audit Committee. Effective procedures in obstetrics suitable for audit. Manchester: RCOG, 1993.

48. Johanson RB, Menon V. Vacuum extraction versus forceps for assisted vaginal delivery (Cochrane Review). The Cochrane Library, Issue 3, 2004. Chichester, UK: John Wiley & Sons, Ltd.

49. Demissie K, Rhoads GG, Smulian JC et al. Operative vaginal delivery and neonatal and infant adverse outcomes: population based retrospective analysis. BMJ 2004;329:20–4.

50. Johanson RB, Heycock E, Carter J, Sultan AH, Walklate K, Jones PW. Maternal and child health after assisted vaginal delivery: five-year follow up of a randomised controlled study comparing forceps and ventouse. Br J Obstet Gynaecol 1999; 106:544–9.

51. Ritgen G. Ueber sein Dammschutzverfahren. Monatschrift fur Geburtskunde 1855;6:21.

52. Myles MF. Textbook for midwives, 9th edn. Edinburgh: Churchill Livingstone, 1981.

53. Dewees WB. Relaxation and management of the perineum during parturition. JAMA 1889;13: 804–8.

54. Floud E. Protecting the perineum in childbirth 2: risk of laceration. Br J Midwifery 1994;2:306–10.

55. Sultan AH, Kamm MA, Hudson CN, Bartram CI. Third degree obstetric anal sphincter tears: risk factors and outcome of primary repair. BMJ 1994; 308:887–91.

56. Fitzpatrick M, McQuillan K, O'Herlihy C. Influence of persistent occiput posterior position on delivery outcome. Obstet Gynecol 2001;98(6):1027–31.

57. Harkin R, Fitzpatrick M, O'Connell PR, O'Herlihy C. Anal sphincter disruption at vaginal delivery: is

recurrence predictable? Eur J Obstet Gynecol Reprod Biol 2003;109(2):149–52.

58. Fynes M, Donnelly V, Behan M, O'Connell PR, O'Herlihy C. Effect of second vaginal delivery on anorectal physiology and faecal incontinence: a prospective study. Lancet 1999;354:983–6.

59. Eason E, Labrecque M, Marcoux S, Mondor M. Anal incontinence after childbirth. CMAJ 2002;166(3): 326–30.

60. MacArthur C, Bick DE, Keighley MRB. Faecal incontinence after childbirth. Br J Obstet Gynaecol 1997;104:46–50.

61. Farrell S, Allen VM, Baskett TF. Anal incontinence in primiparas. JSOGC 2001;23:321–6.

62. Martin S, Labrecque M, Marcoux S, Berube S, Lemieux F, Pinault J-J. The association between perineal trauma and spontaneous perineal tears. J Fam Pract 2001;50:333–7.

63. Payne TN, Carey JC, Rayburn WF. Prior third- or fourth-degree perineal tears and recurrence risks. Int J Gynecol Obstet 1999;64:55–7.

64. Peleg D, Kennedy CM, Merrill D, Zlatnik FJ. Risk of repetition of a severe perineal laceration. Obstet Gynecol 1999;93(6):1021–4.

65. Deering SH, Carlson N, Stitely M, Allaire AD, Satin AJ. Perineal body length and lacerations at delivery. J Reprod Med 2004;49:306–10.

66. Hannah ME, Hannah WJ, Hodnett ED et al. Outcomes at 3 months after planned cesarean vs planned vaginal delivery for breech presentation at term: the international randomized Term Breech Trial. JAMA 2002; 287(14):1822–31.

6
Postpartum Problems and the Role of a Perineal Clinic

Ranee Thakar and Abdul H. Sultan

6.1 Introduction

Over the past century there has been a dramatic fall in maternal morbidity and mortality, especially in the developed countries. Women therefore have high expectations of pregnancy and childbirth and consequently feel disillusioned when complications occur in the postpartum period. Up to 87% of mothers experience at least one health problem in the first 8 weeks postpartum, reducing to 76% 8 weeks to 18 months after delivery.[1] MacArthur et al.[2] found that the majority of symptoms that lasted more than a year after birth were still present 1–8 years later, suggesting that problems arising after childbirth can have long-term consequences on women's health. Common postnatal health problems include tiredness,[1,3,4] headache,[1,3] haemorrhoids,[1,3,4] perineal pain,[1,5] breast conditions,[1] constipation,[1] dyspareunia,[4,6] backache,[7] and urinary[8-10] and anal incontinence.[11-14] However, the majority of women do not consult a health professional even if they feel that they need help.[3] These conditions are more prevalent in primiparas and more likely to occur following instrumental rather than normal vaginal delivery or caesarean section.[1]

In this chapter, management of problems pertaining to the perineum or pelvic floor during pregnancy and the early postpartum period will be discussed.

6.2 Perineal Problems

6.2.1 Perineal Pain

Perineal pain is a common symptom following vaginal delivery, regardless of the presence of perineal trauma. However, the severity of perineal pain is directly proportional to the severity of perineal trauma.[5,15] Perineal pain occurs in 42% of women immediately after delivery but significantly reduces to 22% and 10% at 8 and 12 weeks respectively. Compared to a normal delivery, perineal pain occurs more frequently and persists for a longer period after assisted delivery (forceps, vacuum delivery, vaginal breech delivery).[16] Risk factors include having any perineal stitches (not only episiotomy), primiparity, assisted delivery and using entonox for analgesia in labour.[16]

Perineal pain may be due to soft tissue trauma with or without suturing. The pain becomes exaggerated if there is an associated inflammatory process, which can range from mild inflammation, cellulitis and florid inflammation with wound breakdown to abscess formation. Precipitating factors include lack of aseptic techniques, poor surgical techniques, which can result in poor apposition and/or granulation tissue or a stitch placed inadvertently in the rectal mucosa.

6.2.1.1 Treatment of Perineal Pain

In addition to treating the underlying condition, treatment options used to relieve perineal pain may be divided into local and systemic. Perineal pain is often accompanied with dyspareunia. Figure 6.1 shows a pathway that can be followed for both conditions.

Local Treatment

Although perineal ice packs have been very popular, there is inconclusive evidence regarding their effectiveness. Bathing in water with salt additives (sitz baths) has been traditionally used to relieve perineal wound pain and promote healing. A three-arm randomised controlled trial (*n* = 1,800) examined the effectiveness of adding salt, a 25-ml sachet of Savlon or nothing to the bath water each day for the first 10 days following delivery.[17] At 10 days and at 3 months the prevalence of pain and pattern of wound healing were similar in all the groups. Although bath additives did not enhance healing or reduce pain or dyspareunia, most of the women reported that bathing did provide some relief of the discomfort. Lavender oil added to bath water has been evaluated in a randomised trial and found to be ineffective.[18] Therapeutic ultrasound has been suggested as a means to alleviate perineal pain, but a Cochrane review was inconclusive.[19]

Local anaesthetics that can be applied directly to the perineum include lidocaine, which can be administered as a spray, gel or cream, and Epifoam (anti-inflammatory steroid-based foam containing 1% hydrocortisone acetate and 1% pramoxine hydrochloride). A recent Cochrane review indicated that the evidence for the effectiveness of topically applied anaesthetics is not compelling. The variety of topical anaesthetics used in the eight included trials limited the capacity to pool data, thus making interpretation difficult. The different methods of measuring pain also made comparisons between trials difficult. Furthermore, there has been no evaluation regarding any long-term effects of topically applied anaesthetics.[20]

Systemic Treatment

Oral Analgesics. Paracetamol (acetomenophen) is one of the most commonly used analgesics to relieve mild postnatal perineal pain. This is a sensible choice as it is relatively inexpensive, effective and free of side-effects to the mother and child.[17] As pain increases to moderate and severe levels, stronger analgesics such as opioid analgesics and non-opioid analgesics including non-steroidal anti-inflammatory drugs (NSAIDs) can be considered. However, one must be aware that opioids can cause constipation and NSAIDs can cause gastric irritation, renal failure and haematological problems. In addition, these drugs can be secreted in breast milk.

Suppositories. Rectal analgesia may be preferred in certain situations, e.g. nausea and vomiting and/or gastric irritation. The mother should be informed about the route of administration and verbal consent obtained. About 50% of the drug administered via the rectum will bypass the liver, resulting in faster pain relief and more local

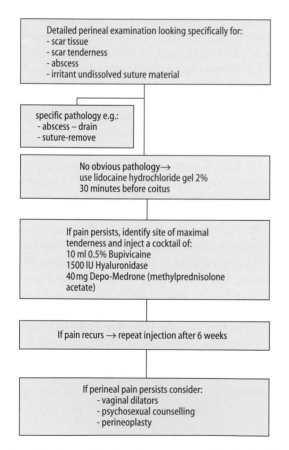

FIGURE 6.1. Suggested regimen for management of perineal pain/dyspareunia.

action.[21] In a systematic review, which set out to assess the effectiveness of analgesic rectal suppositories for perineal pain after childbirth, Hedayati et al.[21] found that compared to placebo women were less likely to experience pain at or close to 24 hours after birth if they received NSAIDs in the form of suppositories such as diclofenac. They also required less additional analgesia in the first 24 hours after birth and this effect was still evident at 48 hours. The effect, if any, on longer-term pain relief and analgesia is not known.

Proven strategies to reduce perineal pain include use of continuous absorbable synthetic sutures[22] and antenatal perineal massage in women who have had a previous vaginal birth.[23]

6.2.2 Perineal Haematoma

Haematomas may be infralevator (vulval, perineal, vaginal) or supralevator (in the broad ligament or paravaginal area). They occur infrequently, with an incidence of between 1:500 and 1:900 vaginal deliveries. Although frequently related to an episiotomy due to an incomplete repair and obliteration of the "dead space", about 20% of cases occur even with an apparently intact perineum due to a concealed ruptured vessel.[24,25] A supralevator haematoma forms in the broad ligament and could be due to an extension of a tear of the cervix, vaginal fornix or uterus. As the haematoma distends, it displaces the uterus contralaterally and bulges into the upper vagina.

With both infralevator and supralevator haematomas, the patient often presents with pain and swelling in the perineal area immediately after delivery or in the postpartum period. However, with a supralevator haematoma, shock may ensue without any obvious swelling. The classical presentation is pain, restlessness, inability to pass urine and rectal tenesmus within a few hours after delivery. On examination there is usually an obvious tender swelling of the perineal area with purple and glistening overlying skin.

Management includes treatment of shock if present. Analgesics, ice packs and pressure dressings can be used if the haematoma is small (less than 5 cm) and not expanding. Surgical evacuation of the infralevator haematoma by incision and drainage should be carried out if the haematoma is large and expanding. The incision should preferably be made in the vagina to avoid scar formation. Often no obvious bleeding points are seen and deep sutures will need to be inserted at the base of the haematoma. It is advisable to leave a drain or pack for at least 24 hours. In contrast to an infralevator haematoma, the management of the supralevator haematoma is largely conservative and a blood transfusion may be necessary. Surgical exploration by laparotomy is usually very frustrating as the bleeding point cannot be identified and the ureter can be injured with the insertion of deep sutures. In this situation, options include evacuation of the clot and packing the cavity for 24 hours or performing an internal iliac artery ligation. The ideal approach when conservative management fails is not to operate, but to involve an intervention radiologist to perform angiographic embolisation of the bleeding vessel.[25]

6.2.3 Perineal Wound Infection

Delay in perineal wound healing due to infection can lead to discomfort, which can contribute to making the entire experience of pregnancy and childbirth very unpleasant. Furthermore, serious complications such as puerperal sepsis[26] and necrotising fasciitis[27] after perineal wound infection have been reported.

It is difficult to quantify the number of women that develop perineal wound infections as there is no standard classification for postpartum perineal wound infection and most studies quoting prevalence are retrospective, observational studies. Furthermore, perineal wound problems are managed in both primary and secondary care, making data collection unreliable. In a survey of 707 women who had spontaneous or assisted vaginal deliveries, Glazener et al.[28] found that 5.5% had perineal wound breakdown. Goldaber et al.[29] undertook a retrospective case review of 390 fourth degree tears in a hospital in Texas, USA and found that 5.4% had postpartum perineal morbidity (1.8% wound dehiscence alone, 2.8% infection and dehiscence, 0.8% infection alone). Women with morbidity were more likely to have experienced shoulder dystocia, endometritis and postpartum pyrexia.

Features of perineal infection include local pain, erythema, exudate, odour, oedema and pyrexia with or without wound breakdown. The care of such women should be transferred to the obstetrician, general practitioner or a specialist perineal clinic. Wound swabs should be taken for culture and sensitivities and antibiotics prescribed. Because there are no randomised studies to develop evidence-based management strategies, there is considerable controversy as to whether perineal wounds should be sutured as soon as possible or let to heal by secondary intention, as the wound may break down further if there is underlying wound infection. Uygur et al.[30] studied 37 women with episiotomy dehiscence (25 underwent early repair and 12 healed by secondary intention). They concluded that with adequate preoperative care such as primary wound cleansing (daily scrubbing and irrigation and intravenous antibiotics), early repair of episiotomy dehiscence is safe and effective. Similarly, in a small randomised study comparing the two methods, Christensen et al.[31] found no significant difference in healing time, hospitalisation and infection between the two groups. However, there was a need for vaginal plastic repair in three of the nine who underwent "open" treatment, i.e. healing by secondary intention.

When third or fourth degree tears break down, it is conventional practice to defer a second attempt at repair for 3–4 months. The delay is considered necessary to ensure adequate blood supply to the margins of the defect and restoration of tissue viability.[32] However, this delay is undesirable (persistent faecal incontinence, effect on sexual intercourse, muscle atrophy, etc.) and therefore early repair after outpatient wound debridement and preparation has been advocated. In a case series of 22 patients who developed wound breakdown within a week of repair of a fourth degree tear, all had a subsequent repair within an average of a further week. None experienced subsequent wound breakdown. One patient developed a small rectoperineal fistula that closed spontaneously after irrigation.[32] In another series of 23 patients (two third and 21 fourth degree tears), a second repair was performed within a mean of 7 days of outpatient debridement and all repairs were successful apart from one rectoperineal fistula that healed spontaneously after 3

months.[33] The authors concluded that forcing women to wait the traditional 3–4 months before repairing such defects may be both cruel and unnecessary and perhaps should be obsolete.

The risk of perineal infection can be minimised by adopting sound surgical principles, and emphasising the importance of good perineal hygiene such as changing sanitary pads regularly and frequent irrigation with a shower.

There are no randomised trials to establish the efficacy of peripartum antibiotics in preventing perineal wound infections.

6.3 Bowel Problems

6.3.1 Anal Fissure

Anal fissure is an ulcer in the squamous epithelium of the anus located just distal to the mucocutaneous junction; it usually occurs in the posterior midline.[34] The mucosa in this area is sensitive to pain due to its somatic nerve supply (see Chapter 1) and therefore can be extremely painful. Anal fissures are believed to be caused by trauma to the anal mucosa, usually after passage of hard, bulky stools. Constipation is the most common predisposing factor, although diarrhoea may also be a cause.[35,36] Atypical fissures (large, irregular, multiple and non-midline) may be caused by inflammatory bowel disease, local or systemic malignancy, venereal infection, trauma, tuberculosis or chemotherapy.[34]

In a prospective study before and after delivery of 163 consecutive women (84 primiparous), Abramowitz et al.[37] reported anal fissures in 15% during the first 2 months postpartum. Others have reported an incidence of 9% during a 6-week follow-up period of primiparous women.[35] Risk factors associated with the development of anal fissure include dyschezia (painful defaecation), heavier babies, long second stage of labour, anal incontinence after delivery,[37] primiparity, forceps deliveries and perineal damage.[38] Caesarean section did not appear to be protective against anal fissure.[35,37]

Anal fissures typically cause episodic pain that occurs during defaecation and for 1–2 hours afterwards. The diagnosis is suspected from the history and frequently confirmed by visual examination of the anal margin. The most consistent finding in typical fissures is spasm of the internal anal sphincter, which is so severe that the pain caused by the fissure is thought to be due to ischaemia of the sphincter.[39] Relief of the spasm has been associated with relief of pain and healing of the fissure without recurrence.

Treatment is aimed at relieving constipation using a high fibre diet along with fibre supplements such as Psyllium seed supplement (Fybogel). Iron preparations should be avoided. Local application of lidocaine in the anal canal can provide effective analgesia. After defaecation, water (preferably a shower) should be used to clean the anus rather than wiping with toilet paper to avoid abrasions. Medical treatments are aimed at relaxing the internal anal sphincter. These include nitroglycerin ointment, calcium channel blockers, either given as tablets or applied topically, and injection of botulinum toxin.[34] In a systematic review, nitroglycerin ointment was found to have a healing rate of about 55%. Combining all analyses in which a placebo was used as the comparison group, the healing rate in the placebo group was found to be 35%. In comparisons of nitroglycerin ointment to botulinum toxin injection or calcium channel blockers, no significant difference in efficacy was found. However, in almost 40% of subjects, nitroglycerin ointment was associated with headache often severe enough to stop treatment.[40] Conservative treatment (stool softeners, laxatives and local anaesthetic cream) has been shown to be successful in 97% of postpartum women.[35,36] There are no data regarding the use of medical treatments for anal fissure during pregnancy. A suggested pathway for the management of anal fissures in postpartum women is shown in Figure 6.2.

Non-pregnant women who fail to respond to these conservative measures are candidates for surgical procedures. However, postpartum anal fissures are associated with low anal canal pressures, and surgical interference with the anal sphincter mechanism must be avoided.[35] For those patients requiring surgery for anal fissure, open and closed partial lateral internal sphincterotomy appear to be equally efficacious. It is less clear whether posterior sphincterotomy should be performed as the primary treatment of anal fissure.[41]

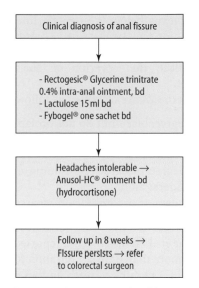

FIGURE 6.2. Management of anal fissures.

6.3.2 Haemorrhoids

Haemorrhoids (piles) are swollen veins at or near the anus. During bowel evacuation, normal haemorrhoids are compressed and drained, facilitating the emptying of the rectum. Haemorrhoids can become symptomatic if there is damage to their structure and/or alteration in function. Associated factors include straining at defaecation, constipation, vascular enlargement secondary to increased intra-abdominal pressure, erect posture and heredity. Several physiological changes during pregnancy may lead to development of haemorrhoids. Constipation is likely to be due to smooth muscle inhibition by high levels of circulating progesterone or by mechanical obstruction by the gravid uterus. Venous engorgement and dilatation may occur during pregnancy as the circulating blood volume is increased by 25–40%. Hormonal changes result in increased laxity of connective tissue, especially in the pelvis.[36] In the postnatal period haemorrhoids are possibly a consequence of pushing in the second stage of labour. Risk factors include instrumental delivery,[1–3] a longer second stage of labour[2] and vaginal delivery of a heavier baby.[2]

Haemorrhoids may be internal or external. Internal haemorrhoids originate from the internal haemorrhoidal plexus above the dentate line and external haemorrhoids originate from the external plexus below the dentate line. Internal haemorrhoids may be classified according to the degree of prolapse, although this may not necessarily reflect the severity of the woman's symptoms.

Haemorrhoids are classified as follows:[42]

1. First degree: bleed but do not prolapse.
2. Second degree: prolapse on straining but reduce spontaneously.
3. Third degree: prolapse on straining and require manual reduction.
4. Fourth degree: prolapsed and incarcerated.

In an observational study of 11,701 women, MacArthur et al.[2] found that 8% reported haemorrhoids of more than 6 weeks' duration for the first time within 3 months of birth and an additional 10% reported these as ongoing or recurrent symptoms. Two thirds reported the presence of haemorrhoids 1–9 years after delivery. Glazener et al.[1] found that 17% of postnatal women reported haemorrhoids (new and recurrent) when questioned in hospital, 22% between delivery and 8 weeks postpartum and 15% after 2 months. The problem can manifest in a wide range of symptoms such as a burning sensation, itching, intermittent bleeding of the anus, varying degrees of leakage of mucus, faeces or flatus, sensation of fullness or a lump, perianal hygienic problems, discomfort and/or pain. The most common symptoms during pregnancy and the puerperium are intermittent bleeding from the anus and pain. Depending on the degree of pain, quality of life could be compromised, affecting the activities of everyday life, such as walking, sitting down, emptying bowels, sleeping, or caring for the family or a new baby. Assessment should include anoscopy and a digital examination in the left lateral position.

Treatment during pregnancy is mainly directed to the relief of symptoms, especially pain control. For many women, symptoms will resolve spontaneously soon after birth, and so any corrective treatment is usually deferred to some time after birth.

Complications of haemorrhoids (acute thrombosis, incarceration of prolapsed internal haemorrhoid, unremitting pain) require more aggressive treatment such as closed excisional haemorrhoidectomy under local anaesthetic.[43]

The treatment for haemorrhoids during pregnancy and the postpartum period should be tailored to the severity of the disease and duration of symptoms. External haemorrhoids require treatment only for acute thrombosis. Internal haemorrhoids are best managed conservatively. Management can be broadly classified as conservative, alternative or surgical.[44,45]

6.3.2.1   Conservative Management

Conservative treatment is based on: (a) dietary modifications (high fibre intake, high liquid intake, stool softeners); (b) stimulants or depressants of the bowel transit (depending on whether the woman has constipation or diarrhoea); (c) local treatments (sitz baths, creams, ointments or suppositories containing anaesthetics, anti-inflammatory drugs, steroids, etc., alone or in combination); (d) drugs of the flavonoid family such as rutosides that cause decreased capillary fragility, improving the microcirculation in venous insufficiency. Most minor haemorrhoidal symptoms can be treated this way.

6.3.2.2   Alternative Management

Alternative treatment is required if the haemorrhoids are severe and non-responsive to conservative treatment. It includes a number of ambulatory interventions that usually do not need anaesthetics, such as injection sclerotherapy, rubber-band ligation, cryotherapy, infrared photocoagulation, laser therapy, etc. Injection sclerotherapy has been used effectively during pregnancy. In one study, 86% of antenatal patients (24 of 28) became asymptomatic by means of injection of 5% phenol in almond oil.[45] No complications occurred and six patients required further injection during the ensuing 30 months.

6.3.2.3   Surgical Management

Surgical treatment includes excision surgery and stapled anopexy. These methods are usually a third-line therapy after other treatments have failed. There are no known trials that have specifically evaluated treatments for severe haemorrhoids during pregnancy and the postpartum period.

6.3.3 Anal Incontinence

The diagnosis and management of anal incontinence are covered in Chapters 8, 11, 12a and 12b).

6.3.4 Constipation

About 80% of people suffer from constipation at some time during their lives, and brief periods of constipation are normal. Widespread beliefs, such as the assumption that everyone should have a movement at least once each day, have led to overuse and abuse of laxatives. Some of the most commonly used definitions include infrequent bowel movements (typically fewer than two bowel actions per week), difficulty in defecation (straining at passing stools for more than 25% of bowel movements or a subjective sensation of hard stools), or the sensation of incomplete bowel emptying.

The prevalence of constipation in pregnancy is reported to be 11–38%.[46] The pathogenesis is not fully understood but It appears to be related to the effect of progesterone on gastrointestinal motility as there is an increase in gut transit time in the second and third trimester compared with both the first trimester and the postpartum period. Fibre supplements are effective, and raise no serious concerns about side-effects to mother or fetus. Stimulant laxatives are more effective than bulk-forming laxatives but are more likely to cause side-effects that reduce their acceptability to patients.

Women complaining of constipation in pregnancy can be treated effectively with daily dietary supplements of fibre in the form of bran or wheat fibre. If these are ineffective, stimulant laxatives may be used.

6.4 Bladder Problems

6.4.1 Postpartum Urinary Retention

There is no standardised definition that qualifies postpartum urinary retention. A commonly used symptom-based definition is the absence of spontaneous voiding of urine within 6 hours of delivery. After caesarean section, if a catheter is used, retention is defined as "no spontaneous voiding within 6 hours after removal of the indwelling catheter".[47] Another commonly used definition is based on the post-void residual bladder volume as estimated by ultrasound or catheterisation. Although most experts agree that residual volumes of less than 50 ml are normal and more than 200 ml are abnormal, little agreement exists on the intervening grey zone.[48] Postpartum urinary retention can be classified into covert and overt forms. The covert form is asymptomatic and recognised by demonstrating an elevated post-void residual measurement of more than or equal to 150 ml, with either ultrasound scanning or catheterisation. Clinically overt postpartum urinary retention refers to the inability to void spontaneously after delivery.[49] Risk factors include nulliparity,[50,51] instrumental delivery,[49,50,52] prolonged first and second stage of labour[51,53] and severe perineal trauma.[51,52] Although there is a lack of consensus in the literature regarding the effect of epidural analgesia on postpartum retention,[48] the Royal College of Obstetricians and Gynaecologists guidelines recommend catheterisation for at least 12 hours following regional anaesthesia.[54]

The incidence of postpartum urinary retention ranges between 0.5% and 14% and varies depending on the definition used.[48] The mother will present with an inability to pass urine associated with acute lower abdominal pain. Occasionally she may complain of continuous leakage of urine in the presence of a large palpable bladder. Other presenting symptoms may be hesitancy, slow or intermittent stream, straining to void and a sense of incomplete emptying. On examination of the abdomen, a suprapubic mass will be palpable. A diagnosis can be made after catheterisation or imaging techniques such as an ultrasound. There is no consensus on the minimal urine volume that constitutes postpartum urinary retention as measured on ultrasound.[55] Ultrasound estimation of post-void residual urine in postpartum women can be measured accurately and is not confounded by the enlarged postpartum uterus.

There is no consensus of opinion on the management of postpartum urinary retention[56] and various treatment regimens have been described.[48,49,51,52] Treatment includes general measures such as administration of oral analgesia, helping the woman to mobilise, ensuring privacy during voiding and having a warm bath. None of the pharmacologic drugs have been studied systematically in postpartum women, as most women would be breastfeeding. If conservative measures fail, it is advisable to insert a urethral catheter and remove it after the bladder has been emptied. If spontaneous voiding fails to occur within 4 hours or if the voided volume is less than 150 ml and/or the post void residual urine is more than 150 ml a Foley catheter should be inserted. A trial without catheter can be attempted after 24–48 hours. The duration of catheterisation is empirical, and no standard has

been agreed to. Burkhart et al.[57] found that no postpartum women with a residual urine volume of less than 700 ml required repeat catheterisation, but repeat catheterisation was required in 14% of patients with 700–999 ml of residual urine. If trial without catheter fails, the woman can be taught intermittent self-catheterisation every 4–6 hours until she is able to void and then until the residual is less than 150 ml. If this is not feasible, send her home with an indwelling catheter for 48 hours and repeat the voiding trial. A suggested regimen for management of postpartum urinary retention is shown in Figure 6.3.

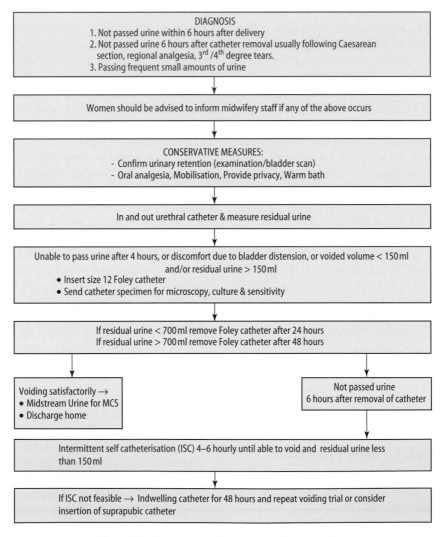

FIGURE 6.3. Management of postpartum urinary retention.

Suprapubic catheterisation may become necessary if the problem becomes chronic and the patient does not wish to per-form intermittent self-catheterisation. Other potential treatment modalities include acupuncture.[58]

Overdistension bladder injury in the postpartum period can be avoided by strict vigilance in ensuring that voiding occurs regularly. Women with potential risk factors, e.g. regional anaesthesia, instrumental delivery, obstetric anal sphincter trauma or severe perineal tears should be catheterised during labour and delivery.

There are very few studies on the sequelae of postpartum urinary retention but published data suggest that this condition returns to normal within a short period and specific treatment is not necessary.[49,50] Yip et al.[59] in a case-controlled study, found that women with postpartum urinary retention did not have a higher incidence of urinary incontinence, frequency nocturia or urgency.

6.4.2   Urinary Incontinence

Childbirth is an established risk factor for urinary incontinence.[60,61] Although vaginal delivery has been implicated as the main contributory factor, the exact mechanism is not known. Pregnancy itself may cause mechanical and/or hormonal changes that can lead to urinary incontinence.

There is evidence that the prevalence of urinary incontinence is highest during pregnancy and decreases in the puerperium.[62,63] Interestingly, stress or urge incontinence during the first pregnancy and puerperium predicts an increased risk of having the symptom 5 years later.[64] In a large community-based epidemiological study, designed to evaluate the risks of incontinence associated with caesarean section and vaginal delivery, Rortveit et al.[65] found that compared to nulliparous women, those who had caesarean section were at higher risk for any incontinence. Vaginal delivery was associated with a greater increase in risk. The risk of moderate or severe incontinence was also higher in the vaginal-delivery group compared to the caesarean section group. As compared with nulliparous status, caesarean section was associated with stress and mixed type of incontinence, whereas vaginal delivery further increased the risk of stress incontinence only.

There was no difference in the prevalence of incontinence in women who underwent elective and emergency caesarean section. The authors suggest that this data should not be used as an argument for increased use of caesarean section, as a very large number of women would have to have a caesarean section to prevent urinary incontinence. Moreover, the decrease in incontinence after caesarean section would apply until 50 years of age, since there was no association of incontinence with mode of delivery in the older age groups.

Current evidence suggests that intensive supervised pelvic floor muscle training should be offered to antenatal women[66] and/or to postnatal high-risk women, i.e. instrumental delivery, large baby, prepregnancy and antenatal stress incontinence, persistent postnatal urinary incontinence, family history of incontinence, prepregnancy obesity, increased bladder neck mobility.[66,67] Unfortunately the early benefits do not seem to persist on long-term follow-up, probably due to reduced compliance.[68]

6.5   Sexual Problems

Recent work on women's sexual health after childbirth has shown that sexual health problems are common. In a cross-sectional study of 796 primiparous women over a 6-month period after delivery, Barrett et al.[6] found that 32% had resumed intercourse within 6 weeks of birth and the majority of respondents (89%) had resumed intercourse within 6 months. Sexual health problems, as recalled by women, increased significantly after childbirth. In the first 3 months, 83% had experienced sexual problems, which declined to 64% at 6 months, although not reaching pre-pregnancy levels of 38%. Dyspareunia in the first 3 months after delivery was significantly associated with vaginal delivery and previous experience of dyspareunia. At 6 months the association with the type of delivery was not significant. However, experience of previous dyspareunia persisted (fourfold) and current breastfeeding was associated with dyspareunia. This suggests that women with dyspareunia prior to pregnancy may have specific needs or issues that could be identified antenatally; appropriate advice and help could be offered. The response rate of this study was 61%, suggesting that the prevalence of these problems is under-reported. In a further analysis of the same cohort of women, Morof et al.[69] found that women who were depressed were less likely to have resumed sexual intercourse by 6 months postpartum and more likely to report sexual health problems than women who were not depressed. However, sexual health problems were common after childbirth in both depressed and non-depressed women and therefore the authors suggest that postnatal sexual morbidity cannot be assumed to be simply a product of the depressed mental state. In a different study, Glazener[70] found that 53% of women experienced sexual problems in the first 8 weeks postpartum and 49% in the subsequent year. Women who reported perineal pain, depression and tiredness experienced problems related to intercourse more often than those who did not. Although sexual problems are common after childbirth, the proportion of women who ask for help or discuss their problem is low.[6,70] Health professionals should therefore include sexual well-being as a part of a women's overall assessment in the postnatal period, which may well extend beyond the traditional 6 weeks after delivery, as 60% of women may not have resumed intercourse at this stage.

Initial assessment involves a detailed history and examination. In the absence of a local pathology, if a psychosexual problem is suspected, referral to a psychosexual counsellor may be helpful. If localised tender scar tissue is identified, we advise women to have sexual intercourse after insertion of lignocaine gel in the vagina. If unsuccessful, a cocktail (10 ml of 0.5% bupivacaine, 1,500 iu of hyaluronidase and 1 ml of Depo-

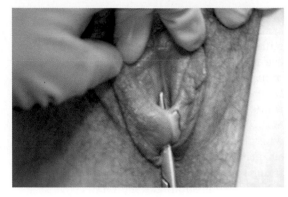

FIGURE 6.5. Fusion of the labia.

Medrone) is injected into the perineum at the site of maximal tenderness (Figure 6.1). Occasionally, women may present with a perineal skin web in the posterior fourchette (Figure 6.4) or fusion of the labia (Figure 6.5). These can be divided after infiltrating the area with a local anaesthetic injection. In women who are breastfeeding, dyspareunia may be due to vaginal dryness. New mothers could be alerted to this side-effect and given advice on the use of lubricants and oestrogen pessaries or creams if necessary, while being reassured about the benefits of breastfeeding.

6.6   Pelvic Organ Prolapse

Injury to the pelvic floor during childbirth is incriminated in the development of pelvic organ prolapse. Other risk factors include defective collagen, race, advancing age, hysterectomy, certain medical illnesses, chronic raised intra-abdominal pressure and states. In a large study in the USA, Swift[71] found an association between gravidity, parity, number of vaginal deliveries, vaginal delivery of a macrosomic infant and an increased pelvic organ prolapse quantification (POPQ) system stage.

In a prospective study conducted to document pelvic organ prolapse throughout the pregnancy, O'Boyle et al.[72] found that the POPQ stage was significantly higher in the third than in the first trimester. They concluded that these findings probably represent normal physiological changes of the pelvic floor during pregnancy, but suggest

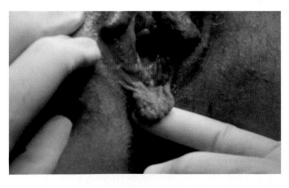

FIGURE 6.4. Perinal skin tag causing dypareunia.

that significant changes may be objectively demonstrated prior to delivery. The effect of delivery on pelvic organ prolapse has been investigated by Sze et al.,[73] who found a prevalence of pelvic organ prolapse in 46% of women (26% had POPQ stage II) at the 36-week antepartum visit. Six weeks postpartum, 83% of women developed prolapse; 52% of these had stage II prolapse. This study directly links the development of prolapse to childbirth. However, this study was small and larger studies are needed to investigate the cause and effect of pregnancy and genital prolapse.

The woman usually presents with a feeling of a lump in the vagina, which may or may not be associated with urinary symptoms. In our practice we use the ring pessary as the first option to relieve the symptom of prolapse in the antenatal and postnatal woman with prolapse. If this is uncomfortable or not retained, we teach the woman to insert a cube pessary herself. There is not enough evidence to suggest the best mode of delivery when a pregnant woman presents with prolapse. Sze et al.,[73] in a small study, demonstrated that elective caesarean section is only partially effective in preventing pelvic organ prolapse. After delivery a decision can be made as to whether the woman wishes to continue with conservative management or plan surgery.

6.7 Perineal Clinic

6.7.1 Background

In a survey of 1,249 women in the postnatal period, Glazener et al.[1] found that all 85% of women who reported at least one health problem in hospital received help or treatment for it. Although just as many had problems on discharge home (87%), a small proportion (69%) were treated, and of the 75% who had a health problem after the first 2 months, just over half received treatment. Reasons for the apparent lack of treatment include that it was inappropriate to ask for help or that professional help was not available, unsatisfactory or ineffective.[1] Perhaps it was perceived that health professionals might only treat women with more severe problems[1] or women may feel that the doctors may be unable to treat this condition or that they can cope with the problem themselves.[74]

The pattern of decreasing help might be due to the natural resolution of the problem or the decrease in severity with time, but might also reflect a lack of recognition of the impact of continuing maternal morbidity by health professionals and mothers themselves.

As these problems are usually of a sensitive nature, women should ideally be seen in a dedicated clinic instead of a busy general clinic. Furthermore, this environment would facilitate childcare and breastfeeding. The establishment of a dedicated one-stop clinic enables provision of evidence-based quality care, by experienced professionals. A dedicated perineal clinic also provides women with an opportunity to be given an explanation of the circumstances under which the perineal injury occurred, and appropriate counselling regarding mode of subsequent delivery. Due to time constraints and inappropriate expertise, explanation and counselling are often suboptimal in a busy postnatal or gynaecology clinic.

Although perineal clinics are now becoming very popular, there appear to be a variety of models of care. In 2002, Fitzpatrick et al.[75] published their experience of the perineal clinic held in the National Maternity Hospital in Dublin. This was a weekly clinic staffed by an obstetric registrar, continence nurse and medical technician and overseen by a consultant obstetrician and colorectal surgeon. Endoanal ultrasound and neurophysiological tests were reported at a later date by a radiologist and neurophysiologist. However, the clinic was not restricted to women of childbearing age, as women up to the age of 77 were included. In North Staffordshire Hospital (Kettle C, personal communication), the perineal clinic is led by a specialist clinical midwife with access to an obstetrician. Endoanal ultrasound and anorectal physiology tests are performed at a separate visit. Complicated cases are discussed at a multidisciplinary meeting (including midwife, colorectal surgeon, physiotherapist and obstetrician).

6.7.2 The Mayday Perineal Clinic

The perineal clinic at Mayday University Hospital, Croydon, UK is run by a consultant urogynaecologist (trained in anal manometry and ultrasound) and a trained nurse/midwife. We have easy access

TABLE 6.1. Reason (main symptom) for postnatal referrals (*n* = 373).

	No. of women	%
OASIS	245	65.7
Dyspareunia	17	4.6
Urinary incontinence	10	2.7
Anal incontinence and faecal urgency	23	6.2
Prolapse	10	2.7
Perineal pain	29	7.8
Haemorrhoids	2	0.5
Wound breakdown/infection	21	5.6
Miscellaneous	16	4.3
	373	100

to a physiotherapist, a continence nurse specialist, a colorectal nurse specialist, colorectal surgeons and a psychosexual counsellor. Integration of multidisciplinary professionals promotes a holistic approach to pelvic floor and perineal problems. Furthermore, in this clinic we accept self-referrals and are easily accessible to general practitioners and midwives to allow fast tracking. This clinic is restricted to childbirth-related problems and includes conditions such as dyspareunia, perineal pain, wound breakdown, infection, prolapse, and urinary incontinence that occur during pregnancy and up to 16 weeks after childbirth. Women who sustain obstetric anal sphincter injuries (OASIS) are seen within 3 months postpartum. In addition pregnant women with previous OASIS are evaluated and counselled regarding mode of delivery (see Chapter 4). The clinic is equipped with facilities for endoanal ultrasound scan and anal manometry to facilitate a one-stop approach.

There were 423 new referrals to the perineal clinic from July 2002 to July 2005. Tables 6.1 and 6.2 show the type of patients seen in the clinic.

TABLE 6.2. Reason (main symptom) for antenatal referrals (*n* = 50).

	No. of women	%
OASIS	39	78
Anal incontinence	8	16
Prolapse	1	2
Urinary incontinence	1	2
Other	1	2
	50	100

6.8 Conclusion

Postpartum problems are clearly an integral part of the care of childbearing women. Ideally, a team of healthcare providers with the knowledge and expertise to care for these women in a single clinic setting should be available to mothers. More research is needed in the management of perineal problems including perineal wounds, OASIS in subsequent pregnancies and perineal pain. A perineal clinic is an ideal setting to advance our knowledge, develop local experts and provide comprehensive care. We have described three models of perineal clinics and each has its merits and limitations. The value of a dedicated perineal clinic is unquestionable but the best model of care will be dependent on local expertise and resources.

References

1. Glazener CM, Abdalla M, Stroud P, Naji S, Templeton A, Russell IT. Postnatal maternal morbidity: extent, causes, prevention and treatment. Br J Obstet Gynaecol 1995;102:282–7.
2. MacArthur C, Lewis M, Knox E. Health after childbirth. London: HMSO, 1991.
3. Brown S, Lumley J. Maternal health after childbirth: results of an Australian population based survey. Br J Obstet Gynaecol 1998;105(2):156–61.
4. Schytt E, Lindmark G, Waldenstrom U. Physical symptoms after childbirth: prevalence and associations with self-rated health. BJOG 2005;112(2):210–17.
5. Albers L, Garcia J, Renfrew M, McCandlish R, Elbourne D. Distribution of genital tract trauma in childbirth and related postnatal pain. Birth 1999;26(1):11–17.
6. Barrett G, Pendry E, Peacock J, Victor C, Thakar R, Manyonda I. Women's sexual health after childbirth. BJOG 2000;107(2):186–95.
7. Thompson JF, Roberts CL, Currie M, Ellwood DA. Prevalence and persistence of health problems after childbirth: associations with parity and method of birth. Birth 2002;29(2):83–94.
8. Hojberg KE, Salvig JD, Winslow NA, Lose G, Secher NJ. Urinary incontinence: prevalence and risk factors at 16 weeks of gestation. Br J Obstet Gynaecol 1999;106(8):842–50.
9. Foldspang A, Mommsen S, Djurhuus JC. Prevalent urinary incontinence as a correlate of pregnancy, vaginal childbirth, and obstetric techniques. Am J Public Health 1999;89(2):209–12.

10. Wilson PD, Herbison RM, Herbison GP. Obstetric practice and the prevalence of urinary incontinence three months after delivery. Br J Obstet Gynaecol 1996;103:154–61.

11. Sultan AH, Kamm MA, Hudson CN, Thomas JM, Bartram CI. Anal sphincter disruption during vaginal delivery. N Engl J Med 1993;329:1905–11.

12. Abramowitz L, Sobhani I, Ganansia R, Vuagnat A, Benifla JL, Darai E et al. Are sphincter defects the cause of anal incontinence after vaginal delivery? Results of a prospective study. Dis Colon Rectum 2000;43(5):590–6.

13. MacArthur C, Bick DE, Keighley MRB. Faecal incontinence after childbirth. Br J Obstet Gynaecol 1997;104:46–50.

14. Chaliha C, Sultan AH, Bland JM, Monga AK, Stanton SL. Anal function: effect of pregnancy and delivery. Am J Obstet Gynecol 2001;185(2):427–32.

15. Macarthur AJ, MacArthur C. Incidence, severity, and determinants of perineal pain after vaginal delivery: a prospective cohort study. Am J Obstet Gynecol 2004;191(4):1199–204.

16. Glazener CM. Women's health after delivery. In: Henderson C, Bick D, eds. Perineal care: an international issue, 1st edn. Salisbury: Quay Books Division, MA Healthcare Ltd, 2005, pp 11–17.

17. Sleep J, Grant A. Relief of perineal pain following childbirth: a survey of midwifery practice. Midwifery 1988;4(3):118–22.

18. Dale A, Cornwell S. The role of lavender oil in relieving perineal discomfort following childbirth: a blind randomized clinical trial. J Adv Nurs 1994;19(1):89–96.

19. Hay-Smith J, Herbison P, Morkved S. Physical therapies for prevention of urinary and faecal incontinence in adults (Cochrane Review). The Cochrane Library, Issue 3, 2004. Chichester, UK: John Wiley & Sons, Ltd.

20. Hedayati H, Parsons J, Crowther CA. Topically applied anaesthetics for treating perineal pain after childbirth. Cochrane Database Syst Rev 2005;2:CD004223.

21. Hedayati H, Parsons J, Crowther CA. Rectal analgesia for pain from perineal trauma following childbirth. Cochrane Database Syst Rev 2003;3:CD003931.

22. Kettle C. Perineal care. Update in Clin Evid 2002;8:1461–74.

23. Labrecque M, Eason E, Marcoux S. Randomized trial of perineal massage during pregnancy: perineal symptoms three months after delivery. Am J Obstet Gynecol 2000;182(1 Pt 1):76–80.

24. Ridgway LE. Puerperal emergency. Vaginal and vulvar hematomas. Obstet Gynecol Clin North Am 1995;22(2):275–82.

25. Villella J, Garry D, Levine G, Glanz S, Figueroa R, Maulik D. Postpartum angiographic embolization for vulvovaginal hematoma. A report of two cases. J Reprod Med 2001;46(1):65–7.

26. Soltesz S, Biedler A, Ohlmann P, Molter G. [Puerperal sepsis due to infected episiotomy wound.] Zentralbl Gynakol 1999;121(9):441–3.

27. Hausler G, Hanzal E, Dagak C, Gruber W. Necrotizing fasciitis arising from episiotomy. Arch Gynecol Obstet 1994;255:153–5.

28. Glazener CMA. Investigation of postnatal experience and care in the Grampian. PhD Thesis, University of Aberdeen, 1999.

29. Goldaber KG, Wendel PJ, McIntire DD, Wendel GD Jr. Postpartum perineal morbidity after fourth-degree perineal repair. Am J Obstet Gynecol 1993;168(2):489–93.

30. Uygur D, Yesildaglar N, Kis S, Sipahi T. Early repair of episiotomy dehiscence. Aust N Z J Obstet Gynaecol 2004;44(3):244–6.

31. Christensen S, Andersen G, Detlefsen GU, Hansen PK. [Treatment of episiotomy wound infections. Incision and drainage versus incision, curettage and sutures under antibiotic cover – a randomized trial.] Ugeskr Laeger 1994;156(34):4829–33.

32. Hankins GD, Hauth JC, Gilstrap LC III, Hammond TL, Yeomans ER, Snyder RR. Early repair of episiotomy dehiscence. Obstet Gynecol 1990;75(1):48–51.

33. Arona AJ, al-Marayati L, Grimes DA, Ballard CA. Early secondary repair of third- and fourth-degree perineal lacerations after outpatient wound preparation. Obstet Gynecol 1995;86(2):294–6.

34. Nelson RL. Treatment of anal fissure. BMJ 2003;327(7411):354–5.

35. Corby H, Donnelly VS, O'Herlihy C, O'Connell PR. Anal canal pressures are low in women with postpartum anal fissure. Br J Surg 1997;84(1):86–8.

36. Medich DS, Fazio VW. Hemorrhoids, anal fissure, and carcinoma of the colon, rectum, and anus during pregnancy. Surg Clin North Am 1995;75(1):77–88.

37. Abramowitz L, Sobhani I, Benifla JL, Vuagnat A, Darai E, Mignon M et al. Anal fissure and thrombosed external hemorrhoids before and after delivery. Dis Colon Rectum 2002;45(5):650–5.

38. Martin JD. Postpartum anal fissure. Lancet 1953;1(6):271–3.

39. Schouten WR, Briel JW, Auwerda JJ, Boerma MO. Anal fissure: new concepts in pathogenesis and treatment. Scand J Gastroenterol Suppl 1996;218:78–81.

40. Nelson R. Non surgical therapy for anal fissure. Cochrane Database Syst Rev 2003;4:CD003431.

41. Nelson R. Operative procedures for fissure in ano. Cochrane Database Syst Rev 2005;2:CD002199.

42. Nisar PJ, Scholefield JH. Managing haemorrhoids. BMJ 2003;327(7419):847–51.

43. Saleeby RG Jr, Rosen L, Stasik JJ, Riether RD, Sheets J, Khubchandani IT. Hemorrhoidectomy during pregnancy: risk or relief? Dis Colon Rectum 1991; 34(3):260–1.

44. Quijano C, Abalos E. Conservative management of symptomatic and/or complicated haemorrhoids in pregnancy and the puerperium. Cochrane Database Syst Rev 2005;3:CD004077.

45. Simmons SC. Ano-rectal disorders in pregnancy. J Obstet Gynaecol Br Commonw 1964;71:960–2.

46. Jewell DJ, Young G. Interventions for treating constipation in pregnancy. Cochrane Database Syst Rev 2001;2:CD001142.

47. Kermans G, Wyndaele JJ, Thiery M, De SW. Puerperal urinary retention. Acta Urol Belg 1986; 54(4):376–85.

48. Yip SK, Sahota D, Pang MW, Day L. Postpartum urinary retention. Obstet Gynecol 2005;106(3): 602–6.

49. Carley ME, Carley JM, Vasdev G, Lesnick TG, Webb MJ, Ramin KD et al. Factors that are associated with clinically overt postpartum urinary retention after vaginal delivery. Am J Obstet Gynecol 2002;187(2): 430–3.

50. Andolf E, Iosif CS, Jorgensen C, Rydhstrom H. Insidious urinary retention after vaginal delivery: prevalence and symptoms at follow-up in a population-based study. Gynecol Obstet Invest 1994;38(1): 51–3.

51. Ching-Chung L, Shuenn-Dhy C, Ling-Hong T, Ching-Chang H, Chao-Lun C, Po-Jen C. Postpartum urinary retention: assessment of contributing factors and long-term clinical impact. Aust N Z J Obstet Gynaecol 2002;42(4):365–8.

52. Glavind K, Bjork J. Incidence and treatment of urinary retention postpartum. Int Urogynecol J Pelvic Floor Dysfunct 2003;14(2):119–21.

53. Yip SK, Brieger G, Hin LY, Chung T. Urinary retention in the post-partum period. The relationship between obstetric factors and the post-partum post-void residual bladder volume. Acta Obstet Gynecol Scand 1997;76(7):667–72.

54. Royal College of Obstetricians and Gynaecologists. Operative vaginal delivery. Guideline no. 26. London: RCOG, 2005.

55. Yip SK, Sahota D, Chang AM. Determining the reliability of ultrasound measurements and the validity of the formulae for ultrasound estimation of

postvoid residual bladder volume in postpartum women. Neurourol Urodyn 2003;22(3):255–60.

56. Zaki MM, Pandit M, Jackson S. National survey for intrapartum and postpartum bladder care: assessing the need for guidelines. BJOG 2004;111(8): 874–6.

57. Burkhart FL, Porges RF, Gibbs CE. Bladder capacity postpartum and catheterization. Obstet Gynecol 1965;26:176–9.

58. Yang DL. Acupuncture therapy in 49 cases of postpartum urinary retention. J Tradit Chin Med 1985;5(1):26.

59. Yip SK, Sahota D, Chang AM, Chung TK. Four-year follow-up of women who were diagnosed to have postpartum urinary retention. Am J Obstet Gynecol 2002;187(3):648–52.

60. Rortveit G, Hannestad YS, Daltveit AK, Hunskaar S. Age- and type-dependent effects of parity on urinary incontinence: the Norwegian EPINCONT study. Obstet Gynecol 2001;98(6):1004–10.

61. Chiarelli P, Brown W, McElduff P. Leaking urine: prevalence and associated factors in Australian women. Neurourol Urodyn 1999;18(6):567–77.

62. Viktrup L, Lose G, Rolff M, Barfoed K. The symptom of stress incontinence caused by pregnancy or delivery in primiparas. Obstet Gynecol 1992;79(6): 945–9.

63. Thorp JM Jr, Norton PA, Wall LL, Kuller JA, Eucker B, Wells E. Urinary incontinence in pregnancy and the puerperium: a prospective study. Am J Obstet Gynecol 1999;181(2):266–73.

64. Viktrup L, Lose G. Lower urinary tract symptoms 5 years after the first delivery. Int Urogynecol J 2000; 11:336–40.

65. Rortveit G, Daltveit AK, Hannestad YS, Hunskaar S. Urinary incontinence after vaginal delivery or cesarean section. N Engl J Med 2003;348(10): 900–7.

66. Adult conservative management [computer program]. Paris: Health Publications Ltd, 2005.

67. Freeman RM. The role of pelvic floor muscle training in urinary incontinence. BJOG 2004;111(Suppl 1):37–40.

68. Glazener CM, Herbison GP, MacArthur C, Grant A, Wilson PD. Randomised controlled trial of conservative management of postnatal urinary and faecal incontinence: six year follow up. BMJ 2005;330(7487): 337.

69. Morof D, Barrett G, Peacock J, Victor CR, Manyonda I. Postnatal depression and sexual health after childbirth. Obstet Gynecol 2003;102(6): 1318–25.

70. Glazener CM. Sexual function after childbirth: women's experiences, persistent morbidity and

lack of professional recognition. Br J Obstet Gynae-col 1997;104(3):330–5.

71. Swift SE. The distribution of pelvic organ support in a population of female subjects seen for routine gynecologic health care. Am J Obstet Gynecol 2000; 183(2):277–85.

72. O'Boyle ALO, O'Boyle JD, Ricks RE, Patience TH, Calhoun B, Davis G. The natural history of pelvic organ support in pregnancy. Int Urogynecol J Pelvic Floor Dysfunct 2003;14:46–9.

73. Sze EH, Sherard GB III, Dolezal JM. Pregnancy, labor, delivery, and pelvic organ prolapse. Obstet Gynecol 2002;100(5 Pt 1):981–6.

74. Bick DE, MacArthur C. Attendance, content and relevance of the six week postnatal examination. Midwifery 1995;11(2):69–73.

75. Fitzpatrick M, Cassidy M, O'Connell RO, O'Herlihy C. Experience with an obstetric perineal clinic. Eur J Obstet Gynecol Reprod Biol 2002;100: 199–203.

7
Female Genital Mutilation

Harry Gordon

7.1 Female Genital Mutilation – Definition

The World Health Organisation (WHO) defines female genital mutilation (FGM) as any procedure that involves partial or total removal of the external female genitalia, or any other injury to the female genital organs for cultural or non-therapeutic reasons.[1]

7.2 History

Various forms of FGM have existed since the fifth century BC.[2] Herodotus (420 BC) stated that Egyptians, Phoenicians, Hittites and Ethiopians practised female genital excision. A Greek papyrus from 163 BC exists in the British Museum, and refers to circumcised girls in Egypt. The term "pharonic circumcision" is still used, and suggests an origin in ancient Egypt. However, no evidence exists of FGM in Egyptian mummies.

The practice of FGM continues to the present day. The WHO suggests that more than 130 million women and girls have undergone genital mutilation, and it continues at a rate of about 2 million each year. The basis for the practice is related to tradition and culture, and not religion. Although common in some Islamic countries, it is not part of Islam and it is not a religious duty. The extent of the cultural importance attached to the procedure is contained in a paper by Jomo Kenyatta published in the 1930s, and related to the Gikuyu of Kenya:

The real argument lies not in the defence of the surgical operation or in its details but in the understanding of a very important fact in the tribal psychology of the Gikuyu – namely that this operation is still regarded as the very essence of an institution which has enormous educational, social, moral and religious implications, quite apart from the operation itself. For the present, it is impossible for a member of the tribe to imagine an initiation without clitoridectomy.[3]

The strength of feeling expressed in this quotation still exists in parts of Africa today, and underlies the difficulty in preventing the mutilation of women and young girls when it is supported by hundreds of years of culture and tradition.

7.3 Incidence

The procedure is carried out in various forms in 26 African countries. The incidence varies, e.g. Somalia and Sudan 100%, Ethiopia 90%, Egypt and Nigeria 50%, Central Africa 20%, Uganda <5%. Furthermore there is also variation in the extent of the mutilation. The classification of the extent of mutilation, as suggested by the WHO, is shown in Table 7.1. However, it must be remembered that traditional circumcisers may show extensive variation in what they actually do.

Female genital mutilation also occurs in parts of the Far East – mainly in Malaysia and Indonesia. Refugees from the affected areas have resulted in genital mutilation coming to the attention of western gynaecologists – mainly involving the more severe forms. The incidence varies not only by country, but also by social class. For example,

TABLE 7.1. WHO classification of genital mutilation.

Type	Synonym	Extent
FGM 1	Sunna	Removal of clitoris or clitoral hood
FGM 2	Excision	Removal of clitoris and part of labia
FGM 3	Infibulation Pharonic circumcision	Removal of clitoris and labia and suture of raw tissues to occlude all but a small area of the introitus
FGM 4	Various, e.g. Gishiri cuts	Pricking, cutting, insertion of corrosives into the vagina (often as a spurious therapeutic measure)

in the Sudan and Somalia the incidence is nearly 100% and is independent of social class. In Nigeria the incidence is around 25%, ranging from 1.9% in the north east to 48% in the south west.[4] It is also heavily biased by age and social class. In other words, there is evidence that genital mutilation is being abandoned by younger, better educated and more affluent women.[5] In the hospital-based study quoted, none of the female infants followed up for at least 9 months had been mutilated. Downward trends in the incidence of mutilation have been observed in the Igbos of Nigeria.[6,7] Igwegbe[5] concluded that at the observed rate of decline, it would take 20 years for the prevalence of 48% to fall to zero among prospective mothers in Nnewu, Nigeria. There is no firm evidence of decline in the incidence of FGM 3 in Somalia and the Sudan.

7.4 Clinical Presentation, Management and Complications

The incidence of serious complications, clinical presentation and management varies with the type (extent) of the mutilation. The outcome also varies according to the available medical facilities. The European and western experience may differ markedly from the African experience. Within Africa, the results for rural and urban populations may also differ. It is therefore best to consider each form of genital mutilation separately.

7.5 FGM 1 (Synonym Sunna)

This involves incision or removal of the hood of the clitoris, or removal of the clitoris (clitoridectomy). This procedure occurs across Africa, and is often regarded as a less traumatic alternative to other forms of mutilation. The main acute complication is haemorrhage, as the dorsal artery of the clitoris is quite large, even in children. Infection and surgical shock may also occur. The operation is usually carried out by a traditional circumciser and no anaesthesia is used. However, in some areas of East Africa where mass circumcisions are common, cold water is used to numb the genital area.

There is certainly a mortality associated with the procedure, but its extent is poorly documented. Once the wound has healed, there are few long-term complications. Para-clitoral epidermal cysts may develop, which may give rise to problems, especially if they are large or infected. Spreading infection may result in contraction at the introitus and cause problems with intercourse and subsequent childbirth. However, most survivors are asymptomatic. The presence of Sunna (FGM 1) may be overlooked at the time of gynaecological or obstetric procedures.

7.6 FGM 2 (Excision)

This is the commonest form of mutilation, and probably accounts for 70–80% of all cases in Africa. This type of mutilation involves the removal of the clitoris, together with excision of part of the labia. This is the most common form of circumcision in West Africa, where FGM 3 is uncommon. The acute complications involve haemorrhage, sepsis, shock, tetanus and urinary retention. Surgical errors may result in vesico-vaginal fistula. Although this is the commonest form of mutilation, it is rarely seen in western gynaecological practice. The reason for this paradox relates to the bias by social class, as the lower social classes are less likely to emigrate to the west. As with FGM 1, there is a significant mortality. However, as with FGM 1, there seem to be few long-term complications among the survivors. Over 10 years at the University College

Hospital in Ibadan, Nigeria, only 39 patients were seen with long-term complications of FGM – mainly FGM 2. The main complications were labial adhesions and para-clitoral epidermal cysts. All were cured by appropriate surgery.[8]

It had been assumed that removal of the clitoris and labia would cause major psychosexual problems, but the recent work of Okonofua et al.[4] showed that female genital cutting of this type did not attenuate sexual feelings or the frequency of early arousal or orgasm. There was some evidence of increased pelvic infection in the circumcised women. There was no evidence in the study that genital mutilation reduced the level of sexual activity – although reducing the rate of promiscuity is often given as a reason for continuing the procedure. There is some anecdotal evidence that spreading infection around the introitus may lead to narrowing and rigidity, causing problems with subsequent childbearing. Unfortunately after FGM, no surgical procedure can restore the genitalia to normality.

7.7 FGM 3 (Infibulation, Pharonic Circumcision)

This type of mutilation is common in the Horn of Africa and uncommon in other parts of Africa. It involves removal of the clitoris and variable amounts of the labia. The raw edges are then sewn across the midline to produce a fibrous barrier. Only a small posterior aperture is left for the passage of urine and menstrual products. The commonest age range for this to be carried out is between 5 and 10 years. In Africa, the procedure is almost universal in Somalia and the Sudan, and common in other parts of the Horn of Africa. The procedure is usually carried out by traditional circumcisers (but in urban areas midwives and doctors may be involved). The child is held by senior female members of the family, while without anaesthesia the clitoris and labia are removed (usually cut with a razor blade) and the raw areas sewn across the midline, leaving only a small orifice posteriorly. Thorns are sometimes used instead of sutures, especially in remote areas. Traditionally, the legs are bound for several days to restrict movement and promote healing. It is

not uncommon for healing to be defective, giving rise to a perforated scar (Figure 7.1).

As for other forms of genital mutilation, the short-term complications are mainly haemorrhage, sepsis, surgical shock and urinary retention. Mortality as high as 10% has been suggested, but there are no good epidemiological data to support this.

Once the initial healing has taken place, long-term complications include recurrent urinary tract infection and vaginal infection. Coital problems and apareunia are common. Psychosexual complications are quoted in the literature, but their extent is poorly documented. Infertility is also quoted – but the high parity of the population suggests that this is not a major issue. The presence of a mechanical barrier at the introitus means that for most women, normal penetrative sexual intercourse will not be possible, but pregnancy

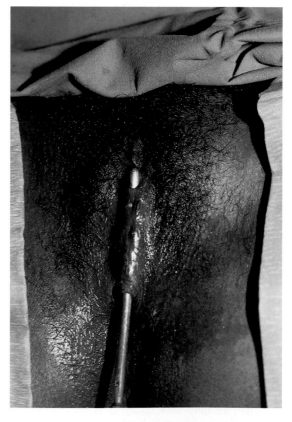

FIGURE 7.1. Female genital mutilation type 3, demonstrating incomplete healing with irregular perforations.

can occur even with a pinhole opening[9,10] and subsequent management of the pregnancy and delivery may be complicated.

For most women who have been subjected to FGM 3, normal penetrative sex is impossible, and an intact circumcision is regarded as a sign of virginity. Uncircumcised women may be unmarriageable. Once married, the circumcision has to be reversed, to permit intercourse. The tradition relating to this may vary. Thus, in North Somalia, where the trend is for a very tight residual orifice, intercourse is impossible. After the marriage, it is common for the bridegroom's mother to inspect and confirm "virginity" and arrange for the traditional circumciser to attend and open up the scar (de-infibulation). In the south of Somalia, where a more open orifice is usually left, the husband is expected to dilate the introitus by forceful intercourse with recourse to cutting only if this fails.

Whereas for FGM 1 and 2, long-term complications are uncommon, FGM 3 results in many long-term problems. Mawad and Hassancin[11] document the extent of this in the Sudan. Over a 3-year study they found that 7% of all obstetric and gynaecological procedures were related to direct complications of genital mutilation (FGM 3): vulval swellings – mainly epidermal cysts, were the commonest reason for surgical intervention.

For those with an intact circumcision or an incomplete reversal, a barrier remains, which would obstruct delivery – this is reversed by a midline anterior episiotomy (anterior incision through the scar) carried out by the midwife or traditional birth attendant in the second stage of labour. In rural areas, if there is a delay in obtaining the services of the birth attendant, delay in delivery may precipitate fetal asphyxia, and extensive maternal perineal damage will commonly occur. In a WHO systematic review of the health complications following FGM there is reference to perinatal mortality related to FGM – especially FGM 3.[12] When considering complications of FGM in Africa, it is difficult to separate genuine complications of FGM from those complications due to inadequate medical resources. Timely intervention to remove the barrier to delivery is usually all that is needed. After delivery, the anterior incision may be left open, except in the Sudan where re-infibulation is usual, recreating some barrier to a future delivery.

7.8 FGM 3: A Western Perspective

When refugees from the Horn of Africa entered Europe and the USA in large numbers, several serious problems confronted the health authorities. The main problem was unfamiliarity with genital mutilation and its results. Often, caesarean section was carried out, as the problems presented for the first time in labour to staff who had never seen the condition and were uncertain how else to proceed. This caused resentment among the mainly Somali community who disliked caesarean section and knew it was not needed.

The first UK clinic for women who had suffered infibulation started at Northwick Park in 1993,[13] supported by funding from the Department of Health and the Foundation for Women's Health Research and Development (FORWARD). Our subsequent experience allowed us to develop a protocol suitable for use in western countries. By the time the first clinic opened, the number of African women delivered in the maternity unit had risen from just over 1% in 1988 to more than 5% in 1994, and these were mainly Somali women.

The main problem was that the women had difficulty in utilising National Health Service primary care. To overcome this, the clinic was established as open access, not requiring referral from a general practitioner. Then those without a family doctor could be helped to join a suitable practice. The women attending could be divided into three groups:

1. Non-pregnant women who needed reversal in order to consummate their (recent) marriages.
2. Women who became pregnant with an intact circumcision.
3. Women with gynaecological complaints where reversal of the circumcision was needed to facilitate investigation.

We can summarise our protocol for each of these groups, and indicate the issues raised for European and western health services.

7.8.1 Non-pregnant Women

Little can be gained from detailed examination – all that is needed is a careful inspection to confirm the extent of the mutilation. Attempts at internal digital examination should be avoided, as they may precipitate distressing flashback memories of the original procedure. The operation is simple, and can be carried out under local anaesthesia. We offer the women a choice of local, spinal or general anaesthetic – and most wish "to be asleep", probably because of memories of the initial painful experience. The extent of the scar can be assessed using a small dilator, and the scar is then incised, keeping strictly to the midline. Bleeding is usually minimal (Figure 7.2). The incision can be bold, until the urethra is exposed. The incision can then be extended with care into the clitoral region. We found that in over 70% of cases, the clitoris was present and undamaged, as shown in Figure 7.2 (in spite of the tradition that the clitoris should be removed).

The raw edges are best closed with fine (3/0–4/0) absorbable sutures. If the area is dry, it is

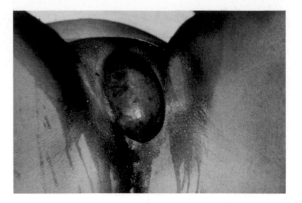

FIGURE 7.3. Large epidermal cyst after circumcision.

tempting to leave the edges unsutured, but there is a tendency to reform labial adhesions and we would advocate haemostatic sutures for all cases. Postoperative analgesia is improved if a long-acting local anaesthetic is injected under the sutured edges (e.g. bupivacaine 0.5% plain).

While the operation is simple in most cases, arrangements must be made to avoid delay on a waiting list. We aim to ensure all cases are operated on within a month of presentation.

In about 5% of cases the situation may be complicated by the presence of epidermal cysts, which may be quite large (Figure 7.3). Excision and reconstruction is usually simple, unless there has been infection or haemorrhage into the cyst. It is not always possible to predict what lies under the scar and in some cases there may be significant tissue loss. Fortunately the skin of the vestibule is very elastic, and with careful dissection it can be stretched to cover the raw area, avoiding skin grafting (Figure 7.4). The anatomy may be significantly distorted. In the case shown in Figure 7.5, the woman could pass urine only if she pressed on her lower abdomen. Examination in the clinic failed to reveal any orifice. Under anaesthetic, the only opening was small and anterior (Figure 7.5). However, when the scar was opened, the clitoris was present and restoration to total normality was achieved. Apart from the cases where the clitoris is intact and present, there are cases where the clitoris has been damaged, usually partial excision leaving a stump of clitoris, which can be reconstructed to leave fairly normal-looking anatomy

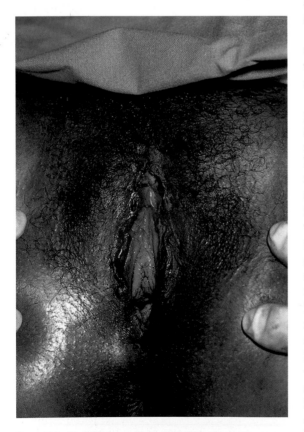

FIGURE 7.2. De-infibulation. Note minimal bleeding and presence of an undamaged clitoris.

– but with an uncertain functional result. Reversal of circumcision is normally a day-care procedure.

The cases we have seen from Africa after de-infibulation usually show incomplete opening, with the clitoris still buried in scar tissue. Few such women complain of any symptoms, but we have encountered two whose complaint was of intensely painful orgasms. In both cases these proved to be related to small neuromas, and were cured by operation. After surgery, the residual labia may be rather attenuated. However, those that we have seen some months after reversal (usually pregnant) showed that significant hypertrophy had occurred and the genital area seemed normal.

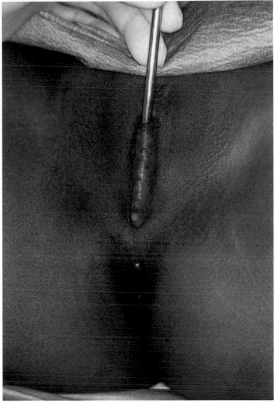

FIGURE 7.5. Healed FGM 3, with no obvious orifice. The woman was able to pass urine only after pressure on the lower abdomen. Small anterior orifice demonstrated with a dilator.

7.8.2 Women Who Are First Seen Pregnant with an Intact Circumcision

Women get pregnant, even with a pinhole opening. In their own country, most would be reversed in the second stage of labour by a traditional birth attendant or a midwife. In rural areas, delay in the anterior incision can cause distress to the baby, and serious perineal damage to the mother including fistulae. After delivery, in the Sudan, the tradition is to reform the introital barrier, though not as tight as before. In Somalia, the area is usually left open.

In western countries, there is no universal familiarity with FGM 3. Many, perhaps most, midwives and junior doctors have never encountered the situation. We would therefore advise reversal in the antenatal period.[10,13] Ideally, avoid the first trimester, lest the woman assumes that a

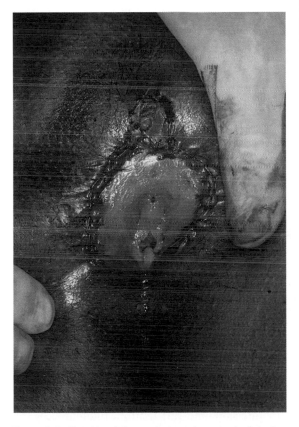

FIGURE 7.4. The skin of the vestibule undercut and stitched to cover the raw area. Note the undamaged clitoris.

spontaneous miscarriage is the result of the operation. Around 20 weeks is ideal, as this tends to be a time of obstetric tranquillity. The procedure can be carried out on a day-care basis, usually under spinal or local anaesthetic – however, some women with bad memories of the initial procedure may insist on general anaesthesia. The procedure is the same as for the non-pregnant woman. The advantage of antenatal reversal is that an experienced operator can deal with the case, a clear sample of urine can be obtained in the antenatal period and the area will be well healed and restored to normal well before the onset of labour.

Some women will refuse antenatal reversal, wishing to follow the traditional practice, and some will just slip through the net. In this latter respect, vaginal examination is no longer routine, and unless directly asked, the women will not tell you that they have been circumcised. It is therefore important to be aware of the groups at risk in the local population. It is important to carry out the reversal as early in labour as possible. This allows adequate assessment in labour, and permits catheterisation if needed. It will often be a midwife unfamiliar with the condition who first sees the women and this is a very stressful situation. If there are women at risk in the local population it is important that a detailed plan is available in the labour ward indicating what must be done. We advise an anterior incision, which is continued forward until the urethra is exposed. This allows maximum room for delivery. Forward extension into the clitoral area may provoke haemorrhage, and does not provide any additional room for delivering the baby. If there are residual problems in the clitoral area, these can be dealt with after the pregnancy – though in our experience few women return for further surgery. Rapid turnover of staff means that constant retraining is advisable to ensure appropriate adherence to protocols. Episiotomy in these cases is controversial. Many European midwives assume that it is needed in all cases – and this is not true. Where antenatal reversal has been carried out, the operation notes should include a note about any residual scarring around the introitus, and a clear statement if an episiotomy should be carried out. If the introitus is returned to normal, a routine episiotomy is not required. Bilateral episiotomy is never indicated in these cases.

The acceptance of antenatal reversal varies. In our first study at Northwick Park Hospital, only 13% of the women still had an intact circumcision at delivery.[13] However, when we moved the clinic to a more deprived area at the Central Middlesex Hospital, the acceptance rate fell to 45% – mainly because the women had assumed that they would all require an episiotomy, and they thought that rather than two "operations" they would prefer both at the same time. In addition, many women wished to follow the tradition of "what was done at home".

In the UK and most European countries, resuture of the perineum to recreate a barrier at the introitus is forbidden by law.

Apart from the UK, large numbers of immigrant women from Somalia and the Horn of Africa are found in Italy (where in Rome alone in 1993 there were 3,800 Somali women[15]), Scandinavia, France and Germany. In 1997 it was estimated that in the USA 168,000 females had undergone or were at risk to have undergone FGM based on the countries of immigration.[16] In the UK and Sweden it is illegal to take a child out of the country to be circumcised elsewhere.

7.8.3 Gynaecological Problems in Women with an Intact Circumcision

In many of these women, the residual opening is so small that adequate examination is impossible. Reversal is then indicated to facilitate adequate examination. Thought should be given to any added procedures that may be needed after reversal – for example hysteroscopy and endometrial biopsy. Then adequate informed consent can be obtained, two separate operations avoided, and adequate anaesthetic planned.

Overall, when dealing with a specific population with genital mutilation, it is worth considering establishing a special clinic, to make maximum use of a translator, and to ensure that the staff are well aware of the cultural and religious issues involved. All the cases that we see in the clinic have been circumcised in their own country.

Mutilation of children in Europe in uncommon. In Paris, three children bled to death after circumcision, and this led to a tightening of the law in France. In 1997 female circumcision became a federal crime in the USA. In the UK some – but probably very few – children may be circumcised. Children who have been circumcised in the west tend to become withdrawn (rather like children who have suffered sexual abuse) and perhaps the most constant physical sign is alteration in micturition. The tight infibulation obstructs the normal flow of urine, and urine is initially retained in the vagina, only draining slowly over some minutes. Circumcised children may therefore be in trouble in primary school for the amount of time they spend in the toilet. If there is worry that children are being circumcised (usually during school holidays), teachers should be alert to the altered behaviour as described.

7.9   FGM 4

This involves a diverse group of otherwise unclassified mutilations. These include pricking, cutting, scraping and burning the genital area. It also includes the introduction of corrosive substances into the vagina. Many of these procedures have a background in traditional healing, rather than only a traditional cultural practice. Like FGM 1 and 2, the results are rarely seen in European practice.

Some of these procedures have particularly serious long-term complications. Gynaetresia is recorded in Ibadan, Nigeria mainly in relation to the use of caustic vaginal pessaries prescribed by traditional healers.[17] The caustic pessaries are prescribed for the treatment of amenorrhoea, infertility, fibroids and vaginal discharge. They are also used in an attempt to procure abortion.

Of the 148 cases documented at University College Hospital, Ibadan, between 1967 and 1996, 106 required extensive vaginoplasty.[17] There was some evidence of a recent increase in the number of cases seen because of an increase in the popularity of alternative medicine. This was considered to be a disorder of great public health concern because its occurrence was based on ignorance and cultural beliefs, and was preventable. These cases are not seen in the west, where vaginal stenosis is seen mainly in relation to colporraphy and irradiation therapy.

Gishiri cuts are another potentially dangerous form of FGM 4. These are incisions into (usually) the anterior vagina carried out by traditional healers to treat a variety of conditions including obstructed labour, infertility, dyspareunia, amenorrhoea, goitre and backache. In one study from Nigeria,[18] 13% of vesico-vaginal fistulae were caused by Gishiri cuts.

7.10   Conclusion

Female genital mutilation includes a number of harmful traditional practices, which are a danger to health and an abuse of young women and children. Every effort is being made by the WHO, governments and other organisations to eliminate FGM in all its forms, with variable success. The complications will be with us for decades and it is important that health professionals are aware of the best therapeutic options available.

References

1. World Health Assembly. Geneva: World Health Organization, 1997.
2. Elchalal W, Ben Ami, Gillis R et al. Ritualistic female genital mutilation, current status and future outlook. Obstet Gynecol Sur 1997;52:643–51.
3. Kenyatta J. Initiation of boys and girls in the traditional life of the Gikuyu. Kenway Publications, 1935, pp 131–54.
4. Okonofua FE, Larsen V, Oronsaye F et al. The association between female genital cutting and correlates of sexual and gynaecological morbidity in Elo State Nigeria. Br J Obstet Gynaecol 2002;109:1089–96.
5. Igwegbe AO, Egbuonu I. The prevalence and practice of female genital mutilation in Nnewi, Nigeria. The impact of female education. J Obstet Gynecol 2000;20:520–2.
6. Adinma JIB. Current status of female circumcision among Nigerian Igbos. West African J Med 1997;16:227–31.
7. Meneru JA. Female circumcision among Igbos of Nigeria; trends. Nigerian J Med 1991;1:55–60.
8. Adekunle AO, Fakokunde FA, Odukogbe AA et al. Post circumcision vulval complications in Nigerians. J Obstet Gynecol 1999;19:632–5.
9. Modawi S. The impact of social and economic changes in female circumcision. Sudan Med Assn Cong Ser 1974;1:242–54.
10. MacCaffrey M, Jankowska A, Gordon H. Management of female genital mutilation: the Northwick

Park Hospital experience. Br J Obstet Gynaecol 1995;102:787–90.

11. Mawad NM, Hassanein OM. Female circumcision: three years experience of common complications in patients treated in Khartoum teaching hospitals. J Obstet Gynaecol 1994:14:40–3.

12. World Health Organization. A systematic review of health complications following female genital mutilation. Genaeva: WHO, 1998, pp 49–51.

13. Gordon H. Female genital mutilation (female circumcision). The Diplomate 1998;5:86–90.

14. Essen B, Bodker B, Sjoberg NO et al. Is there an association between female circumcision and perinatal death? Bull WHO 2002;80:629–32.

15. Porseri Porta R, Coppola S, Nobili F et al. Survey of the deliveries of immigrant women from developing countries in the second Institute of Gynaecology and Obstetrics, University of Rome "La Sapienza", Italy. J Obstet Gynaecol 1997;17:346–8.

16. Jones W, Smith J, Kieke B et al. Female genital mutilation/female circumcision. Who is at risk in the US? Public Health Rep 1997;112:368–77.

17. Arowojolu AO, Okunlola MA, Adekunle AO et al. Three decades of acquired gynaetresia in Ibadan: clinical presentation and management. J Obstet Gynaecol 2001;21:375–8.

18. Tahzib F. Epidemiological determinants of vesicovaginal fistulas. Br J Obstet Gynaecol 1983;90:387–91.

8
Pathophysiology of Anal Incontinence

Peter J. Lunniss and S. Mark Scott

8.1   Introduction

It would be beyond the aim of this chapter, and probably also the reader's interest, to proffer a highly detailed description of our current knowledge of the mechanisms underlying anal continence and defaecation. Nevertheless, to understand disturbance of these functions, it is important to appreciate that although continence is dependent to a large degree upon the functional integrity of the lowest sphincter of the gastrointestinal tract,[1,2] and that this is the structure most threatened by obstetric trauma,[1-5] the ability of an individual to retain rectal contents and only allow their passage when desired, results from a multitude of factors in addition to the anal sphincter complex.[1,4-7] Such factors include the physical nature of the hindgut contents, the speed at which they are delivered there, and the ability of the hindgut to accommodate that which is delivered to it.[1,2,4,6,7]

Our knowledge of the mechanisms underlying the "suprasphincteric" components to continence remains somewhat rudimentary, but they are known to depend upon the biomechanical properties of the gut tube itself, the integrated function of the enteric and autonomic nervous systems, and spinal and cerebral connections.[1,2,4,6,7] Appreciation of the dynamic nature of the anal sphincter complex itself is similarly important, this structure providing an airtight seal at all times other than when the owner is happy that it may open; such a function depends upon not only structural integrity, but also reflexes that allow coordinated activity with structures above, and "plasticity", rather than acting as a passive barrier.

Continence, for the majority of our days and nights, is largely controlled by subconscious processes, with a myriad of reflexes occurring at multiple levels; it is only when recruitment reaches a threshold that awareness of lower gut activity reaches consciousness, enabling the owner to make decisions about whether to respond by visiting the lavatory, or whether it may be possible to defer defaecation until a more socially convenient time.

Western patterns of living have somewhat interfered with such a balanced process. Our eating habits may not be conducive to optimal gut motor activity, and certainly the perceived necessity of ridding the bowel of its contents (through straining) before the more important activities of the day (work), and before the decision that defaecation should occur has been triggered from the bowel itself, or repeatedly suppressing the natural desire to defaecate until the sanctuary of one's own lavatory at home is reached, may, over time, have a detrimental effect upon the efficiency of such a complex process.

8.2   Continence Mechanisms

Normal bowel continence is maintained by the structural and functional integrity of the anus, rectum, sigmoid colon and adjoining pelvic floor musculature,[5] and is a complex process involving integration of somatic and visceral muscle function with sensory information under local, spinal and central control. The various factors required for normal continence are listed in Table 8.1 and

TABLE 8.1. Factors contributing to the maintenance of continence.

Component	Routine assessment
Sphincteric	
Structural	
Internal anal sphincter	Yes
External anal sphincter	Yes
Conjoined longitudinal muscle	No
Vascular anal cushions	No
Longitudinal anal muscle folds	No
Functional	
Anal resting tone	Yes
Anal canal/high pressure zone length	Yes
Resting anal pressure gradient	Yes
Voluntary anal squeeze pressure	Yes
Anal sensation	Yes
Anal motility	No
Rectoanal inhibitory ("sampling") reflex	Yes
Rectoanal contractile reflex	Yes
Neurological	
Pudendal nerve	Yes
Sympathetic (hypogastric) nerves	No
Parasympathetic (pelvic) nerves	No
Suprasphincteric	
Structural	
Levator ani	
Puborectalis	Yes
Iliococcygeus	No
Pubococcygeus	No
Perineal resting position/level of descent	No
Rectal	
Capacity	Yes
Curvatures/transverse folds	No
Flap valve effect of the anterior wall	No
Endopelvic musculofascial support	No
Rectosigmoid sphincter	No
Functional	
Tonic levator ani contraction	No
Anorectal angle	No
Rectosigmoid angle	No
Postural pelvic floor reflex	No
Rectal sensation	Yes
Rectal tone	No
Rectal compliance	Yes
Rectosigmoid motility	No
Anorectal pressure gradient	No
Rectosigmoid pressure gradient	No
Rectosigmoid high pressure zone	No
Stool consistency	No
Stool volume	No
Gastrointestinal/colonic motility	No
Neurological	
Pudendal nerve	Yes
Sympathetic nerves	No
Parasympathetic nerves	No
Afferent nerves	No
Intrinsic (enteric) nerves	No
Other	
Normal rectal evacuation	Yes
Psycho-behavioural factors	Yes

simplified in Figure 8.1.[8] The anal sphincters are not by themselves responsible for providing a barrier to the involuntary loss of faecal contents. Although the high pressure zone of the internal and external anal sphincters is of primary importance with regard to closure of the anal canal,[5–7] the contribution of other muscular and non-muscular components should not be underestimated. The sphincter muscles alone cannot entirely close the anal lumen,[9,10] and approximately 15% of the basal anal canal resting tone is generated by the expansile vascular anal cushions,[11] which, along with secondary anal mucosal folds,[5,12] provide a hermetic seal. The importance of these structures becomes evident in patients with either prolapsing haemorrhoids (where the mucocutaneous junction, which provides a barrier against mucus and liquid faecal leakage, may be displaced beyond the anal verge[6]) or following haemorrhoidectomy, where faecal soiling is not uncommon.[1,13] The role of the conjoined longitudinal muscle is poorly understood and widely ignored.[14]

It is also becoming increasingly accepted that the levator ani group of muscles, comprising the iliococcygeus, pubococcygeus and puborectalis, is integral to the continence mechanism.[4,15] The levator ani is the largest of the pelvic floor muscles, and supports the pelvic viscera and prevents excessive perineal descent through a state of tonic contraction, mediated via the postural reflex of the pelvic floor.[6,15] Traction of the puborectalis sling maintains the anorectal junction at an angle of approximately 90°,[5,16] likely helping to obstruct the outlet, possibly by a flap-valve effect[6,12] (although this concept has been disputed[17]). Levator ani failure is now recognised as being of aetiological importance in the development of incontinence.[15,18,19] Other suprasphincteric structures involved in the maintenance of continence are the endopelvic musculofascial support system of the anorectal complex,[19] and the perineal and anococcygeal bodies.[12] It is possible that the curvatures and transverse folds of the rectum may also contribute,[4,20] with the anterior rectal wall possibly acting as a "plug" at the anorectal junction (the flap-valve effect).[12] A further, again widely ignored, functional apparatus likely important to continence is the so-called "rectosigmoid sphincter",[21–23] which serves to regulate the passage of stool into the rectum.[21,22]

FIGURE 8.1. The mechanism of maintaining continence and defaecation. *IAS* Internal anal sphincter,
EAS external anal sphincter. (Reproduced with permission from Blackwell Publishing, Sultan and
Nugent.[8])

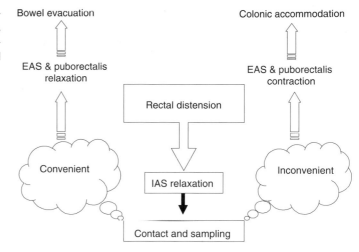

Overall, continence is dependent on the normal
function of each of these structural units, and an
appropriate, coordinated interplay between them.
In simple terms, as long as the combination of
these factors results in anal canal pressure being
greater than that in the rectum, continence is
maintained.[10,24,25] This rectoanal pressure gradient
is further supplemented by a longitudinal pressure gradient within the anal canal (the highest
pressure being found toward the anal verge;[26,27]
this gradient is typically reversed or reduced in
those patients with passive faecal incontinence[27,28]),
and also by a retrograde pressure gradient from
the rectum (higher resting pressures) to the
sigmoid (lower resting pressures).[29,30] This latter
pressure differential, in combination with the
existence of a high pressure zone at the rectosigmoid junction,[22] compatible with a rectosigmoid
sphincter,[21,23] presumably helps to retard untimely
flow of faeces from the sigmoid. Disruption of
these rectosigmoid pressure gradients has been
implicated in the pathophysiology of incontinence, where unhindered passage of stool into the
rectum may serve to overwhelm its reservoir
function.[30]

With regard to the anal sphincters and puborectalis, function is mediated by tonic contractile
activity, under both neurogenic and myogenic
control (primarily the internal anal sphincter, but
also the external anal sphincter and puborectalis[6,10,11,15]), voluntary contraction of the striated
musculature,[10] and various reflex mechanisms,

involving both intrinsic and extrinsic neural pathways.[6,10] These include the rectoanal inhibitory
reflex, which can be induced by distending the
rectum,[6,31,32] or occurs in vivo in response to rectal
contraction or filling (the anal "sampling reflex",
which allows equalisation of rectal and anal pressures, bringing rectal contents into contact with
the upper anal epithelium[10,33]), and the reciprocal
rectoanal contractile reflex, a compensatory contraction of the external anal sphincter in response
to increases in rectal pressure, so that anal pressure still exceeds that of the rectum.[10,31] The rectoanal contractile reflex appears to be heavily
modulated by conscious mechanisms, in that it is
closely associated with rectal perception;[34] the
reflex may be absent if there is no sensation, and
the duration of the response is related to the
duration of perception. It has been suggested,
therefore, that an inappropriate external anal
sphincter response (i.e. delayed or absent contraction) to increases in rectal pressure may result
in faecal incontinence.[34]

With regard to innervation of the pelvic floor,
which ultimately subserves these reflex activities,
it is extremely important to remember that the
pudendal nerve is only one of several nerves that
mediate sensorimotor function. Innervation is
also provided by both sympathetic and parasympathetic extrinsic components of the autonomic
nervous system (via the inferior mesenteric, superior hypogastric and inferior hypogastric [pelvic]
plexuses), afferent neurons, and by the complex

neural architecture of the enteric nervous system, intrinsic to the bowel wall.[6,32,35-37] Although pudendal nerve damage has received preferential attention with regard to the pathoaetiology of incontinence (both faecal and urinary),[3-5,32,38-42] it should not be forgotten that other neural components present may also be susceptible to injury during obstetric (and also iatrogenic, or other) trauma. Indeed, it has recently been postulated that disruption of the inferior hypogastric plexus during difficult intrapartum episodes may damage both extrinsic and intrinsic nerves innervating the pelvic viscera, and as such contributes to pelvic floor dysfunction, and the development of symptoms such as urgency and altered sensory function,[43] which are common in patients with faecal incontinence.[30,44-46]

Other factors central to the preservation of continence are rectal sensorimotor function (notably compliance, capacity, sensation and motility), colonic transit, which is inextricably linked to stool consistency;[47] and central nervous system control.[4,6,7,12,32] In terms of rectal function, the mechanism of compliance (the ability of the rectum to adapt to an imposed stretch, defined more accurately as the "volume response to an imposed pressure"[48]) enables rectal contents to be accommodated, which allows defaecation to be delayed. Under normal conditions, the viscoelastic properties of the rectal wall allow it to maintain a low intraluminal pressure during filling, so that continence is not threatened.[49,50] If rectal compliance is impaired, however, small volumes during filling can generate high intraluminal pressures that may overwhelm the resistance of the (perhaps functionally compromised) anal sphincter complex,[32] resulting in incontinence.[6,49,51,52] Reduced compliance may thus be associated with attenuated reservoir function, coupled with decreased rectal capacity and heightened sensory perception, leading to symptoms of urgency and frequency of defaecation,[30,45,46] as well as urge incontinence. Conversely, increased compliance (hypotonic rectum), as seen in conditions of megarectum, may result in the loss of a sense of urgency, faecal impaction and overflow incontinence.[51,53]

Intact anorectal sensation is similarly crucial to the maintenance of continence, in that it provides a warning of impending defaecation, and also allows discrimination of rectal contents.[1,32] In addition, the ability of the patient to perceive distension of the rectum, caused by the arrival of stool or flatus, appears necessary for an appropriate "guarding" reflex contraction of the external anal sphincter.[34] However, the mechanisms and neural pathways involved in rectal sensory function remain poorly understood. Impaired (blunted) rectal sensation (i.e. hyposensitivity) may lead to excessive accumulation of stool, resulting in faecal impaction and "overflow" incontinence, in the absence of an appropriate "compensatory" sphincteric response.[54-56] Conversely, heightened rectal sensation (hypersensitivity) is usually allied to reduced rectal compliance, and has been demonstrated in up to 50% of patients with urge faecal incontinence.[44,46] In such patients, rectal hypersensitivity is associated with increased bowel frequency, a reduced ability to defer defecation, increased pad usage, and negative lifestyle effects.[46] As for intact anal sensory function, although this is essential for the "sampling" of rectal contents, its importance, per se, in the preservation of continence has been questioned.[32]

There is increasing awareness that specific colorectal contractile activities may also contribute to normal continence and defaecation, and that disturbance of these motility patterns may be implicated in the pathophysiology of incontinence. High amplitude propagated contractions (HAPCs) are the major motor correlates of mass intraluminal movement,[57,58] and there is a clear association with both the urge to defecate[59] and faecal expulsion.[60,61] Studies in constipation have shown that HAPC frequency and amplitude are reduced, providing one possible pathophysiological mechanism for the symptoms reported by such patients.[62,63] Conversely, therefore, it is possible that exaggerated HAPC activity may underlie symptomatology in a proportion of patients with incontinence. In such cases, the arrival of copious quantities of liquid stool (reported as diarrhoea[64]) due to rapid hindgut transit may, on occasion, overwhelm the reservoir capacity of the rectum.[30] Recent reports appear to support this hypothesis.[65,66] Furthermore, regular cyclical bursts of phasic pressure waves, called rectal or colonic motor complexes depending upon the recording site, are evident on prolonged manometric studies.[66–69] These subconscious motor patterns predominate in the rectosigmoid, where they are thought to represent localised segmental activity,[67,68] acting as a "braking" mechanism to untimely flow of colonic contents,[68] so keeping the rectum empty.[67] It has been proposed that these motor complexes may be used as a marker of enteric neuromotor function, as their presence is independent of intact extrinsic innervation.[70] Recent studies have shown that motor complex frequency is significantly elevated in patients with urge incontinence;[67,71] whether this represents a protective mechanism to increased flow of colonic contents and/or reflects a true intrinsic hindgut dysmotility is unclear at present.

Finally, given that faecal incontinence and "constipation" frequently coexist, and that, indeed, rectal evacuatory dysfunction may underlie the involuntary loss of bowel contents, notably post-defaecation faecal seepage,[56,72 74] a comprehension of the normal process of defaecation should also be considered fundamental to the clinical management of patients with incontinence. As with the mechanisms responsible for the preservation of continence, the process of faecal expulsion involves a complex sequence of events that integrates the central, somatic, autonomic and enteric nervous systems, although the mechanism of the integration of these components is still poorly understood.[75] Important factors include: integrity of anorectal sensorimotor function, allowing conscious awareness of rectal filling, and the sampling of luminal contents, but also the ability to defer defaecation if socially inconvenient; propulsive colorectal contractile activities, both prior to, and temporally associated with rectal evacuation;[60,61] inhibition of tonic pelvic floor activity, allowing relaxation of the puborectalis and straightening of the anorectal angle; reflex and voluntary relaxation of the external anal sphincter, together with prolonged relaxation of the internal anal sphincter, which enables anal pressure to fall, concomitant with coordinated straining manoeuvres, involving descent of the diaphragm, contraction of the abdominal and chest wall muscles, contraction of the pelvic floor muscles and forced expiration against a closed glottis (the Valsalva manoeuvre), which raises intra-abdominal pressure (and hence intrapelvic pressure), thus facilitating faecal expulsion by reversal of the normal rectoanal pressure gradient; and, a "closing reflex", which occurs upon completion of defaecation, involving temporary contraction of the puborectalis and external sphincter to restore the anorectal angle, thus allowing the internal sphincter to recover its tone and close the anal canal. The mechanisms involved in defaecation are reviewed in depth elsewhere.[6,12,75–79]

8.3 Pathophysiology of Obstetric Hindgut Trauma

Despite the complexity of mechanisms involved in continence (Table 8.1), our knowledge of those factors implicated in anal incontinence following childbirth is fairly rudimentary, with clinical research centred predominantly on sphincteric function alone. Thus, the effects of childbirth on central processing, colorectal sensorimotor function, colonic transit, etc. remain essentially unexplored, and appropriate research may go some way to explain the often suboptimal results of surgical strategies aimed at restoring anatomy alone.[7] The physiological evaluation of women whose continence has been compromised by childbirth has revealed two predominant insults: structural and neurological.[1–5] Until the advent of endoanal ultrasound, the majority of such patients were labelled as having "neurogenic" faecal incontinence.[80] It is now known that isolated neuropathy (unilateral or bilateral) as a cause of incontinence is rare (about 10% in our, and others',[81] experience), and that structural sphincteric damage is the main pathogenic mechanism in the majority.[82–84]

8.3.1 Manometric Changes Associated with Delivery

One of the goals of manometry is to provide objective evaluation of anal sphincter function, which is reflective of the combined effects of those structural and functional components (principally, but not exclusively, the internal and external anal sphincters) involved in the "sphincteric" contribution to continence (see previously). One consistent finding from such studies is that anal squeeze pressure is significantly decreased following spontaneous and instrumental vaginal delivery. Although such a decrease is restricted to those with either incontinence[85] or evidence of sphincteric damage[86,87] in some reports, the majority of studies have shown a deleterious effect of vaginal childbirth on anal squeeze pressures, irrespective of postpartum continence status or sphincter integrity.[88–96] Indeed, Reiger et al.[91] showed that squeeze pressure was attenuated in a group of 18 primiparous women at 4–6 weeks, even though there was no evidence of sphincter rupture on ultrasound, and pudendal nerve function was normal.[91] In terms of anal resting tone, published findings are more contradictory; although some prospective studies show significantly decreased resting pressures postpartum compared to antepartum,[81,88,92,95] others show no change in resting tone,[87,90,91] or report that a decrease is confined to those in whom structural defects are found at ultrasound,[86] those who have had an instrumental delivery,[89] or only those who become incontinent.[85] It is important to note, from a clinical viewpoint, however, that there may be considerable overlap in pressures between those with postpartum symptoms of incontinence and those without. Nevertheless, it appears that poorest anal sphincter function (either squeeze pressures or resting tone) is found in those women with endosonographically confirmed sphincter defects.[89,95] In general, postpartum follow-up in most published studies is short, typically 3–6 months, and longer-term follow-up has shown a recovery in sphincter pressures in a proportion of women,[92] although those who remain incontinent represent a group with persistent weak sphincter function.[97] Fynes et al.[93] studied a group of women through two pregnancies, and showed a significant decrease in resting tone and squeeze pressures after the first delivery, and further smaller, though still significant decreases in both measures following the second delivery.[93] This finding was corroborated by Fornell et al.,[98] who demonstrated that anal sphincter function deteriorates further over time, and with subsequent vaginal deliveries.

Caesarean section, performed either electively, or as an emergency in early labour appears, from the results of most studies, to afford protection against anal structural damage and sphincter dysfunction, as both resting and squeeze pressures are unchanged.[81,88,89,93,99] However, when performed as an emergency in late labour, Caesarean section may be associated with significantly reduced squeeze pressures (in the absence of anal structural defects), which indicates neurological injury to the anal sphincter mechanism.[93,99]

8.3.2 Anal Sphincter Trauma

The seminal study of Sultan et al.[88] reported a 13% incidence of anal incontinence or faecal urgency in 79 primiparous women following vaginal delivery, and a 4% incidence of new symptoms among 48 multiparous mothers[88] (refer also to Chapters 2 and 4). Of perhaps greater significance was the incidence of sphincter defects observed at endoanal ultrasound following delivery, with 35% of primiparous, and 4% of multiparous women noted to have defects resulting from vaginal delivery (with only two of 150 women having recognised tears of the anal sphincter at the time of delivery), and a strong association demonstrated between presence of a defect and development of symptoms.[88] Table 8.2 summarises those studies ($n \geq$ 59 subjects) in which sphincter integrity has been assessed by ultrasound, highlighting the relationship of "new" sphincter defects to the development of incontinence symptoms,[87–89,93,97,100–103] and shows a remarkably consistent incidence of structural damage to the anal sphincter complex, which is covert in the majority. However, Bayesian calculation has suggested that for a woman presenting with faecal incontinence postpartum, the probability of her having a sphincter defect is ~80%.[42] The high incidence of covert (occult) sphincter damage as a result of vaginal delivery provides the background for the development of symptoms later in life[40–42,104,105] when other risk factors (specific and non-specific) impact (see above).

The external anal sphincter is the structure most threatened during vaginal delivery, and disruption may result, of course, from extension of perineal trauma (either tear or episiotomy). Table 8.3 clearly demonstrates that in women with ultrasonographic confirmation of sphincter defects, approximately 90% involve the external anal sphincter,[87,97,100–103] either in isolation, or com-

TABLE 8.2. Incidence of anal sphincter damage following vaginal delivery: studies utilising endoanal ultrasonography.

Author	Date	Number P	Number M	New sphincter defect % P	New sphincter defect % M%	Newly symptomatic (new defect) %	Newly symptomatic (no defect) %
Sultan et al.[88]	1993	79	48	35	8	41	1.3
Fynes et al.[93]*	1999	59	59	34[†]	5	68	0
Abramowitz et al.[100]	2000	96	106	26	13	23	6.7
Faltin et al.[101]	2000	150	0	28	–	37	6.8
Chaliha et al.[89]	2001	130	0	·-45[††]	–	–	–
Belmonte-Montes et al.[102]	2001	98	0	29	–	75	0
Nazir et al.[97]	2002	80	0	26	–	–	–
Pinta et al.[87]	2004	75	0	23	–	47	–
Damon et al.[103]	2005	197	0	34[†]	–	71	4.5
Summary data: median		96		29		44	1.3
(range)		(35–197)		(20–45)		(0–75)	(0–6.8)

*Same cohort studied through first two vaginal deliveries.
[†]No prenatal assessment performed, therefore defects may have pre-existed, i.e. possible overestimate.
[†]Accurate denominator not documented: 58 defects in 125–130 patients (i.e. 44–46%).
P Primiparous, M multiparous.

bined with rupture of the internal anal sphincter. Isolated internal anal sphincter defects are much less common, accounting for 10% or less of all defects in the majority of studies.[87,97,100–103] In the absence of an overt tear (i.e. an intact perineum), it is presumed that such isolated defects in the internal anal sphincter result from shearing forces imposed during delivery and are probably of no clinical significance.[88]

It can be noted from Table 8.2 that a small percentage of women develop new symptoms of incontinence, despite apparent sphincter integrity. Several explanations may contribute towards this: under-reporting of endosonographic defects,

incomplete specificity of ultrasound, and the results of a recent home interview questionnaire study,[106] which has questioned the totally "protective" link between elective (as distinct from a prelabour emergency procedure) caesarean section and anal continence. This raises the possibility of suprasphincteric or neurophysiological insults as having clinical effects. The significance of the findings of Williams et al.[107] that anal sphincter morphology changes as a result of atraumatic delivery (reduced anterior external anal sphincter length), but with no correlation with results of manometry or function, is unclear.

TABLE 8.3. Type of anal sphincter disruption identified on endoanal ultrasound.

Author	Date	Number of defects	Isolated IAS defect %	Isolated EAS defect %	Combined IAS/EAS defect %	All EAS defects %
Sultan et al.[88]	1993	28	46	18	36	56
Abramowitz et al.[100]	2000	39	10	85	5	90
Faltin et al.[101]	2000	42	5	71	24	95
Chaliha et al.[89]	2001	59	17	59	24	83
Belmonte-Montes et al.[102]	2001	28	0	66	34	100
Nazir et al.[97]	2002	14	7	79	14	93
Pinta et al.[87]	2004	17	12	65	23	88
Damon et al.[103]	2005	66	0	74	26	100
Summary data: median		33.5	8.5	68.5	24	91.5
(range)		(14–66)	(0–46)	(18–85)	(5–36)	(56–100)

IAS Internal anal sphincter, EAS external anal sphincter.

8.3.3 Neurophysiological Damage

In the late 1970s, Parks et al.[108] and Neill and Swash,[109] using histological and neurophysiological techniques, were the first to propose that faecal incontinence was caused by injury to the pudendal or perineal nerves, as evidenced by external anal sphincter and puborectalis denervation,[108] with subsequent muscle reinnervation.[109] Ensuing studies confirmed that such denervation/reinnervation injury occurred following vaginal delivery.[38,110] The branches of the pudendal nerve, which contain both motor and sensory fibres, are vulnerable to stretch or compression injury, which may occur during childbirth,[38,39,111–115] when descent of the pelvic floor and progression of the fetal head toward the pelvic outlet may stretch the nerve as it emerges from Alcock's canal, where its course is relatively fixed along the pelvic sidewall.[2] Multiparity, instrumental delivery (notably forceps), protracted second stage, anal sphincter tears and high birth weight are identified risk factors.[38,86,88,93,116] In respect of parity, first vaginal delivery appears, from the results of prospective studies, to be the most injurious to sphincter[93,117–119] and neural[93,113] integrity alike, with damage to the pudendal nerves being cumulative with successive deliveries.[93,95,111,112,115,116] Importantly, studies assessing pudendal nerve function in patients undergoing emergency versus elective caesarean section have shown that a section performed after the onset of labour (especially during the later stages) does not protect against neural damage,[88,99,110] especially on the left side,[88,99,113] although the significance of this is unclear. An association between pudendal neuropathy and symptoms of incontinence acquired following childbirth has been shown in some,[39,81,96,112,120] but not all[88] studies.

The most widely available technique for the evaluation of pudendal nerve function is assessment of the nerve terminal motor latency (PNTML), which is a measurement of the conduction time from stimulation of the pudendal nerve at the level of the ischial spine, to the evoked external anal sphincter contraction; this is achieved using a disposable glove-mounted stimulating and recording electrode (see Chapter 9). Prolonged latencies are a surrogate marker of pudendal neuropathy, and are used as a measure of demyelination (and also axonal injury), and have been demonstrated in 16–30% of primiparous women at around 6 weeks following childbirth.[81,88,93,99,120] However, frequency is dependent upon the threshold used to define the upper limit of normality for PNTML; accordingly, higher incidences have been reported using a "cut-off" of 2.2 ms,[120] whereas lower published incidences have used a threshold for normality of 2.4 ms.[81,88,93] In addition, PNTMLs appear to recover with time:[38,88,94,113] Snooks et al.[38] showed that 60% of women with prolonged latencies at 2–3 days following childbirth had normal PNTMLs at 2 months; similarly, Sultan et al.[88] demonstrated that of women who had prolonged latencies at 6 weeks after vaginal delivery, PNTMLs had recovered to normal in 67% at 6 months. Likewise, disturbed anal sensation (a marker of pudendal afferent function), as demonstrated by decreased mucosal sensitivity to electrostimulation,[121] which has been shown by some,[122] but not others[89,96] to occur following childbirth, may also revert to normal with time.[122] Nevertheless, although such studies suggest that the nerve may recover from initial injury, it is feasible that with multiparity,[93,95,111,112,115,116] perhaps chronic straining at stool,[115,123,124] and indeed ageing,[125] neuropathy may be cumulative and thence become an independent risk factor resulting in symptoms;[95] it may certainly constitute one of the multiple aetiologies contributing to incontinence in parous women presenting in later life.[1,40,41,104,105] The importance of a unilateral pudendal neuropathy[126] remains unclear and inadequately researched.

It has been suggested that alternative tests, such as quantitative electromyography and assessment of sacral reflexes (e.g. clitoral-anal reflex, urethral-anal reflex), are required to demonstrate more subtle nerve injury not detectable by evaluation of PNTML alone.[127–130] Using such methods, Fitzpatrick et al.[130] recently investigated 83 women with postpartum incontinence, and identified three patterns of abnormal pudendal nerve function attributable to obstetric events, with evidence of pudendal nerve demyelination, axonal neuropathy with or without reinnervation, and a mixed demyelinating and axonal neuropathy.[130]

8.3.4 Other Mechanisms

Because of the close interaction (both structural and functional) between the anus and rectum, it is possible that sphincter dysfunction (through mechanical disruption, neurogenic weakness or both) may have an effect on suprasphincteric mechanisms, such as rectal sensorimotor behaviour (e.g. sensitivity, compliance, contractility, tone, etc.). In patients with urge faecal incontinence, an association between both internal and external anal sphincter defects and rectal hypersensitivity has indeed been identified;[44–46,66] however, the only prospective study to date that has assessed rectal sensory thresholds to simple volumetric balloon distension following vaginal delivery found no effect in the cohort studied,[95] although individual values, especially in those with reduced postpartum anal pressures, were not reported.[105] It is equally possible that childbirth, especially if complicated, may have consequences on the components of the continence mechanism, which we are currently unable to test or measure in the physiology laboratory (Table 8.1); this might further explain the sometimes suboptimal functional outcome following surgical management.[7]

8.4 Summary

The complexity of the processes of continence and defaecation is reflected by an incomplete understanding of pathophysiological mechanisms related to childbirth. Vaginal delivery, especially the first and if complicated, is associated with a substantial risk of the early onset of symptoms of incontinence, thought to be primarily structural (mechanical sphincter trauma) in aetiology. The much higher prevalence of female faecal incontinence in later life may reflect the additive effects of covert obstetric trauma, progressive pudendal neuropathy consequent upon further deliveries and straining, other insults (often surgical) and ageing. The effects of vaginal delivery on other components contributing to continence (enteric, spinal, cerebral) have not been adequately studied. Elective caesarean section before the onset of labour protects against mechanical sphincter trauma but not incontinence. Long-term prospective detailed studies of large cohorts of women are not practical and thus the strength of evidence reported in the literature will continue to have limitations.

References

1. Rao SS. Pathophysiology of adult fecal incontinence. Gastroenterology 2004;126(Suppl 1):S14–22.
2. Madoff RD, Parker SC, Varma MG et al. Faecal incontinence in adults. Lancet 2004;364:621–32.
3. Kamm MA. Obstetric damage and faecal incontinence. Lancet 1994;344:730–3.
4. Bharucha AE. Fecal incontinence. Gastroenterology 2003;124:1672–85.
5. Rao SS. Diagnosis and management of fecal incontinence. Am J Gastroenterol 2004;99:1585–604.
6. Rasmussen OØ. Anorectal function. Dis Colon Rectum 1994;37:386–403.
7. Gladman MA, Scott SM, Williams NS. Assessing the patient with fecal incontinence. An overview. In: Zbar AP, Pescatori M, Wexner SD, eds. Complex anorectal disorders – investigation and management. London: Springer-Verlag London Ltd, 2005, pp 547–94.
8. Sultan AH, Nugent K. Pathophysiology and non-surgical treatment of anal incontinence. Br J Obstet Gynaecol 2004;111(Suppl 1):84–90.
9. Gibbons CP, Trowbridge EA, Bannister JJ et al. Role of anal cushions in maintaining continence. Lancet 1986;1:886–8.
10. Read NW, Sun WM. Anorectal manometry. In: Henry MM, Swash M, eds. Coloproctology and the pelvic floor, 2nd edn. Oxford: Butterworth-Heinemann Ltd, 1992, pp 119–45.
11. Lestar B, Penninckx F, Kerrimans R. The composition of the anal basal pressure. An in vivo and in vitro study in man. Int J Colorect Dis 1989;4:118–22.
12. Sagar PM, Pemberton JH. The assessment and treatment of anorectal incontinence. Adv Surg 1996;30:1–20.
13. Read MG, Read NW, Haynes WG et al. A prospective study of the effect of haemorrhoidectomy on sphincter function and faecal continence. Br J Surg 1982;69:396–8.
14. Lunniss PJ, Phillips RK. Anatomy and function of the anal longitudinal muscle. Br J Surg 1992;79:882–4.
15. Azpiroz F, Fernandez-Fraga X, Merletti R, Enck P. The puborectalis muscle. Neurogastroenterol Motil 2005;17(Suppl 1):68–72.

16. Mahieu P, Pringot J, Bodart P. Defecography: I. Description of a new procedure and results in normal patients. Gastrointest Radiol 1984;9: 247–51.

17. Bannister JJ, Gibbons C, Read NW. Preservation of faecal continence during rises in intra-abdominal pressure: is there a role for the flap valve? Gut 1987;28:1242–5.

18. Fernandez-Fraga X, Azpiroz F, Malagelada JR. Significance of pelvic floor muscles in anal incontinence. Gastroenterology 2002;123:1441–50.

19. Eguare EI, Neary P, Crosbie J et al. Dynamic magnetic resonance imaging of the pelvic floor in patients with idiopathic combined fecal and urinary incontinence. J Gastrointest Surg 2004;8:73–82.

20. Shafik A, Doss S, Ali YA et al. Transverse folds of rectum: anatomic study and clinical implications. Clin Anat 2001;14:196–203.

21. Ballantyne GH. Rectosigmoid sphincter of O'Beirne. Dis Colon Rectum 1986;29:525–31.

22. Wadhwa RP, Mistry FP, Bhatia SJ et al. Existence of a high pressure zone at the rectosigmoid junction in normal Indian men. Dis Colon Rectum 1996;39:1122–5.

23. Shafik A, Doss S, Asaad S et al. Rectosigmoid junction: anatomical, histological, and radiological studies with special reference to a sphincteric function. Int J Colorectal Dis 1999;14:237–44.

24. Rasmussen OO, Sorensen M, Tetzschner T et al. Anorectal pressure gradient in patients with anal incontinence. Dis Colon Rectum 1992;35:8–11.

25. Williamson ME, Lewis WG, Holdsworth PJ et al. Decrease in the anorectal pressure gradient after low anterior resection of the rectum. A study using continuous ambulatory manometry. Dis Colon Rectum 1994;37:1228–31.

26. Taylor BM, Beart RW, Phillips SF. Longitudinal and radial variations of pressure in the human anal sphincter. Gastroenterology 1984;86:693–7.

27. Stojkovic SG, Balfour L, Burke D et al. Role of resting pressure gradient in the investigation of idiopathic fecal incontinence. Dis Colon Rectum 2002;45:668–73.

28. Lindsey I, Jones OM, Smilgin-Humphreys MM et al. Patterns of fecal incontinence after anal surgery. Dis Colon Rectum 2004;47:1643–9.

29. Smith AN, Varma JS, Binnie NR et al. Disordered colorectal motility in intractable constipation following hysterectomy. Br J Surg 1990;77:1361–5.

30. Cooper ZR, Rose S. Fecal incontinence: a clinical approach. Mt Sinai J Med 2000;67:96–105.

31. Bannister JJ, Read NW, Donnelly TC et al. External and internal anal sphincter responses to rectal distension in normal subjects and in patients with idiopathic faecal incontinence. Br J Surg 1989;76: 617–21.

32. Diamant NE, Kamm MA, Wald A et al. American Gastroenterological Association medical position statement on anorectal testing techniques. Gastroenterology 1999;116:732–60.

33. Miller R, Bartolo DC, Cervero F et al. Anorectal sampling: a comparison of normal and incontinent patients. Br J Surg 1988;75:44–7.

34. Sun WM, Read NW, Miner PB. Relation between rectal sensation and anal function in normal subjects and patients with faecal incontinence. Gut 1990;31:1056–61.

35. Knowles CH, Scott SM, Lunniss PJ. Slow transit constipation: a disorder of pelvic autonomic nerves? Dig Dis Sci 2001;46:389–401.

36. Kaiser AM, Ortega AE. Anorectal anatomy. Surg Clin North Am 2002;82:1125–38.

37. Berthoud HR, Blackshaw LA, Brookes SJ et al. Neuroanatomy of extrinsic afferents supplying the gastrointestinal tract. Neurogastroenterol Motil 2004;16(Suppl 1):28–33.

38. Snooks SJ, Setchell M, Swash M et al. Injury to innervation of pelvic floor sphincter musculature in childbirth. Lancet 1984;2:546–50.

39. Tetzschner T, Sorensen M, Rasmussen OO et al. Pudendal nerve damage increases the risk of fecal incontinence in women with anal sphincter rupture after childbirth. Acta Obstet Gynecol Scand 1995;74:434–40.

40. Fitzpatrick M, O'Herlihy C. The effects of labour and delivery on the pelvic floor. Best Pract Res Clin Obstet Gynaecol 2001;15:63–79.

41. Lunniss PJ, Gladman MA, Hetzer FH et al. Risk factors in acquired faecal incontinence. J R Soc Med 2004;97:111–16.

42. Oberwalder M, Dinnewitzer A, Baig MK et al. The association between late-onset fecal incontinence and obstetric anal sphincter defects. Arch Surg 2004;139:429–32.

43. Quinn M. Obstetric denervation-gynaecological reinnervation: disruption of the inferior hypogastric plexus in childbirth as a source of gynaecological symptoms. Med Hypotheses 2004;63: 390–3.

44. Sun WM, Donnelly TC, Read NW. Utility of a combined test of anorectal manometry, electromyography, and sensation in determining the mechanism of "idiopathic" faecal incontinence. Gut 1992;33:807–13.

45. Williams NS, Ogunbiyi OA, Scott SM et al. Rectal augmentation and stimulated gracilis anal neosphincter: a new approach in the management

of fecal urgency and incontinence. Dis Colon Rectum 2001;44:192–8.

46. Chan CL, Scott SM, Williams NS et al. Rectal hypersensitivity worsens stool frequency, urgency, and lifestyle in patients with urge faecal incontinence. Dis Colon Rectum 2005;48:134–40.

47. Degen LP, Phillips SF. How well does stool form reflect colonic transit? Gut 1996;39:109–13.

48. Gregersen H, Kassab G. Biomechanics of the gastrointestinal tract. Neurogastroenterol Motil 1996;8:277–97.

49. Ihre T. Studies on anal function in continent and incontinent patients. Scand J Gastroenterol 1974; 25(Suppl):1–64.

50. Arhan P, Faverdin C, Persoz B et al. Relationship between viscoelastic properties of the rectum and anal pressure in man. J Appl Physiol 1976;41: 677–82.

51. Felt-Bersma RJ, Sloots CE, Poen AC et al. Rectal compliance as a routine measurement: extreme volumes have direct clinical impact and normal volumes exclude rectum as a problem. Dis Colon Rectum 2000;43:1732–8.

52. Siproudhis L, Bellissant E, Pagenault M et al. Fecal incontinence with normal anal canal pressures: where is the pitfall? Am J Gastroenterol 1999;94: 1556–63.

53. Siproudhis L, Bellissant E, Juguet F et al. Perception of and adaptation to rectal isobaric distension in patients with faecal incontinence. Gut 1999;44: 687–92.

54. Buser WD, Miner PB Jr. Delayed rectal sensation with fecal incontinence. Successful treatment using anorectal manometry. Gastroenterology 1986;91:1186–91.

55. Lubowski DZ, Nicholls RJ. Faecal incontinence associated with reduced pelvic sensation. Br J Surg 1988;75:1086–8.

56. Gladman MA, Scott SM, Chan CL et al. Rectal hyposensitivity: prevalence and clinical impact in patients with intractable constipation and fecal incontinence. Dis Colon Rectum 2003;46:238–46.

57. Torsoli A, Ramorino ML, Ammaturo MV et al. Mass movements and intracolonic pressures. Am J Dig Dis 1971;16:693–6.

58. Cook IJ, Furukawa Y, Panagopoulos V et al. Relationships between spatial patterns of colonic pressure and individual movements of content. Am J Physiol Gastrointest Liver Physiol 2000;278: G329–41.

59. Narducci F, Bassotti G, Gaburri M et al. Twenty four hour manometric recording of colonic motor activity in healthy man. Gut 1987;28:17–25.

60. Kamm MA, van der Sijp JR, Lennard-Jones JE. Colorectal and anal motility during defaecation. Lancet 1992;339:820.

61. Bampton PA, Dinning PG, Kennedy ML et al. Spatial and temporal organization of pressure patterns throughout the unprepared colon during spontaneous defecation. Am J Gastroenterol 2000; 95:1027–35.

62. Bassotti G, Gaburri M, Imbimbo BP et al. Colonic mass movements in idiopathic chronic constipation. Gut 1988;29:1173–9.

63. Rao SS, Sadeghi P, Beaty J et al. Ambulatory 24-hour colonic manometry in slow-transit constipation. Am J Gastroenterol 2004;99:2405–16.

64. Whitehead WE, Wald A, Norton NJ. Treatment options for fecal incontinence. Dis Colon Rectum 2001;44:131–44.

65. Bouchoucha M, Devroede G, Faye A et al. Importance of colonic transit evaluation in the management of fecal incontinence. Int J Colorectal Dis 2002;17:412–17.

66. Chan CLH, Lunniss PJ, Wang D et al. Rectal sensorimotor dysfunction in patients with urge fecal incontinence: evidence from prolonged manometric studies. Gut 2005;54:1263–72.

67. Orkin BA, Hanson RB, Kelly KA. The rectal motor complex. J Gastrointest Motil 1989;1:5–8.

68. Rao SS, Welcher K. Periodic rectal motor activity: the intrinsic colonic gatekeeper? Am J Gastroenterol 1996;91:890–7.

69. Hagger R, Kumar D, Benson M et al. Periodic colonic motor activity identified by 24-h pancolonic ambulatory manometry in humans. Neurogastroenterol Motil 2002;14:271–8.

70. Spencer NJ. Control of migrating motor activity in the colon. Curr Opin Pharmacol 2001;1: 604–10.

71. Santoro GA, Eitan BZ, Pryde A et al. Open study of low-dose amitriptyline in the treatment of patients with idiopathic fecal incontinence. Dis Colon Rectum 2000;43:1676–81.

72. Rex DK, Lappas JC. Combined anorectal manometry and defecography in 50 consecutive adults with fecal incontinence. Dis Colon Rectum 1992;35:1040–5.

73. Rao SS, Ozturk R, Stessman M. Investigation of the pathophysiology of fecal seepage. Am J Gastroenterol 2004;99:2204–9.

74. Scarlett Y. Medical management of fecal incontinence. Gastroenterology 2004;126(Suppl 1):S55–63.

75. Duthie GS, Bartolo DCC. Faecal continence and defaecation. In: Henry MM, Swash M, eds. Coloproctology and the pelvic floor. Pathophysiology

and management, 2nd edn. London: Butterworths, 1992, pp 86–97.

76. Cherry DA, Rothenberger DA. Pelvic floor physiology. Surg Clin North Am 1988;68:1217–30.

77. Kumar D, Wingate DL. Colorectal motility. In: Henry MM, Swash M, eds. Coloproctology and the pelvic floor. Pathophysiology and management. 2nd edn. London: Butterworths, 1992, pp 72–85.

78. Gordon PH. Anorectal anatomy and physiology. Gastroenterol Clin North Am 2001;30:1–13.

79. Thorson AG. Anorectal physiology. Surg Clin North Am 2002;82:1115–23.

80. Kiff ES, Swash M. Slowed conduction in the pudendal nerves in idiopathic (neurogenic) faecal incontinence. Br J Surg 1984;71:614–16.

81. Donnelly V, Fynes M, Campbell D et al. Obstetric events leading to anal sphincter damage. Obstet Gynecol 1998;92:955–61.

82. Kamm MA. Faecal incontinence. BMJ 1998;316: 528–32.

83. Law PJ, Kamm MA, Bartram CI. Anal endosonography in the investigation of faecal incontinence. Br J Surg 1991;78:312–14.

84. Nielsen MB, Hauge C, Pedersen JF et al. Endosonographic evaluation of patients with anal incontinence: findings and influence on surgical management. Am J Roentgenol 1993;160: 771–5.

85. Damon H, Henry L, Bretones S et al. Postdelivery anal function in primiparous females: ultrasound and manometric study. Dis Colon Rectum 2000; 43:472–7.

86. Zetterstrom J, Mellgren A, Jensen LL et al. Effect of delivery on anal sphincter morphology and function. Dis Colon Rectum 1999;42:1253–60.

87. Pinta TM, Kylanpaa ML, Teramo KA et al. Sphincter rupture and anal incontinence after first vaginal delivery. Acta Obstet Gynecol Scand 2004; 83:917–22.

88. Sultan AH, Kamm MA, Hudson CN et al. Analsphincter disruption during vaginal delivery. N Engl J Med 1993;329:1905–11.

89. Chaliha C, Sultan AH, Bland JM et al. Anal function: effect of pregnancy and delivery. Am J Obstet Gynecol 2001;185:427–32.

90. Fornell EK, Berg G, Hallbook O et al. Clinical consequences of anal sphincter rupture during vaginal delivery. J Am Coll Surg 1996;183:553–8.

91. Rieger N, Schloithe A, Saccone G et al. The effect of a normal vaginal delivery on anal function. Acta Obstet Gynecol Scand 1997;76:769–72.

92. Rieger N, Schloithe A, Saccone G et al. A prospective study of anal sphincter injury due to childbirth. Scand J Gastroenterol 1998;33:950–5.

93. Fynes M, Donnelly V, Behan M et al. Effect of second vaginal delivery on anorectal physiology and faecal continence: a prospective study. Lancet 1999;354:983–6.

94. Lee SJ, Park JW. Follow-up evaluation of the effect of vaginal delivery on the pelvic floor. Dis Colon Rectum 2000;43:1550–5.

95. Willis S, Faridi A, Schelzig S et al. Childbirth and incontinence: a prospective study on anal sphincter morphology and function before and early after vaginal delivery. Langenbecks Arch Surg 2002;387:101–7.

96. Hojberg KE, Hundborg HH, Ryhammer AM et al. The impact of delivery on anorectal function in women with and women without anal incontinence – a prospective study. Int Urogynecol J Pelvic Floor Dysfunct 2003;14:38–45.

97. Nazir M, Carlsen E, Nesheim BI. Do occult anal sphincter injuries, vector volume manometry and delivery variables have any predictive value for bowel symptoms after first time vaginal delivery without third and fourth degree rupture? A prospective study. Acta Obstet Gynecol Scand 2002; 81:720–6.

98. Fornell EU, Matthiesen L, Sjodahl R et al. Obstetric anal sphincter injury ten years after: subjective and objective long term effects. BJOG 2005;112: 312–16.

99. Fynes M, Donnelly VS, O'Connell PR et al. Cesarean delivery and anal sphincter injury. Obstet Gynecol 1998;92:496–500.

100. Abramowitz L, Sobhani I, Ganansia R et al. Are sphincter defects the cause of anal incontinence after vaginal delivery? Results of a prospective study. Dis Colon Rectum 2000;43:590–8.

101. Faltin DL, Boulvain M, Irion O et al. Diagnosis of anal sphincter tears by postpartum endosonography to predict fecal incontinence. Obstet Gynecol 2000;95:643–7.

102. Belmonte-Montes C, Hagerman G, Vega-Yepez PA et al. Anal sphincter injury after vaginal delivery in primiparous females. Dis Colon Rectum 2001;44:1244–8.

103. Damon H, Bretones S, Henry L et al. Long-term consequences of first vaginal delivery-induced anal sphincter defect. Dis Colon Rectum 2005; 48:1772–6.

104. Sultan AH, Stanton SL. Occult obstetric trauma and anal incontinence. Eur J Gastroenterol Hepatol 1997;9:423–7.

105. Nygaard IE, Rao SS, Dawson JD. Anal incontinence after anal sphincter disruption: a 30-year retrospective cohort study. Obstet Gynecol 1997; 89:896–901.

106. Hartmann K, Viswanathan M, Palmieri R et al. Outcomes of routine episiotomy: a systematic review. JAMA 2005;293:2141–8.

107. Williams AB, Bartram CI, Halligan S et al. Alteration of anal sphincter morphology following vaginal delivery revealed by multiplanar anal endosonography. BJOG 2002;109:942–6.

108. Parks AG, Swash M, Urich H. Sphincter denervation in anorectal incontinence and rectal prolapse. Gut 1977;18:656–65.

109. Neill ME, Swash M. Increased motor unit fibre density in the external anal sphincter muscle in ano-rectal incontinence: a single fibre EMG study. J Neurol Neurosurg Psychiatry 1980; 43:343–7.

110. Allen RE, Hosker GL, Smith AR et al. Pelvic floor damage and childbirth: a neurophysiological study. Br J Obstet Gynaecol 1990;97:770–9.

111. Snooks SJ, Swash M, Henry MM et al. Risk factors in childbirth causing damage to the pelvic floor innervation. Int J Colorectal Dis 1986;1:20–4.

112. Snooks SJ, Swash M, Mathers SE et al. Effect of vaginal delivery on the pelvic floor: a 5-year follow-up. Br J Surg 1990;77:1358–60.

113. Sultan AH, Kamm MA, Hudson CN. Pudendal nerve damage during labour: prospective study before and after childbirth. Br J Obstet Gynaecol 1994;101:22–8.

114. Tetzschner T, Sorensen M, Jonsson L et al. Delivery and pudendal nerve function. Acta Obstet Gynecol Scand 1997;76:324–31.

115. Rieger N, Wattchow D. The effect of vaginal delivery on anal function. Aust N Z J Surg 1999;69: 172–7.

116. Pollack J, Nordenstam J, Brismar S et al. Anal incontinence after vaginal delivery: a five-year prospective cohort study. Obstet Gynecol 2004;104: 1397–402.

117. Eason E, Labrecque M, Marcoux S et al. Anal incontinence after childbirth. CMAJ 2002;166: 326–30.

118. Richter HE, Brumfield CG, Cliver SP et al. Risk factors associated with anal sphincter tear: a comparison of primiparous patients, vaginal births after cesarean deliveries, and patients with previous vaginal delivery. Am J Obstet Gynecol 2002; 187:1194–8.

119. Christianson LM, Bovbjerg VE, McDavitt EC et al. Risk factors for perineal injury during delivery. Am J Obstet Gynecol 2003;189:255–60.

120. Zetterstrom J, Lopez A, Holmstrom B et al. Obstetric sphincter tears and anal incontinence: an observational follow-up study. Acta Obstet Gynecol Scand 2003;82:921–8.

121. Roe AM, Bartolo DC, Mortensen NJ. New method for assessment of anal sensation in various anorectal disorders. Br J Surg 1986;73:310–12.

122. Cornes H, Bartolo DC, Stirrat GM. Changes in anal canal sensation after childbirth. Br J Surg 1991; 78:74–7.

123. Kiff ES, Barnes PR, Swash M. Evidence of pudendal neuropathy in patients with perineal descent and chronic straining at stool. Gut 1984;25: 1279–82.

124. Engel AF, Kamm MA. The acute effect of straining on pelvic floor neurological function. Int J Colorectal Dis 1994;9:8–12.

125. Jameson JS, Chia YW, Kamm MA et al. Effect of age, sex and parity on anorectal function. Br J Surg 1994;81:1689–92.

126. Lubowski DZ, Jones PN, Swash M et al. Asymmetrical pudendal nerve damage in pelvic floor disorders. Int J Colorectal Dis 1988;3:158–60.

127. Osterberg A, Graf W, Edebol Eeg-Olofsson K et al. Results of neurophysiologic evaluation in fecal incontinence. Dis Colon Rectum 2000;43:1256–61.

128. Thomas C, Lefaucheur JP, Galula G et al. Respective value of pudendal nerve terminal motor latency and anal sphincter electromyography in neurogenic fecal incontinence. Neurophysiol Clin 2002;32:85–90.

129. Gregory WT, Lou JS, Stuyvesant A et al. Quantitative electromyography of the anal sphincter after uncomplicated vaginal delivery. Obstet Gynecol 2004;104:327–35.

130. Fitzpatrick M, O'Brien C, O'Connell PR et al. Patterns of abnormal pudendal nerve function that are associated with postpartum fecal incontinence. Am J Obstet Gynecol 2003;189:730–5.

9
Investigations of Anorectal Function

S. Mark Scott and Peter J. Lunniss

9.1 Introduction

When investigation of the anorectum is appropriate (i.e. those patients in whom empirical conservative measures have failed, concurrent disease has been excluded, and there is a significant impact of symptoms on quality of life), assessment should be carried out in the context of global pelvic floor evaluation, aimed at both morphology/anatomy and function. The former can be evaluated by physical examination, but in more detail by imaging (static or dynamic), and the latter by clinical history and examination, but in more detail by tests of physiology. It is important that assessment is combined with an understanding of the sufferer's expectations of treatment.

With the advance of diagnostic technology, it is now accepted that in the field of functional bowel disorders, symptom-based assessment, although important, is unsatisfactory as the sole means of directing therapy. The symptom repertoire of the gut is limited and relatively non-specific, such that similar symptom profiles may reside in differing pathoaetiologies and pathophysiologies.[1] In a field of practice in which normal physiological function is so complex (that of defaecation and continence), and in which pathoaetiology on a structural basis is only partly understood (e.g. mechanical sphincter trauma may be demonstrable by endoanal ultrasound, but suboptimal function only, reported after "successful" surgical repair[2]), reliance on clinical symptoms alone as a basis for taxonomy is now obsolete. A robust taxonomy based on underlying pathophysiology must therefore be paramount.[1]

The multifactorial pathoaetiology of female incontinence, incurred either simultaneously (e.g. neuropathy and sphincter disruption[3–5]) or sequentially, means that directed therapy requires comprehensive assessment of all understood and measurable components that contribute towards continence, including tests of suprasphincteric as well as sphincteric function.

9.2 Investigations

Incorporating the findings from clinical history, physical examination and investigations allows the cause of incontinence to be elucidated, coexisting pathology to be excluded, and a decision regarding choice of suitable, rather than empirical therapy to be made on an individual basis. It must be stressed, however, that the results of any individual tests have to be integrated within the clinical scenario, and not be interpreted in isolation. Several studies have looked at the clinical impact of anorectal physiological investigation in patients with faecal incontinence and demonstrated that the information provided markedly improved diagnostic yield[6,7] and directly influenced a change in management in a significant proportion of cases.[6–9]

There are many complementary investigations for the assessment of anorectal structure and function (Table 9.1). Ideally, an evaluation of all components of the continence mechanism, as outlined previously (see Table 8.1), should be performed. However, although many tests are now established in clinical practice (e.g. anorectal

TABLE 9.1. Tests available for the assessment of anorectal and colonic function in patients with faecal incontinence

Investigation	Modality Assessed	Clinical Use
Anorectal manometry	(i) anal sphincter function	Established
Traditional	(ii) rectoanal reflexes	Established
	(iii) rectal sensation	Established
	(iv) rectal compliance	Established
	(v) rectal evacuation (balloon expulsion test)	Established
	(vi) continence to liquid (saline continence test)	Established
Prolonged ambulatory	anorectal / rectosigmoid motility	Research
Vector volume	anal sphincter function / pressure profile	Research
Barostat studies	(i) rectal sensation	Established
	(ii) rectal compliance	Established
	(iii) rectal tone	Research
	(iv) rectal wall tension	Research
	(v) rectal capacity	Research
	(vi) rectal motility	Research
Impedance planimetry	Rectal biomechanical properties	Research
Endo-anal ultrasound		
2-Dimensional	imaging of the anal sphincters/associated structures	Established
3-Dimensional	imaging of the anal sphincters/associated structures	Research
Endo-anal MRI	imaging of the anal sphincters/associated structures	Research
Neurophysiological		
Nerve conduction	pudendal nerve terminal motor latency	Established – limited value
Electromyography	(i) motor unit potentials	Established – limited value
	(ii) fibre density	Established – limited value
Evoked potentials	(i) motor	Research
	(ii) somatosensory	Research
Other	anocutaneous reflex	Established – limited value
Other	clitoral-anal reflex	Established limited – value
	strength-duration test (muscle innervation)	Research
Anorectal sensation		
Anal	(i) mucosal electrosensitivity	Established – limited value
	(ii) mucosal thermosensitivity	Research
Rectal	(i) mucosal electrosensitivity	Established – limited value
	(ii) mucosal thermosensitivity	Research
Evacuation proctography		
Fluoroscopy	rectal evacuatory function	Established – limited value
Scintigraphy	rectal evacuatory function	Research
Dynamic MRI	rectal evacuatory function/pelvic organ movement	Research
Colonic transit studies		
Radio-opaque markers	global colonic transit	Established
Scintigraphy	segmental colonic transit	Established – limited value

manometry, endoanal ultrasound, etc.), the clinical value of some is controversial (e.g. neurophysiological techniques), and others (e.g. vector-volume manometry, prolonged rectosigmoid manometry, magnetic resonance imaging, etc.) currently remain as research techniques, limited to a few specialist centres. Consequently only a proportion of the factors contributing to the preservation of continence are routinely assessed. Nevertheless, the diagnostic yield undoubtedly improves, the broader the series of tests per-

formed,[8] and thus it is our firm belief that all patients should undergo as thorough an assessment as is available, performed in a structured and systematic manner.

The patient should be fully informed about the details of the procedures; this will also enhance patient cooperation. Written consent should be obtained prior to commencement of the studies. Although some centres advocate rectal preparation using enemas and/or cathartics, this is not a necessity and can usually be avoided unless scybalous stool is expected or detected upon digital examination. The patient should be asked to void residual urine and faeces before the study starts. Sedatives are not required and should be avoided. Manometric procedures should not be carried out within 5 minutes of anorectal palpation (digital examination) or longer if an enema has been administered, in order to allow sphincter activity to return to basal levels.[10]

Imaging techniques are described in Chapter 10.

9.3 Established Methodologies

9.3.1 Anorectal Manometry

The human finger is a poor pressure-measuring device, and digital examination alone is not accurate enough for the diagnostic assessment of anal sphincter function.[11] In addition, it is not possible to assess other important components of the continence mechanism by this method, notably colorectal sensorimotor function or rectoanal reflex activity.

Anorectal manometry is the best established and the most widely available investigative tool. In patients with faecal incontinence, manometric evaluation commonly encompasses a series of measurements designed to test for:

1. Deficits in anal sphincter function
2. The presence or absence of rectoanal reflexes
3. Rectal sensory function and compliance.

In addition, a manometric assessment may also include components designed to assess defaecatory function, namely:

1. Expulsion of a rectal balloon
2. Saline continence test
3. Rectoanal pressure relationships during bearing down/straining manoeuvres (this test has not found routine use for patients with faecal incontinence).

The apparatus required consists of four major components: (1) an intraluminal pressure-sensing catheter (water-perfused, or with mounted solid-state microtransducers, air- or water-filled microballoon(s), or a sleeve sensor); (2) pressure transducers; (3) a balloon for inflation within the rectum (either integral to the catheter assembly or fixed to an independent catheter); (4) the amplification/recording/display system. Unfortunately, the biggest pitfall with anorectal manometry is the lack of uniformity regarding such equipment and technique. As a consequence, comparison of results between centres is problematic. Each individual institution is therefore encouraged to develop its own control values (preferably sex and age stratified) or, if using normative data from the literature, adopt similar methodology, such that a particular result may be compared with the appropriate normal range.[11–13] Currently, a six-sensor probe (either water-perfused or solid-state) is recommended[13] with a balloon (preferably non-latex) of not less than 4 cm tied to the end. One pressure sensor, and a lumen opening to allow for inflation, should be located inside the balloon. The remaining five sensors should be arranged radially and spaced 1 cm apart.[13]

9.3.1.1 Anal Sphincter Function

The objectives of assessment are to identify the functional anal canal length and to record the maximum resting anal canal pressure and voluntary anal squeeze pressure (Figures 9.1 and 9.2). As noted above, however, there is marked variability in reported pressures, affected by:

1. The intraluminal pressure sensor itself
2. The assessment technique: station pull-through,[14,15] (the recommended method[12,16]) continuous pull-through[17,18] or stationary[19]
3. Catheter diameter
4. Orientation of the recording ports/sensors
5. Patient posture
6. Perfusion rate (for perfused-tube catheters)
7. The distending medium (air or water: for microballoons)
8. Size of the microballoon
9. The rate of withdrawal (for rapid pull-through technique).

The two most important considerations are probably catheter diameter and radial and longitudinal variations in pressure within the anal canal.[20,21] Large bore probes can distort the anal canal and falsely record high pressures; a positive correlation exists between catheter diameter and maximum anal resting and squeeze pressures.[17] Anterior quadrant pressures are lower in the

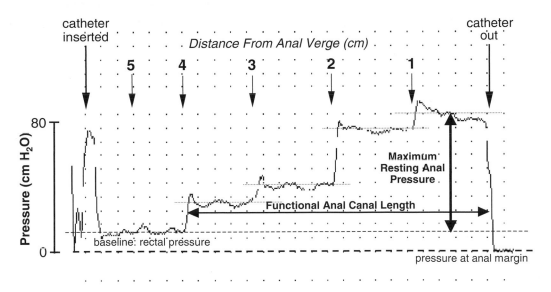

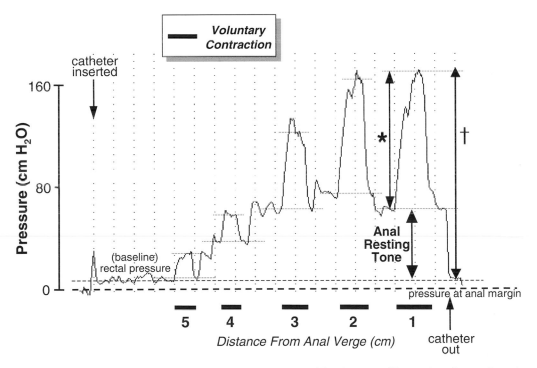

FIGURE 9.1. Functional anal canal length and maximum resting pressure. With the patient at rest, the pressure-sensitive recording device (in this case a water-filled microballoon) is pulled through the anal canal from the rectum. Pressures are allowed to stabilise at each station (denoted by the fine dotted lines). In this patient, a maximum resting pressure of 85 cmH$_2$O is recorded, 1 cm from the anal verge. The functional anal canal length is 4 cm.

FIGURE 9.2. Maximum anal squeeze pressure/increment. By asking the patient to contract their anal canal musculature during a station pull-through procedure, the maximum voluntary squeeze pressure (†) or increment (*) at a given distance from the anal verge can be determined. In this patient, a maximum squeeze increment of 105 cmH$_2$O is recorded 1 cm from the anal verge.

proximal anal canal than those in the other three quadrants, whereas posterior quadrant pressures are lower in the distal anal canal. In the mid anal canal, radial pressures are equivalent in all quadrants.[21] Variation in radial and longitudinal pressures is also related to sex differences.[18] Given such functional asymmetry of the anal sphincters, pressures should be calculated by averaging values recorded in all four quadrants.[22]

The functional anal canal length is defined as the length of the anal canal over which resting pressure exceeds that of rectum by >5 mmHg,[18,19,23] or alternatively, as the length of the anal canal over which pressures are greater than half of the maximal pressure at rest.[14] The length of the functional anal canal is usually shorter in incontinent patients than in normal control subjects[23] (Figure 9.3). The clinical significance of this measure, however, has recently been questioned.[12]

Maximal resting anal pressure is defined as the difference between intrarectal pressure and the highest recorded anal sphincter pressure at rest.[13,18] Pressure at the level of the anal margin can alternatively be used as the zero baseline.[19] The maximal pressure is generally recorded 1–2 cm cephalad to the anal verge (Figure 9.1), which corresponds to the condensation of smooth muscle fibres of the internal anal sphincter. Anal resting tone is subject to pressure oscillations caused by slow waves, of amplitude 5–25 cmH$_2$O, occurring at a frequency of 6–20/min,[15,17] or high-amplitude "ultra-slow" waves, 30–100 cmH$_2$O in magnitude, occurring at 0.5–2/min[20] (although the latter are rarely observed in patients with low resting pressures). Symptoms of passive faecal incontinence correlate with low resting anal tone[24] (Figure 9.4) and often a reversal of the anal pressure gradient.[25] This is typically due to internal anal sphincter rupture (e.g. secondary to obstetric trauma[25,26] or iatrogenic injury[25,27]), but may also be secondary to smooth muscle degeneration.[28] However, patients with very low basal pressures may be fully continent, and thus measurement of resting tone, though of pathophysiological significance in patients with incontinence, must be considered in combination with other functional findings.[12]

The measure of a patient's ability to squeeze their striated anal musculature can be calculated as the maximal voluntary anal squeeze pressure (the difference between intrarectal pressure, or the pressure at the level of the anal margin, and the highest recorded pressure during anal squeeze),[13] or the maximal voluntary anal squeeze increment

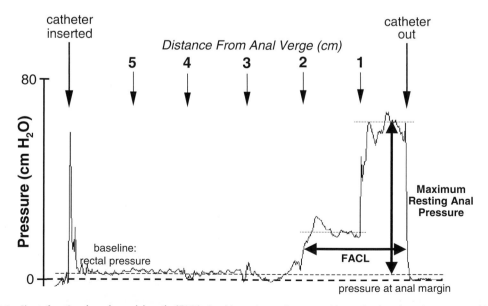

FIGURE 9.3. Short functional anal canal length (*FACL*). In this patient with faecal incontinence, an increase in pressure above that of rectal (baseline) pressure is only observed at 1–2 cm from the anal verge, with maximal anal resting pressure (67 cmH$_2$O) being recorded in the last 1 cm. Steady-state is denoted by the fine dotted lines.

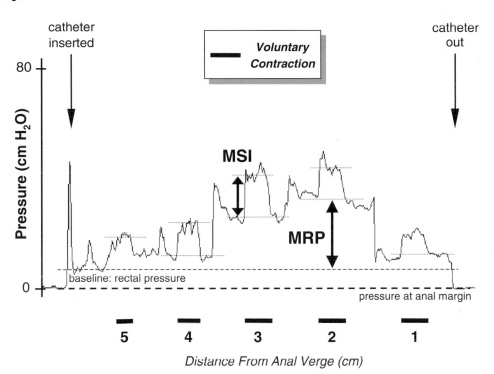

FIGURE 9.4. Attenuated anal resting and squeeze pressures. In this patient presenting with symptoms of both passive and urge faecal incontinence, both maximum anal resting pressure (*MRP*) and

maximum anal squeeze increment (*MSI*) are abnormally low (33 and 15 cmH₂O, respectively). The fine dotted lines denote steady-state.

(the difference between resting pressure at any given level of the anal canal, and the highest recorded pressure during anal squeeze);[12,19] the latter is probably a better determinant of anal squeeze function (Figure 9.2). The squeeze response normally consists of an initial peak, followed by a decrease to "steady-state level", followed by a decline toward resting (baseline) pressure.[15] The measurement of highest recorded pressure may be taken as the true maximum pressure at any point during the squeeze manoeuvre (usually the initial peak), or as the maximum steady-state pressure. The duration of the sustained squeeze can be defined as the time interval at which the subject can maintain squeeze pressure at ≥50% of the maximum squeeze pressure.[13]

Symptoms of urge or stress faecal incontinence often correlate with low anal squeeze pressures[24] (Figure 9.4), with the major causative factor being obstetric injury.[3,26] In addition, squeeze duration is reduced[29] and "fatigue rate" is significantly shortened[30] in incontinent patients compared to controls (Figure 9.5). However, though low or

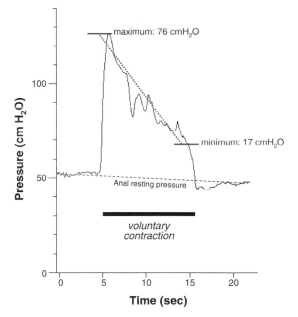

FIGURE 9.5. External anal sphincter fatiqability. In this patient with urge faecal incontinence, the voluntary squeeze increment rapidly "decays" with time during an anal squeeze manoeuvre. The fatigue index is the coefficient of maximum squeeze pressure and gradient of decay.

poorly sustained voluntary anal squeeze pressures imply external anal sphincter (EAS) weakness, standard manometry alone cannot differentiate between compromised muscle integrity, impaired innervation, or both (or indeed a poorly compliant patient[12]) as a cause of that weakness. Anal squeeze pressure has been shown to be reasonably sensitive and specific for discrimination of patients with faecal incontinence;[31] nevertheless, the correlation between anal canal pressures and incontinence is not perfect[32] given the wide range of normal values and the contribution of those various other factors crucial to anorectal continence. This is compounded by the fact that simply recording maximum pressures may not reflect global sphincter function along its length, a problem that might be overcome by recording pressures at several points along the anal canal, but which then makes comparison with normal more difficult due to the complex radial and longitudinal pressure profiles that exist within the anal canal.

Overall, anal resting tone is probably less susceptible to artefact than the measurement of squeeze pressures, which is dependent upon the patient's understanding and ability to comply with instructions.[12,16] However, recording of both measures has been shown to be highly reproducible in the same subject on separate days.[33] At present, there is no accepted method for the evaluation of puborectalis contractile activity.[12]

9.3.1.2 Rectoanal Reflex Activity

Relaxation of the caudad anus in response to rectal distension, the rectoanal inhibitory reflex,[34] is thought to allow rectal contents to be sampled by the sensory area of the anal canal, thus allowing discrimination between flatus and faecal matter, i.e. "fine-tuning" of the continence mechanism. It is an intramural reflex mediated by the myenteric plexus, and modulated via the spinal cord.[17] The rectoanal inhibitory reflex can be simply measured by concomitantly recording resting anal pressures during rapid inflation of the rectal balloon (i.e. mimicking a sudden arrival of faecal bolus).[12] The amplitude and duration of the drop in pressure (relaxation) are correlated with

the distending volume, in that the greater the distension volume, the greater the fall in anal pressure, and the more sustained the response.[35] However, although differences in reflex parameters have been shown between incontinent patients and healthy subjects,[36,37] the clinical significance of these findings is unclear.

As stressed previously, one aspect of the continence mechanism is that anal pressure needs to exceed rectal pressure. During transient increases in intra-abdominal or intrarectal pressure, preservation of this positive anal to rectal pressure gradient is maintained by a compensatory multisynaptic sacral reflex, the rectoanal contractile reflex, which results in a contraction of the EAS. This protective mechanism prevents faecal leakage during activities such as coughing.[14] Investigation of the rectoanal contractile reflex requires simultaneous monitoring of intrarectal and anal pressures during a sudden increase in intra-abdominal/intrapelvic pressure caused by blowing up a balloon placed in the rectum, or by having the patient cough to test the "cough reflex".[12,19,31] This test is also useful for further evaluation of EAS function, especially in those patients with apparently attenuated voluntary anal squeeze pressures in whom poor compliance is suspected.[12] Under normal circumstances, intra-anal pressure should exceed intrarectal pressure. An abnormal reflex response, but normal squeeze pressures indicate neural damage of the sacral arc, either of the spinal sacral segments or the pudendal nerves;[12] such patients usually suffer from urge incontinence. Both the reflex response and voluntary squeeze pressures are absent in patients with lesions of the cauda equina or sacral plexus.[4,31]

9.3.1.3 Rectal Sensation

Rectal sensory function is most commonly quantified using balloon distension, during which the patient is instructed to volunteer a range of sensations: first sensation, constant (flatus) sensation (optional), desire to defaecate, and maximum toleration.[38] The distending volume (and/or pressure) at each of these sensory thresholds should be recorded. Two techniques are used for inflation: (1) ramp (continual); or (2) intermittent, which can be either phasic (volumes injected and then withdrawn)[39] or stepwise (volumes are maintained between inflations)[40] in nature. It has been suggested that a ramp inflation technique is superior to that of intermittent distension in assessing rectal sensation.[39,41] Unfortunately, the results of this investigation are probably influenced more by differences in methodology than that of any other anorectal physiological technique. Sensory responses are altered by:

1. The type of inflation
2. The distending medium (air or water)
3. The speed of inflation[39]
4. The material, e.g. the size and shape of the balloon
5. The distance of the balloon from the anal verge
6. The position of the patient.

However, despite large intersubject variation, several studies have reported a high degree of reproducibility with regard to recorded sensory thresholds,[39,42,43] notably for maximum tolerable volume.[17] It is probable that sensory threshold pressures, as opposed to volumes, are an even more robust measure,[33] but their use is less practical in the clinical setting.

The purpose of any clinically useful test, including tests of rectal sensation, is to allow an individual patient to be clearly placed within, or be discriminated from, the normal population. Accordingly, once normal ranges have been determined in healthy control subjects, abnormalities of rectal sensitivity may be defined on the basis of aberrant values in comparison to those normal ranges. Sensory thresholds reduced below the normal range imply heightened sensory awareness and can be termed rectal hypersensitivity, while elevated sensory thresholds related to impaired or blunted rectal sensory function can be termed rectal hyposensitivity.[44] Both abnormalities have been reported in patients with faecal incontinence. Those with rectal hypersensitivity typically complain of urgency/urge incontinence and increased frequency of defaecation.[26,35,45,46] Those with significant blunting of the ability to sense distension may have passive (overflow) incontinence.[47-50]

Other methods of assessing rectal sensitivity are described below.

9.3.1.4 Rectal Compliance

Compliance, which reflects rectal capacity and distensibilty, may be measured in conjunction with the evaluation of sensory thresholds (Figure 9.6). Though feasible using conventional manometry, rectal compliance can be most accurately assessed using a programmable barostat (see below), which minimises both observer bias and error.[15] Employing an intermittent balloon distension technique, intraballoon (intrarectal) volumes and pressures must be recorded concomitantly.[13] Measurement by means of latex (or equivalent) balloons requires correction to account for their intrinsic elasticity.[12,13] Oversized polyethylene bags are favoured; provided that the range of volumes used for the study remains below 90% of the maximum volume of the bag, polyethylene can be regarded as infinitely compliant, in that its own properties have no influence on the internal pressure (i.e. large volumes can be accommodated without an increase in intrabag pressure, until the volume injected is >90% of the maximum bag volume).[51] Rectal compliance describes the pressure/volume relationship, and is (perhaps simplistically) calculated as change in volume divided by change in pressure ($\Delta V/\Delta P$).[11,12,19] However, for technical and physiological reasons, the pressure/

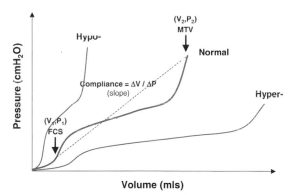

FIGURE 9.6. Pressure-volume relationships during rectal distension. Rectal compliance is calculated from the slope (denoted by the dashed line) over that part of the curve between first constant sensation (FCS: V_1, P_1) and maximum tolerable volume (MTV: V_2, P_2), and is defined as $\Delta DV/\Delta P$. In a patient with rectal hypocompliance (stiff rectal wall), the curve is shifted to the left, and the slope steepens; conversely, in a patients with rectal hypercompliance, the curve shifts to the right, and the slope is shallower.

volume curve is non-linear, and thus calculating a single value to describe the slope of that curve (i.e. ascribing a linear measurement for compliance) is imprecise.[11,13] It is more accurate to express compliance values as a graphical plot of all volumes tested,[11,13] although this is rather cumbersome in practice. Alternatively, compliance can be approximated to an exponential function.[16] Irrespective of the methodology employed, however, measurement of compliance has been shown to be highly reproducible.[33,42]

9.3.1.5 Balloon Expulsion Test

Evaluation of a patient's ability to expel a filled balloon from the rectum is a simple method of assessing (simulated) defaecation dynamics. Inflation volume (either water at 37°C or air) of the catheter-mounted balloon is typically 50 ml[19,52] and need not exceed 150 ml.[53] The patient can then be transferred to a commode and instructed to expel the balloon. The time taken for expulsion should be recorded and intraballoon pressure can be monitored concomitantly to evaluate changes in intrarectal pressure. Asymptomatic subjects can expel the balloon in a median of 50 s (range 10–300)[19] with an increase in intra-abdominal pressure of >80 cmH$_2$O.[19,52] Despite generating similar increases in intra-abdominal/pelvic pressure on straining as normal subjects, patients with constipation are often unable to expel a filled balloon,[54] which may be secondary to functional (variably termed paradoxical pelvic floor contraction, pelvic floor dyssynergia or anismus) or mechanical outlet obstruction. Understandably, however, some patients find this test extremely embarrassing, which may inhibit normal evacuation, leading to a gross overdiagnosis of functional outlet obstruction.[55,56] Evacuation proctography remains the gold-standard method for investigating the process of rectal evacuation[5] (see below). In patients with faecal incontinence, most have no problems expelling the balloon.[4] However, in those presenting with faecal seepage, many demonstrate impaired evacuation,[48] suggesting that a disorder of defaecation may underlie their symptoms. The balloon expulsion test may be incorporated into therapeutic biofeedback programmes.[4]

9.3.1.6 Saline Continence Test

This investigation is designed to evaluate the continence mechanism by reproducing a situation simulating diarrhoea.[19,57] The test may be useful in providing objective proof/evidence of faecal incontinence, and also in assessing improvement in continence following conservative medical or surgical therapy.[4] The aims are to determine: (i) the efficiency (resistance) of the anal sphincters, and (ii) the capacity of the rectum/defaecation mechanism. With the patient lying in the left-lateral position, a fine bore (~2 mm) plastic tube is introduced 8–10 cm into the rectum. The patient should then be seated on a commode, and the tube attached to an infusion pump. Saline at 37°C can then be infused into the rectum at a steady flow rate of 60 ml/min up to a maximum of either 800 ml[19] or 1.5 litres[57,58] (the former is quicker and enhances the sensitivity and specificity of the test[19]). The subject should be instructed to retain the fluid for as long as possible. Leaked saline may be collected in a graduated vessel located in the bowl of the commode. Measurements taken are: (i) volume infused at onset of first leak, (ii) volume of first leak, and (iii) total volume leaked at the end of the study period. If simultaneous monitoring of rectal and anal pressure changes is performed, anorectal reflex activity (inhibitory and contractile reflexes) can be identified.[20]

Normal subjects are able to retain a volume in excess of 1.5 litres without any significant leakage of saline.[8,57] Significant leakage is defined as a leak of >10[57] or 15 ml.[4] The volume of saline retained at the end of the study is calculated as the difference between the volume infused and the volume leaked. Patients with a weak sphincter mechanism or with reduced rectal capacity/compliance can retain a lesser volume of fluid than normal asymptomatic subjects.[58,59] In patients with faecal incontinence, leakage starts after infusion of only 250–600 ml, with volume retention of 500–1,000 ml.[58]

9.3.2 Barostat Studies

A major recent innovation in the field of anorectal physiological investigation is the establishment of the computerised barostat as the method of choice, in favour of traditional manometric techniques for the evaluation of various components of rectal sensorimotor function.[12,15,16] The fact that that this device was developed 20 years ago[60] gives an indication of the time it may take for a research technique to be accepted in clinical practice. Primarily, the barostat is used for accurate assessment of pressure/volume relationships (and hence compliance) during the measurement of rectal sensitivity;[13,51] however, it can also be employed for the study of other parameters of visceral sensation, reflex activity, wall tension and capacity, and changes in rectal tone or phasic activity over a prolonged period (although these modalities remain within the realms of research at present).[51,61] In simple terms, the barostat is a pneumatic device that maintains a constant pressure within an air-filled bag situated in the rectum, by a feedback mechanism that rapidly aspirates air from the bag when the rectum contracts, and injects air when the rectum relaxes. The volume of air aspirated/injected is proportional to the magnitude of contraction/relaxation. The use of the barostat has the following advantages:

1. The infinitely compliant, oversized bag (see above) is attached at both ends to the catheter, which ensures distension in the circumferential axis by eliminating axial migration into the sigmoid colon.

2. Simultaneous acquisition of volume and pressure data is possible, and thus it is not subject to the same limitations as volume-based (simple balloon) distension techniques.[51]

3. The distension is computerised, which allows distension parameters known to affect visceral sensitivity (see above), such as rate and pattern of inflation,[39] to be tightly controlled and standardised using the associated computer software. In addition, the influence of response bias may be minimised by employing the use of (pseudo-) random distension sequences.[51] This improves reproducibility and removes some observer bias.[11]

In regard to the measurement of sensation/compliance, either phasic (ascending methods of limits)[15] or stepwise (staircase)[16] isobaric distension paradigms may be employed. Good repro-ducibility for both measures has been reported.[33,62] In patients with faecal incontinence, studies have been limited thus far,[32,63] but have confirmed alterations in compliance (and sensation) in some subjects. The major limitation with the barostat is its expense, which may preclude its widespread use, in view of the relative low cost of traditional manometry.

9.3.3 Transit Studies

In patients with symptoms of constipation and incontinence, gastrointestinal (predominantly colonic) transit studies provide an objective confirmation of a subjective complaint of infrequent defaecation and enable a distinction between normal and slow colonic transit.[11] Stool frequency, as reported by the patient, is an unreliable measure for defining constipation.[64] Radio-opaque marker studies, with plain abdominal films taken 3–5 days later, are an adequate screening test for detecting transit abnormalities;[65–67] the simplest method is a modification of that originally described by Hinton et al.,[65] and involves the patient swallowing 50 markers (radio-opaque feeding tube, cut up into 2-mm slices) contained in a gelatin capsule. A single abdominal x-ray is taken 96h later.[68,69] The patient is instructed to discontinue laxative medication for the duration of the study. The study is considered abnormal if >20% of markers remain.[66,68,69] For accurate assessment of segmental colonic transit, however, more complex marker studies,[66,67] or radionuclide scintigraphy is required.[68,70,71] A comprehensive description of such methods is given in detail elsewhere.[72,73] Irrespective of methodology, if a delay in colonic transit is identified, the management strategy can be altered accordingly.

Conversely, rapid gastrointestinal transit may result in diarrhoea and underlie symptoms of urgency and frequency of defaecation in patients with incontinence.[74] Evaluation of accelerated transit is feasible using radio-opaque markers,[75] but is best appreciated with scintigraphy.[76] However, methodologies need to be refined and more robust normative data need to be acquired.

9.4 Established Methodologies: Contentious Clinical Value

9.4.1 Electrophysiology

9.4.1.1 Pudendal Nerve Terminal Motor Latency

The pudendal nerve is a mixed nerve providing efferent and afferent pathways to the EAS, urethral sphincter, perineal musculature, mucosa of the anal canal and perineal skin. The branches of the pudendal nerve that course over the pelvic floor are vulnerable to stretch injury, which may result in muscle weakness and consequently incontinence. Prior to the advent of endoanal ultrasound, the majority of cases of idiopathic or neurogenic faecal incontinence were believed to be a result of pudendal nerve injury.[77] However, it is now recognised that structural damage to the anal sphincters rather than pudendal neuropathy is the underlying pathogenic mechanism in most patients[78,79] and true isolated neuropathy may be rare.[80]

Pudendal nerve terminal motor latency (PNTML) is a measurement of the conduction time from stimulation of the pudendal nerve at the level of the ischial spine to the EAS contraction. This is achieved using disposable glove-mounted stimulating and recording electrodes (St Mark's pudendal electrode) connected to a suitable recorder. To ensure that all motor fibres within the nerve are stimulated, a supramaximal stimulus should be applied. Prolonged latencies are used as a surrogate marker of pudendal neuropathy, and have been demonstrated in incontinent patients who have suffered obstetric trauma[81–83] (Figure 9.7), have abnormal perineal descent[84] (perhaps due to excessive straining at stool[85]), have rectal prolapse,[86] or have a recognised neurological disorder.[87] However, the value, and indeed the validity, of pudendal nerve latency testing has come under increasing scrutiny,[4,11,12,22] given that most patients are now recognised as having identifiable muscle damage or degeneration.[28,78] Although grouped data show that incontinent patients with bilaterally prolonged PNTMLs have reduced anal squeeze pressures compared to controls[88] (thus supporting the concept that a neuropathic process impairs EAS function[88]), the sensitivity and specificity of this test is poor; many patients with delayed latencies have squeeze pressures within the normal range and vice versa.[88,89] This lack of agreement is likely to be due to methodological limitations:

1. Pudendal nerve terminal motor latency increases with age, independent of continence status.[90,91]
2. Pudendal nerve terminal motor latency reflects the function of the fastest conducting motor fibres and thus normal latencies may be recorded in a damaged nerve, as long as some fast-conducting fibres remain.[90]
3. The test is operator dependent[5,22] and may be technically difficult to perform in some patients, notably those with a high body mass index or a long anal canal.
4. Reproducibility of the test is unknown.[22]

In conclusion, recording PNTML may contribute little to the management of individual patients with faecal incontinence; for example, it does not appear to be predictive of surgical success in restoring continence.[11,22] The routine use of PNTML measurement is thus now questioned;[88] indeed, recent consensus reports have stated that, on the evidence to date, this technique is no longer to be advocated.[11,12,22] Unilateral prolongation of PNTMLs has been regarded historically as of little clinical significance,[91] but with evidence of laterality of pudendal nerve innervation of the EAS,[92] this perhaps merits further investigation.

9.4.1.2 Electromyography

In patients with incontinence, pelvic floor electromyography (EMG) can be used in a variety of ways.[11,93] The primary purposes are to:

1. Map the sphincter to identify areas of injury or congenital abnormality
2. Determine striated muscle function (i.e. whether the muscle contracts or relaxes appropriately, based on recruitment of firing motor units)
3. Assess denervation-reinnervation potentials, indicative of neural injury.

In addition, EMG can be combined with other tests of motor function (e.g. manometry, proctography[94]) to provide an integrated assessment.

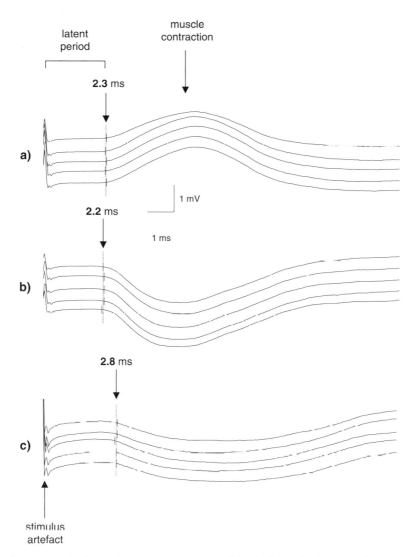

FIGURE 9.7. Pudendal nerve terminal motor latency. The latency is measured as the time from stimulation of the pudendal nerve at the level of the ischial spine to the onset of external anal sphincter contraction. Recordings (five separate stimuli) from (**a**) the right and (**b**) the left pudendal nerves of an asymptomatic volunteer show latencies within the normal range, whereas in (**c**), left pudendal nerve terminal motor latencies are prolonged, indicative of neuropathy, in a patient with urge faecal incontinence.

Studies of EMG activity can be performed using a needle electrode (either a concentric needle, which samples approximately 30 motor units simultaneously, or a single-fibre electrode, which samples only one motor unit at a time), a skin electrode, placed on the perianal skin, or an anal plug electrode. The choice of recording electrode is dependent upon the modality under study. Needle electrodes are usually favoured and are inserted transcutaneously without anaesthesia into the EAS (usually at multiple sites) and the puborectalis. Concentric needle electrodes enable various parameters of motor unit potentials (duration, amplitude, percentage polyphasia and recruitment) to be measured at rest, and during moderate voluntary muscle contraction.[16,93] These parameters may be altered (e.g. motor unit potential duration is prolonged, number of polyphasic motor unit potentials is increased, etc.) in partially denervated muscle where there has been attempted reinnervation.[93] Alternatively, using single-fibre electrodes, fibre density can be calculated, which is an index of motor unit grouping, a consequence of denervation and subsequent reinnervation.[93,95] For either method, 20 motor unit potentials are traditionally recorded at each site.[95] Single-fibre EMG has been shown to be highly repeatable.[96] In the striated anal musculature of patients with faecal incontinence, both motor unit potential activity (duration, amplitude, polyphasic nature) and fibre density have been shown to be increased, in comparison to controls.[89,93,95,97–99]

It has recently been suggested that the results of anal sphincter EMG are more sensitive, and more closely related to the anal functional status, as assessed on manometry, than measurement of PNTMLs.[97–99] However, the routine use of EMG studies for the assessment of patients with faecal incontinence is diminishing in clinical practice, given patient discomfort, the widespread availability of endoanal ultrasonography, and the fact that interpretation may require specialised training and experience.

The clinical relevance of other electrophysiological techniques, including the strength-duration test[100] (a minimally invasive technique for the measurement of muscle innervation) and motor[101] and somatosensory[102] evoked potentials remains controversial.

9.4.2 Anorectal Sensation

9.4.2.1 Anal Sensation

The epithelium of the anal canal has a rich sensory nerve supply made up of both free and organised nerve endings. The modalities of anal sensation can be defined precisely, with stimuli such as touch, pain and temperature being readily appreciated.[11,103] Such exquisite sensitivity allows for the sampling of rectal contents and enables discrimination between flatus and faeces. Anal mucosal sensation can be quantified using a catheter-mounted bipolar ring electrode inserted into the anal canal (anal mucosal electrosensitivity).[104] A current is passed through the electrode and steadily increased until sensation threshold (usually reported as a "prickling" feeling) is noted by the patient.[104] Mucosal sensitivity may be impaired in patients with faecal incontinence.[104–106] This impairment has been shown to persist long-term following a traumatic vaginal deliv-

ery.[107] Although such findings have contributed to our understanding of the pathophysiology of faecal incontinence, the diagnostic value of this test and its influence on management are limited.[11,106] An alternative measure for anal sensation is using thermal stimulation via specialised thermoprobes.[43,108] Again, this technique has not found routine use in clinical practice.

9.4.2.2 Rectal Sensation

Similar methods have been used for the assessment of rectal sensation.[43,109] Such techniques carry theoretical advantages over distension-based protocols in that they are thought to test purely the afferent (sensory) pathway by excitation of mucosal receptors, rather than a composite of rectal sensory function and wall biomechanics.[11] However, both electro- and thermostimulation techniques have been criticised as "non-physiological",[16,110] and their use is primarily restricted to research laboratories.

9.4.3 Evacuation Proctography

Passive (overflow) incontinence, or post-defaecation leakage may occur secondary to disorders of rectal evacuation.[47,48,111] Evacuation proctography may thus be useful to exclude outlet obstruction due to anatomy (e.g. large rectocoele, intussusception, megarectum, etc.)[111–113] or function (e.g. pelvic floor dyssynergia, etc.).[47,114] In addition, given the incidence of new-onset rectal evacuatory dysfunction following continence-restoring procedures,[115–117] proctography may be considered in the clinical work-up of patients with incontinence being considered for surgery. Any abnormalities revealed and deemed significant may be amenable to concurrent surgical correction, or adjunctive postoperative conservative therapy (e.g. a bowel retraining programme).

Proctography is a simple, dynamic radiological technique,[118] which provides morphological information regarding the rectum and anal canal. It involves fluoroscopic imaging of the process, rate and completeness of rectal emptying following insertion of enough barium paste (mimicking stool) to give the patient a sustained desire to defaecate.[119] The patient is seated upright on a radiolucent commode during lateral screening.

There are several limitations to this technique, however, which render the clinical usefulness uncertain:

1. It is not a normal study of defaecation.
2. It is not performed in response to the spontaneous desire to defaecate.
3. Patients' embarrassment of the nature and setting of the test may inhibit normal evacuation (leading to overdiagnosis of functional outlet obstruction;[55,56] see above).
4. Inter-observer agreement may be poor.[120]
5. There is a large degree of overlap in results between patients and controls.[121,122]
6. Normal rates of emptying vary widely.[122]

To reduce radiation exposure, scintigraphic proctography utilising a gamma-camera[123,124] can be carried out, substituting a radionuclide compound (usually [99M]Tc) for barium. Although quantitative measures of rectal evacuation are improved, anatomical resolution is greatly inferior.

Proctography, as well as assessing rectal evacuatory function, may be used to determine objectively the ability to retain stool. However, a much simpler and more practical way is the "porridge continence test" (equivalent to the saline continence test, but using a closer approximation of stool consistency[11]). After instillation of porridge (pseudostool), several manoeuvres can be requested of the patient (e.g. coughing, walking, climbing stairs, etc.). This test may be especially useful in patients who have been defunctioned with a proximal stoma, and who therefore cannot volunteer continence symptoms at that time.

9.4.4 Perineometry

The pelvic floor normally descends <1.5 cm during straining in association with anal relaxation. Excessive perineal descent (>3 cm) is closely related to faecal incontinence and is likely associated with traction of the pudendal nerve.[74] Descent of the perineum, relative to the ischial tuberosity, can be measured using the perineometer.[125] This test, however, has fallen out of favour, as reproducibility is poor,[12] and it grossly underestimates movement of the pelvic floor as compared to radiological measurement (which it was designed to replace).[126]

Recently, the perineal dynamometer was developed specifically to assess levator ani contraction.[127] This technique has yet to find common use.

9.4.5 Reflex Testing

9.4.5.1 Anocutaneous Reflex Test

Lightly scratching the perianal skin will elicit contraction of the EAS, termed the "anocutaneous reflex", or the "anal wink".[74] This reflex has its afferent and efferent pathways in the pudendal nerve and arcs via the sacral cord. When positive, the anal wink indicates an intact pathway and functioning sacral cord. However, it can be inhibited voluntarily, or may appear absent if the patient is tense, and thus to date there are no data to support its routine clinical use.[13] However, in the setting of acute onset of faecal incontinence, an absent anal wink may direct the clinician to further evaluate the patient's spinal cord for lesions or disc protrusions causing cauda equina syndrome.

9.4.5.2 Clitoral-anal Reflex Test

As an alternative to evaluation of pudendal nerve terminal motor latencies (see previously), which only assesses the short distal segment of the nerve, the clitoral-anal reflex, a multisynaptic sacral reflex, allows assessment of both pudendal afferent sensory and motor functions. The afferent limb of the reflex arc is the clitoral branch of the pudendal nerve, and the efferent limb is via the inferior haemorrhoidal branch; the reflex is integrated at the S2–S2 level of the spinal cord.[99,128,129]

Electrical stimulation is applied periclitorally; the sensory threshold is volunteered by the patient, and the clitoral-anal reflex latency recorded either via a fine needle electrode placed in the EAS,[128] or surface electrodes positioned at the mucocutaneous junction of the anal mucosa.[98,129]

In one recent study, comprehensive neurophysiological assessment in women with postpartum faecal incontinence, which included assessment of the clitoral-anal reflex, showed four patterns of abnormal pudendal nerve function: demyelinating (involving increased sensory threshold of the clitoral-anal reflex); axonal (normal reflex parameters); mixed demyelinating and axonal neuropathy (increased sensory thresholds and prolonged latencies); and a more widespread polyneuropathy (also involving abnormal reflex parameters), inconsistent with obstetric damage, and attributable to lumbosacral disease/injury.[128] Indeed it has been suggested that the test would be most clinically useful in cauda equina or conus medullaris syndromes.[129]

9.5 Non-established (Research) Methodologies

9.5.1 Ambulatory Manometry

Prolonged assessment of anorectal, rectosigmoid or colonic motor activity may provide further invaluable information regarding the pathophysiology of faecal incontinence; such techniques are gaining more widespread use.[130] To date, the majority of studies have been limited to the pelvic colon by a retrograde (per rectal) approach.[45,130-133] However, recent technological advances have facilitated pan-colonic investigation.[134-136] For the study of rectosigmoid motility, a manometric catheter, incorporating several solid-state pressure microtransducers, is stationed intraluminally at flexible sigmoidoscopy (unprepared bowel), so that recording sites lie within the sigmoid, rectum and anal canal.[131] The catheter is connected to a portable, solid-state recording system, which allows monitoring of intraluminal pressure changes under normal physiological conditions, over prolonged periods, in ambulant subjects. This is particularly useful in patients in whom symptoms are intermittent, where an extended recording period may enable symptom episodes (e.g. urgency, incontinence) to be correlated with pressure events.[15,130]

In patients presenting with incontinence, prolonged manometric studies have shown that transient internal anal sphincter relaxation or sampling reflexes (equalisation of rectal and anal canal pressures) occur more frequently than in control subjects, and that duration of relaxation is longer.[137] Symptoms of urgency or urge incontinence may be associated with high-amplitude contractions of the rectosigmoid,[45,131,138] or

increased periodic rectal motor activity,[131,133] suggesting that rectal hypercontractility may contribute to the pathogenesis of this condition. However, studies of rectosigmoid or colonic motility are time-intensive and technologically challenging, notably in terms of data interpretation and analysis. Consequently, there is a relative paucity of data on normal motor function, and until this is expanded, our understanding of motility disorders affecting the large bowel and anorectum will remain inadequate. The clinical value of prolonged ambulatory manometry therefore remains unproven and studies should at present be limited to specialty centres.[15,130]

9.5.2 Vector Volume Manometry (Vectography)

This technique is designed to assess the circumferential symmetry of anal canal pressures.[139,140] A multichannel manometric catheter with radially-orientated side holes (typically eight orifices, set 45° apart) is utilised. With the patient at rest or during sustained, voluntary contraction of the anal canal musculature, an automated, continuous pull-through technique is used, following which a computer-derived, three-dimensional pressure profile of the anal canal can be obtained[14,15] (Figure 9.8). Cross-sectional analysis permits accurate localisation of pressure defects and allows differentiation between global and sector pressure deficits in patients with incontinence.[141] Sphincter asymmetry, which indicates sphincter injury, may be a useful parameter for assessing the competence of anal sphincter function[142,143] (Figure 9.8). However, as with electrode mapping of the anal sphincter, use of vector volume manometry has largely been superseded by endoanal ultrasonography.

9.5.3 Impedance Planimetry

An alternative methodology for studying biomechanical properties of the rectal wall is impedance planimetry, which combines rectal balloon inflation with measurement of intrabag (i.e. intraluminal) impedance[144,145] and may give a better appreciation of capacity (cross-sectional area) and tension-strain relationships in comparison to studies utilising the barostat.

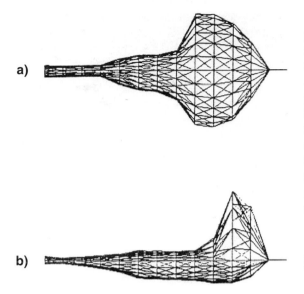

a)

b)

FIGURE 9.8. Anal pressure profile as recorded by vector volume manometry. In a normal asymptomatic volunteer (**a**), the pressure profile is relatively symmetrical, whereas in a patient with faecal incontinence (**b**), vectography demonstrates sphincter pressure asymmetry, indicative of sphincter damage, as well as reduction in functional length. (Reproduced with permission from Rao.[140])

9.6 Summary

Faecal incontinence is a common, yet underappreciated condition, whose physical and psychosocial consequences may be devastating. In the majority of patients, symptoms occur secondary to disordered function of the anorectum (both sphincteric and suprasphincteric components), and in females are most often acquired following obstetric trauma. Specialist referral for assessment of colorectal/anorectal function is not required for all patients with faecal incontinence, as the majority with mild to moderate symptoms will successfully respond to simple medical management. However, those patients with intractable and sufficiently severe symptoms, in whom such measures have failed, warrant rigorous clinical evaluation at a tertiary centre. The modern management of patients with faecal incontinence should involve a multidisciplinary team of professionals, reflecting the multifaceted approach to the different aspects of patient assessment, education, support and treatment.

In recent years, with the advent of anorectal physiological investigations, a more detailed understanding of the pathophysiological mechanisms underlying faecal incontinence is evolving. As several physiological abnormalities may be present, it is recommended that patients with intractable symptoms should undergo a structured, comprehensive series of tests in order to evaluate systematically all aspects of anorectal function. The results of these tests will help to suggest appropriate, rather than empirical management, both non-surgical and, in particular, surgical.

References

1. Camilleri M, Talley NJ. Pathophysiology as a basis for understanding symptom complexes and therapeutic targets. Neurogastroenterol Motil 2004;16:135–42.
2. Gearhart S, Hull T, Floruta C et al. Anal manometric parameters: predictors of outcome following anal sphincter repair? J Gastrointest Surg 2005; 9:115–20.
3. Kamm MA. Obstetric damage and faecal incontinence. Lancet 1994;344:730–3.
4. Rao SS. Diagnosis and management of fecal incontinence. Am J Gastroenterol 2004;99:1585–604.
5. Madoff RD, Parker SC, Varma MG et al. Faecal incontinence in adults. Lancet 2004;364:621–32.
6. Keating JP, Stewart PJ, Eyers AA et al. Are special investigations of value in the management of patients with fecal incontinence? Dis Colon Rectum 1997;40:896–901.
7. Vaizey CJ, Kamm MA. Prospective assessment of the clinical value of anorectal investigations. Digestion 2000;61:207–14.
8. Rao SS, Patel RS. How useful are manometric tests of anorectal function in the management of defecation disorders? Am J Gastroenterol 1997;92: 469–75.
9. Liberman H, Faria J, Ternent CA et al. A prospective evaluation of the value of anorectal physiology in the management of fecal incontinence. Dis Colon Rectum 2001;44:1567–74.
10. Corrazziari E. Anorectal manometry: a round table discussion. Gastroenterol Int 1989;2: 115–17.
11. Diamant NE, Kamm MA, Wald A et al. American Gastroenterological Association medical position statement on anorectal testing techniques. Gastroenterology 1999;116:732–60.

12. Azpiroz F, Enck P, Whitehead WE. Anorectal functional testing: review of collective experience. Am J Gastroenterol 2002;97:232–40.

13. Rao SS, Azpiroz F, Diamant N et al. Minimum standards of anorectal manometry. Neurogastroenterol Motil 2002;14:553–9.

14. Jorge JMN, Wexner SD. Anorectal manometry: techniques and clinical applications. Southern Med J 1993;86:924–31.

15. Sun WM, Rao SSC. Manometric assessment of anorectal function. Gastroenterol Clin North Am 2001;30:15–32.

16. Bharucha AE. Outcome measures for fecal incontinence: anorectal structure and function. Gastroenterology 2004;126(Suppl 1):S90–8.

17. Rasmussen OØ. Anorectal function. Dis Colon Rectum 1994;37:386–403.

18. McHugh SM, Diamant NE. Anal canal pressure profile: a reappraisal as determined by rapid pullthrough technique. Gut 1987;28:1234–41.

19. Rao SSC, Hatfield R, Soffer E et al. Manometric tests of anorectal function in healthy adults. Am J Gastroenterol 1999;94:773–83.

20. Read NW, Sun WM. Anorectal manometry. In: Henry MM, Swash M, eds. Coloproctology and the pelvic floor, 2nd edn. Oxford: Butterworth-Heinemann Ltd, 1992, pp 119–45.

21. Taylor BM, Beart RW, Phillips SF. Longitudinal and radial variations of pressure in the human anal sphincter. Gastroenterology 1984;86:693–7.

22. Bharucha AE. Fecal incontinence. Gastroenterology 2003;124:1672–85.

23. Nivatvongs S, Stern HS, Fryd DS. The length of the anal canal. Dis Colon Rectum 1981;24:600–1.

24. Engel AF, Kamm MA, Bartram CI et al. Relationship of symptoms in faecal incontinence to specific sphincter abnormalities. Int J Colorect Dis 1995;10:152–5.

25. Lindsey I, Jones OM, Smilgin-Humphreys MM et al. Patterns of fecal incontinence after anal surgery. Dis Colon Rectum 2004;47:1643–9.

26. Lunniss PJ, Gladman MA, Hetzer FH et al. Risk factors in acquired faecal incontinence. J R Soc Med 2004;97:111–16.

27. Felt-Bersma RJ, van Baren R, Koorevaar M et al. Unsuspected sphincter defects shown by anal endosonography after anorectal surgery. A prospective study. Dis Colon Rectum 1995;38:249–53.

28. Vaizey CJ, Kamm MA, Bartram CI. Primary degeneration of the internal anal sphincter as a cause of passive faecal incontinence. Lancet 1997;349:612–15.

29. Chiarioni G, Scattolini C, Bonfante F et al. Liquid stool incontinence with severe urgency: anorectal function and effective biofeedback treatment. Gut 1993;34:1576–80.

30. Telford KJ, Ali AS, Lymer K et al. Fatigability of the external anal sphincter in anal incontinence. Dis Colon Rectum 2004;47:746–52.

31. Sun WM, Donnelly TC, Read NW. Utility of a combined test of anorectal manometry, electromyography, and sensation in determining the mechanism of 'idiopathic' faecal incontinence. Gut 1992;33:807–13.

32. Siproudhis L, Bellissant E, Pagenault M et al. Fecal incontinence with normal anal canal pressures: where is the pitfall? Am J Gastroenterol 1999;94:1556–63.

33. Bharucha AE, Seide B, Fox JC et al. Day-to-day reproducibility of anorectal sensorimotor assessments in healthy subjects. Neurogastroenterol Motil 2004;16:241–50.

34. Gowers WR. The automatic action of the sphincter ani. Proc R Soc Lond 1877;26:77–84.

35. Sun WM, Read NW, Miner PB. Relation between rectal sensation and anal function in normal subjects and patients with faecal incontinence. Gut 1990;31:1056–61.

36. Sangwan YP, Coller JA, Schoetz DJ et al. Spectrum of abnormal rectoanal reflex patterns in patients with fecal incontinence. Dis Colon Rectum 1996;39:59–65.

37. Kaur G, Gardiner A, Duthie GS. Rectoanal reflex parameters in incontinence and constipation. Dis Colon Rectum 2002;45:928–33.

38. Farthing MJG, Lennard-Jones JE. Sensibility of the rectum to distension and the anorectal distension reflex in ulcerative colitis. Gut 1978;19:64–9.

39. Sun WM, Read NW, Prior A et al. Sensory and motor responses to rectal distention vary according to rate and pattern of balloon inflation. Gastroenterology 1990;99:1008–15.

40. Whitehead WE, Schuster MM. Anorectal physiology and pathophysiology. Am J Gastroenterol 1987;82:487–97.

41. Keighley MRB, Henry MM, Bartolo DCC et al. Anorectal physiology measurement: report of a working party. Br J Surg 1989;76:356–7.

42. Varma JS, Smith AN. Reproducibility of the proctometrogram. Gut 1986;27:288–92.

43. Chan CL, Scott SM, Birch MJ et al. Rectal heat thresholds: a novel test of the sensory afferent pathway. Dis Colon Rectum 2003;46:590–5.

44. Gladman MA, Scott SM, Williams NS. Assessing the patient with fecal incontinence. An overview. In: Zbar AP, Pescatori M, Wexner SD, eds. Complex anorectal disorders – investigation and management. London: Springer-Verlag London Ltd, 2005, pp 547–94.

45. Williams NS, Ogunbiyi OA, Scott SM et al. Rectal augmentation and stimulated gracilis anal neosphincter: a new approach in the management of fecal urgency and incontinence. Dis Colon Rectum 2001;44:192–8.

46. Chan CL, Scott SM, Williams NS et al. Rectal hypersensitivity worsens stool frequency, urgency, and lifestyle in patients with urge faecal incontinence. Dis Colon Rectum 2005;48:134–40.

47. Gladman MA, Scott SM, Chan CL et al. Rectal hyposensitivity: prevalence and clinical impact in patients with intractable constipation and fecal incontinence. Dis Colon Rectum 2003;46:238–46.

48. Rao SS, Ozturk R, Stessman M. Investigation of the pathophysiology of fecal seepage. Am J Gastroenterol 2004;99:2204–9.

49. Lubowski DZ, Nicholls RJ. Faecal incontinence associated with reduced pelvic sensation. Br J Surg 1988;75:1086–8.

50. Hoffmann BA, Timmcke AE, Gathright JB Jr et al. Fecal seepage and soiling: a problem of rectal sensation. Dis Colon Rectum 1995;38:746–8.

51. Whitehead WE, Delvaux M, The Working Team. Standardization of barostat procedures for testing smooth muscle tone and sensory thresholds in the gastrointestinal tract. Dig Dis Sci 1997;42:223–41.

52. Meunier PD, Gallavardin D. Anorectal manometry: the state of the art. Dig Dis 1993;11:252–64.

53. Stendal C. Practical guide to gastrointestinal function testing. Oxford; Blackwell Science, 1997, pp 214–24.

54. Read NW, Timms JM, Barfield LJ et al. Impairment of defecation in young women with severe constipation. Gastroenterology 1986;90:53–60.

55. Schouten WR, Briel JW, Auwerda JJ et al. Anismus: fact or fiction? Dis Colon Rectum 1997;40:1033–41.

56. Voderholzer WA, Neuhaus DA, Klauser AG et al. Paradoxical sphincter contraction is rarely indicative of anismus. Gut 1997;41:258–62.

57. Haynes WG, Read NW. Ano-rectal activity in man during rectal infusion of saline: a dynamic assessment of the anal continence mechanism. J Physiol 1982;330:45–56.

58. Read NW, Haynes WG, Bartolo DCC et al. Use of anorectal manometry during rectal infusion of saline to investigate sphincter function in incontinent patients. Gastroenterology 1983;85:105–13.

59. Rao SSC, Read NW, Stobhart JAH et al. Anorectal contractility under basal conditions and during rectal infusion of saline in ulcerative colitis. Gut 1988;29:769–77.

60. Azpiroz F, Malagelada JR. Physiological variations in canine gastric tone measured by an electronic barostat. Am J Physiol 1985;248:G229–37.

61. van der Schaar PJ, Lamers CBHW, Masclee AAM. The role of the barostat in human research and clinical practice. Scand J Gastroenterol 1999; 34(Suppl 230):52–63.

62. Spetalen S, Jacobsen MB, Vatn MH et al. Visceral sensitivity in irritable bowel syndrome and healthy volunteers: reproducibility of the rectal barostat. Dig Dis Sci 2004;49:1259–64.

63. Gladman MA, Dvorkin LS, Lunniss PJ et al. Rectal hyposensitivity: a disorder of the rectal wall or the afferent pathway? An assessment using the barostat. Am J Gastroenterol 2005;100:106–14.

64. Ashraf W, Park F, Lof J et al. An examination of the reliability of reported stool frequency in the diagnosis of idiopathic constipation. Am J Gastroenterol 1996;91:26–32.

65. Hinton JM, Lennard-Jones JE, Young AC. A new method for studying gut transit times using radioopaque markers. Gut 1969;10:842–7.

66. Arhan P, Devroede G, Jehannin B et al. Segmental colonic transit time. Dis Colon Rectum 1981;24:625–9.

67. Metcalf AM, Phillips SF, Zinsmeister AR et al. Simplified assessment of segmental colonic transit. Gastroenterology 1987;92:40–7.

68. Roberts JP, Newell MS, Deeks JJ et al. Oral [111In]DTPA scintigraphic assessment of colonic transit in constipated subjects. Dig Dis Sci 1993; 38:1032–9.

69. Bassotti G, Chiarioni G, Vantini I et al. Anorectal manometric abnormalities and colonic propulsive impairment in patients with severe chronic idiopathic constipation. Dig Dis Sci 1994;39:1558–64.

70. Krevsky B, Malmud LS, D'Ercole F et al. Colonic transit scintigraphy. A physiologic approach to the quantitative measurement of colonic transit in humans. Gastroenterology 1986;91:1102–12.

71. Scott SM, Knowles CH, Lunniss PJ et al. Scintigraphic assessment of colonic transit in patients with slow transit constipation arising de novo (chronic idiopathic) and following pelvic surgery or childbirth. Br J Surg 2001;88:405–11.

72. Lennard-Jones JE. Transit studies. In: Kamm MA, Lennard-Jones JE, eds. Constipation. Petersfield: Wrightson Biomedical Publishing Ltd, 1994, pp 125–36.

73. Parkman HP, Miller MA, Fisher RS. Role of nuclear medicine in evaluating patients with suspected gastrointestinal motility disorders. Semin Nucl Med 1995;25:289–305.

74. Cooper ZR, Rose S. Fecal incontinence: a clinical approach. Mt Sinai J Med 2000;67:96–105.

75. Bouchoucha M, Devroede G, Faye A et al. Importance of colonic transit evaluation in the

management of fecal incontinence. Int J Colorectal Dis 2002;17:412–17.

76. Bonapace ES, Maurer AH, Davidoff S et al. Whole
gut transit scintigraphy in the clinical evaluation
of patients with upper and lower gastrointestinal symptoms. Am J Gastroenterol 2000;95:
2838–47.

77. Kiff ES, Swash M. Slowed conduction in the
pudendal nerves in idiopathic (neurogenic) faecal
incontinence. Br J Surg 1984;71:614–16.

78. Kamm MA. Faecal incontinence. BMJ 1998;316:
528–32.

79. Nielsen MB, Hauge C, Pedersen JF et al. Endosonographic evaluation of patients with anal
incontinence: findings and influence on surgical
management. Am J Roentgenol 1993;160:771–5.

80. Vaizey CJ, Kamm MA, Nicholls RJ. Recent
advances in the surgical treatment of faecal incontinence. Br J Surg 1998;85:596–603.

81. Snooks SJ, Swash M, Henry MM et al. Risk
factors in childbirth causing damage to the pelvic
floor innervation. Int J Colorectal Dis 1986;1:
20–4.

82. Sultan AH, Kamm MA, Hudson CN. Pudendal
nerve damage during labour: prospective study
before and after childbirth. Br J Obstet Gynaecol
1994;101:22–8.

83. Tetzschner T, Sorensen M, Jonsson L et al. Delivery and pudendal nerve function. Acta Obstet
Gynecol Scand 1997;76:324–31.

84. Jones PN, Lubowski DZ, Swash M et al. Relation
between perineal descent and pudendal nerve
damage in idiopathic faecal incontinence. Int J
Colorectal Dis 1987;2:93–5.

85. Snooks SJ, Barnes PR, Swash M et al. Damage to
the innervation of the pelvic floor musculature in
chronic constipation. Gastroenterology 1985;89:
977–81.

86. Pfeifer J, Salanga VD, Agachan F et al. Variation
in pudendal nerve terminal motor latency
according to disease. Dis Colon Rectum 1997;
40:79–83.

87. Pinna Pintor M, Zara GP, Falletto E et al. Pudendal
neuropathy in diabetic patients with faecal incontinence. Int J Colorectal Dis 1994;9:105–9.

88. Hill J, Hosker G, Kiff ES. Pudendal nerve terminal
motor latency measurements: what they do and do
not tell us. Br J Surg 2002;89:1268–9.

89. Wexner SD, Marchetti F, Salanga VD et al. Neurophysiologic assessment of the anal sphincters. Dis
Colon Rectum 1991;34:606–12.

90. Cheong DM, Vaccaro CA, Salanga VD et al. Elec-
trodiagnostic evaluation of fecal incontinence.
Muscle Nerve 1995;18:612–19.

91. Rasmussen OO, Christiansen J, Tetzschner T et al.
Pudendal nerve function in idiopathic fecal incontinence. Dis Colon Rectum 2000;43:633–6.

92. Hamdy S, Enck P, Aziz Q et al. Laterality effects of
human pudendal nerve stimulation on corticoanal
pathways: evidence for functional asymmetry. Gut
1999;45:58–63.

93. Swash M. Electromyography in pelvic floor disorders. In: Henry MM, Swash M, eds. Coloproctology and the pelvic floor, 2nd edn. Oxford:
Butterworth-Heinemann Ltd, 1992, pp 184–95.

94. Womack NR, Williams NS, Holmfield JH et al.
New method for the dynamic assessment of anorectal function in constipation. Br J Surg 1985
;72:994–8.

95. Neill ME, Swash M. Increased motor unit fibre
density in the external anal sphincter muscle
in ano-rectal incontinence: a single fibre EMG
study. J Neurol Neurosurg Psychiatry 1980;43:
343–7.

96. Rogers J, Laurberg S, Misiewicz JJ et al. Anorectal
physiology validated: a repeatability study of the
motor and sensory tests of anorectal function. Br
J Surg 1989;76:607–9.

97. Osterberg A, Graf W, Edebol Eeg-Olofsson K et al.
Results of neurophysiologic evaluation in fecal
incontinence. Dis Colon Rectum 2000;43:1256–
61.

98. Thomas C, Lefaucheur JP, Galula G et al. Respective value of pudendal nerve terminal motor
latency and anal sphincter electromyography in
neurogenic fecal incontinence. Neurophysiol Clin
2002;32:85–90.

99. Gregory WT, Lou JS, Stuyvesant A et al. Quantitative electromyography of the anal sphincter after
uncomplicated vaginal delivery. Obstet Gynecol
2004;104:327–35.

100. Telford KJ, Faulkner G, Hosker GL et al. The
strength duration test: a novel tool in the identification of occult neuropathy in women with
pelvic floor dysfunction. Colorectal Dis 2004;
6:442–5.

101. Pelliccioni G, Scarpino O, Piloni V. Motor evoked
potentials recorded from external anal sphincter
by cortical and lumbo-sacral magnetic stimulation: normative data. J Neurol Sci 1997;149:69–
72.

102. Speakman CT, Kamm MA, Swash M. Rectal
sensory evoked potentials: an assessment of
their clinical value. Int J Colorectal Dis 1993;8:
23–8.

103. Duthie HL, Gairns FW. Sensory nerve-endings
and sensation in the anal region of man. Br J Surg
1960;47:585–95.

104. Roe AM, Bartolo DC, Mortensen NJ. New method for assessment of anal sensation in various anorectal disorders. Br J Surg 1986;73: 310–12.

105. Rogers J, Henry MM, Misiewicz JJ. Combined sensory and motor deficit in primary neuropathic faecal incontinence. Gut 1988;29:5–9.

106. Felt-Bersma RJ, Poen AC, Cuesta MA et al. Anal sensitivity test: what does it measure and do we need it? Cause or derivative of anorectal complaints. Dis Colon Rectum 1997;40: 811–16.

107. Cornes H, Bartolo DC, Stirrat GM. Changes in anal canal sensation after childbirth. Br J Surg 1991;78: 74–7.

108. Miller R, Bartolo DC, Cervero F et al. Anorectal temperature sensation: a comparison of normal and incontinent patients. Br J Surg 1987;74: 511–15.

109. Kamm MA, Lennard-Jones JE. Rectal mucosal electrosensory testing – evidence for a rectal sensory neuropathy in idiopathic constipation. Dis Colon Rectum 1990;33:419–23.

110. Meagher AP, Kennedy ML, Lubowski DZ. Rectal mucosal electrosensitivity – what is being tested? Int J Colorectal Dis 1996;11:29–33.

111. Rex DK, Lappas JC. Combined anorectal manometry and defecography in 50 consecutive adults with fecal incontinence. Dis Colon Rectum 1992; 35:1040–5.

112. Mellgren A, Bremmer S, Johansson C et al. Defecography. Results of investigations in 2,816 patients. Dis Colon Rectum 1994;37:1133–41.

113. Agachan F, Pfeifer J, Wexner SD. Defecography and proctography. Results of 744 patients. Dis Colon Rectum 1996;39:899–905.

114. Wald A. Outlet dysfunction constipation. Curr Treat Options Gastroenterol 2001;4:293–7.

115. Mander BJ, Wexner SD, Williams NS et al. Preliminary results of a multicentre trial of the electrically stimulated gracilis neoanal sphincter. Br J Surg 1999;86:1543–8.

116. Malouf AJ, Norton CS, Engel AF et al. Long-term results of overlapping anterior anal-sphincter repair for obstetric trauma. Lancet 2000;355: 260–5.

117. Altomare DF, Dodi G, La Torre F et al. Multicentre retrospective analysis of the outcome of artificial anal sphincter implantation for severe faecal incontinence. Br J Surg 2001;88:1481–6.

118. Mahieu P, Pringot J, Bodart P. Defecography: I. Description of a new procedure and results in normal patients. Gastrointest Radiol 1984;9: 247–51.

119. Chan CL, Scott SM, Knowles CH et al. Exaggerated rectal adaptation – another cause of outlet obstruction. Colorectal Dis 2001;3:141–2.

120. Muller-Lissner SA, Bartolo DC, Christiansen J et al. Interobserver agreement in defecography – an international study. Z Gastroenterol 1998;36: 273–9.

121. Shorvon PJ, McHugh S, Diamant NE et al. Defecography in normal volunteers: results and implications. Gut 1989;30:1737–49.

122. Freimanis MG, Wald A, Caruana B et al. Evacuation proctography in normal volunteers. Invest Radiol 1991;26:581–5.

123. Papachrysostomou M, Stevenson AJ, Ferrington C et al. Evaluation of isotope proctography in constipated subjects. Int J Colorectal Dis 1993;8: 18–22.

124. Hutchinson R, Mostafa AB, Grant EA et al. Scintigraphic defecography: quantitative and dynamic assessment of anorectal function. Dis Colon Rectum 1993;36:1132–8.

125. Henry MM, Parks AG, Swash M. The pelvic floor musculature in the descending perineum syndrome. Br J Surg 1982;69:470–2.

126. Oettle GJ, Roe AM, Bartolo DC et al. What is the best way of measuring perineal descent? A comparison of radiographic and clinical methods. Br J Surg 1985;72:999–1001.

127. Fernandez-Fraga X, Azpiroz F, Malagelada JR. Significance of pelvic floor muscles in anal incontinence. Gastroenterology 2002;123:1441–50.

128. Fitzpatrick M, O'Brien C, O'Connell PR et al. Patterns of abnormal pudendal nerve function that are associated with postpartum fecal incontinence. Am J Obstet Gynecol 2003;189:730–5.

129. Wester C, FitzGerald MP, Brubaker L et al. Validation of the clinical bulbocavernosus reflex. Neurourol Urodyn 2003;22:589–91.

130. Scott SM. Manometric techniques for the evaluation of colonic motor activity: current status. Neurogastroenterol Motil 2003;15:483–513.

131. Chan CLH, Lunniss PJ, Wang D et al. Rectal sensorimotor dysfunction in patients with urge fecal incontinence: evidence from prolonged manometric studies. Gut 2005;54:1263–72.

132. Rao SS, Welcher K. Periodic rectal motor activity: the intrinsic colonic gatekeeper? Am J Gastroenterol 1996;91:890–7.

133. Santoro GA, Eitan BZ, Pryde A et al. Open study of low-dose amitriptyline in the treatment of patients with idiopathic fecal incontinence. Dis Colon Rectum 2000;43:1676–81.

134. Cook IJ, Furukawa Y, Panagopoulos V et al. Relationships between spatial patterns of colonic

pressure and individual movements of content. Am J Physiol Gastrointest Liver Physiol 2000;278: G329–41.

135. Bampton PA, Dinning PG, Kennedy ML et al. Spatial and temporal organization of pressure patterns throughout the unprepared colon during spontaneous defecation. Am J Gastroenterol 2000;95:1027–35.

136. Hagger R, Kumar D, Benson M et al. Periodic colonic motor activity identified by 24-h pancolonic ambulatory manometry in humans. Neurogastroenterol Motil 2002;14:271–8.

137. Roberts JP, Williams NS. The role and technique of ambulatory anal manometry. Baillieres Clin Gastroenterol 1992;6:163–78.

138. Herbst F, Kamm MA, Morris GP et al. Gastrointestinal transit and prolonged ambulatory colonic motility in health and faecal incontinence. Gut 1997;41:381–9.

139. Perry RE, Blatchford GJ, Christensen MA et al. Manometric diagnosis of anal sphincter injuries. Am J Surg 1990;159:112–16.

140. Rao SSC. Manometric evaluation of defecation disorders: part II. Fecal incontinence. The Gastroenterologist 1997;5:99–111.

141. Zbar AP, Kmiot WA, Aslam M et al. Use of vector volume manometry and endoanal magnetic resonance imaging in the adult female for assessment of anal sphincter dysfunction. Dis Colon Rectum 1999;42:1411–18.

142. Williams N, Barlow J, Hobson A et al. Manometric asymmetry in the anal canal in controls and patients with fecal incontinence. Dis Colon Rectum 1995;38:1275–80.

143. Jorge JM, Habr-Gama A. The value of sphincter asymmetry index in anal incontinence. Int J Colorectal Dis 2000;15:303–10.

144. Dall FH, Jorgensen CS, Houe D et al. Biomechanical wall properties of the human rectum. A study with impedance planimetry. Gut 1993;34:1581–6.

145. Krogh K, Mosdal C, Gregersen H et al. Rectal wall properties in patients with acute and chronic spinal cord lesions. Dis Colon Rectum 2002;45: 641–9.

10
Imaging of the Anal Sphincter

Clive Bartram and Abdul H. Sultan

10.1 Introduction

Radiologic imaging of the perineum and sphincteric complex has been a process of evolution in which technical developments from the perineal and endoanal ultrasound, to the newer modalities of three-dimensional (3D) imaging[1,2] and endocoil magnetic resonance imaging (MRI),[3] have allowed finer details of the perineal anatomy to be unravelled. Endoanal ultrasound was developed in the early 1990s[4] as a simple method for imaging the sphincter complex as a complement to manometric studies, so that both the structural and functional aspects of the anal sphincter could be investigated. While the technique may seem relatively simple, the sonographic anatomy of the perineal region has proven to be surprisingly complex.[5,6]

10.2 Technique

Standard linear endocavity endfire probes placed on the perineum can image the sphincters,[7,8] and transperineal 3D volume sonography shows the levators and anal sphincter during the dynamics of pelvic floor movement.[9] However, most of the work described in this section has been undertaken with the B-K Medical endoprobe (Sandoften 9, 2820 Gentofte, Denmark), a mechanically rotated 10-MHz single crystal within a plastic cone with a 17-mm outer diameter filled with degassed water. The latest 3D B-K Medical 2050 endoprobe (Figure 10.1) is a sealed unit, requiring covering with a condom, liberally coated inside and outside with ultrasound gel, to maintain sterility and achieve good acoustic coupling. This probe contains two mechanically rotated crystals placed back to back, and is a multifrequency unit that is probably best run at 12 MHz. The older 1850 endoprobe uses a single fixed 10-MHz transducer (type 6004) protected by a hard TPX plastic cone that needs to be filled carefully with degassed water to prevent bubbles.

Women should be examined in the prone position (unless pregnant), as this minimises deformity of the upper canal and puborectalis.[10] The left lateral or prone position may be used in men as the longer canal and different arrangement of the proximal sphincter do not distort the anatomy to the same extent as in women. The probe should be gently inserted and rotated so that the rectovaginal septum is anterior, then withdrawn until the "U" shape of the puborectalis is visible. Either a complete dataset along the length of the canal for 3D analysis is obtained using the automated drive system that is an integral part of the 2050 system, or the probe is slowly withdrawn down the canal as multiple images are taken to record an overview of the sphincters at all levels (Figure 10.2), with more detailed imaging of any pathology. The advantage of the 3D system is that the dataset allows multiplanar imaging and immediate examination, whereas with two-dimensional imaging only the stored images are available for review.

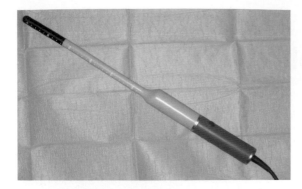

FIGURE 10.1. The B-K Medical 2050 3D probe.

10.3 Normal Anatomy

The anus has two structures that are either an integral part of the sphincters or form the support mechanism for the anus: sphincteric and perineal. The sphincteric structure has a four-layer pattern (Figure 10.3) generated either by the different acoustic reflectivity of the layers, or by interface reflections from junctions of layers of different acoustic impedance, such as muscle and fat. The layers are (starting with those medially):

1. *Subepithelium* (moderately reflective): The mucosa is not identified. The muscularis submucosae ani may be seen as a thin low reflective band with the upper subepithelium. Large vascular channels may be seen anteriorly and posteriorly and traced up to the anal cushions.

2. *Internal anal sphincter* (low reflectivity): This well-defined ring is a useful landmark for the sonographic anatomy. It is about 2 mm thick, becoming thicker with age. It may be thinned anteriorly and is not always symmetric in thickness. Minor changes may reflect a contraction within the smooth muscle, but any marked change in thickness is abnormal. The length may be measured on 3D studies as a mean of 34 mm,[4,11] terminating 8 mm (15 mm in males) proximal to the anal verge. It is derived from the circular smooth muscle of the rectum, with the change to internal sphincter denoted by an increase in thickness.

3. *Longitudinal layer* (low to moderately reflective): This is a complex structure, consisting of fibroelastic tissue from the pubocervical fascia, smooth muscle from the longitudinal layer of rectum and striated muscle of the puboanalis. The muscle fibres fuse in the upper part of the canal, and disappear before the termination of the internal sphincter, so that low reflective muscle fibre bundles are seen in the upper longitudinal layer and moderately reflective fibroelastic tissue only in the lower part.

4. *External sphincter*: This striated muscle is of low to moderate reflectivity.

The internal sphincter is easy to distinguish from the longitudinal layer and subepithelium. Interface reflections are the key to differentiating the outer border of the longitudinal layer from the

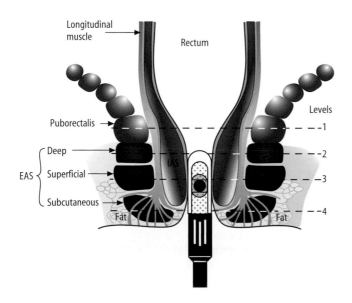

FIGURE 10.2. Schematic representation of the anorectum demonstrating levels of imaging.
EAS = External anal sphincter
IAS = Internal anal sphincter

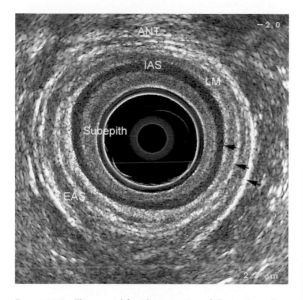

FIGURE 10.3. The normal four-layer pattern of the anal canal on axial endosonography in the normal orientation with anterior (*ANT*) uppermost. The subepithelium (*Subepith*) is moderately reflective, the internal anal sphincter (*IAS*) a well-defined low-reflective ring, the longitudinal layer a mixture of muscle (*LM*) and fibroelastic tissue of varying reflectivity, and the external anal sphincter (*EAS*) of low reflectivity. Note the interface reflections (*black arrows*) between the IAS and the LM, the LM and the EAS and at the outer border of the EAS.

inner external sphincter, and the outer external sphincter from the ischioanal fat.

The structures that contribute to the sphincteric anus and its support include the rectum, the levator ani with its fascia, and the perineal muscles. Although the anatomic detail varies between the sexes, only women will be described. The puborectalis forms a "U"-shaped sling around the upper anus at the anorectal junction, and fuses laterally and posteriorly with the deep external sphincter. Fibres from the medial puborectalis run into the longitudinal layer and are termed the puboanalis. Just superficial to the puborectalis, the transverse perineii fuse with the anterolateral aspect of the external sphincter. Anteriorly, the perineal body consists largely of fibroelastic tissue and is relatively uniform and low in reflectivity. The fusion of the transverse perineii with the external sphincter creates an anterior muscle bundle that is shorter than the posterior external sphincter with sides that slope down to a midline junction (Figure 10.4). At the upper puborectalis level there is no muscle anteriorly, just the low reflective fibro-

elastic tissue of the perineal body. The striated muscle of the external sphincter comes in from the side at the lower border of the puborectalis as the probe is withdrawn, fusing in the midline with the transverse perineii.

The external sphincter may be divided into three parts: (i) the deep part can be seen coming forward from each side of the puborectalis as

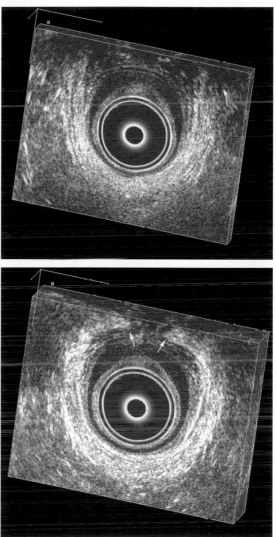

FIGURE 10.4. **a** Axial view at the puborectalis level with the perineal structures anteriorly; **b** at a lower level with the external anal sphincter coming in (*arrows*) symmetrically from the side, and **c** when the external anal sphincter is an intact ring. **d** Coronal slice from the three-dimensional dataset showing the axial levels a–c and the sloping sides of the external anal sphincter (*black arrows*).

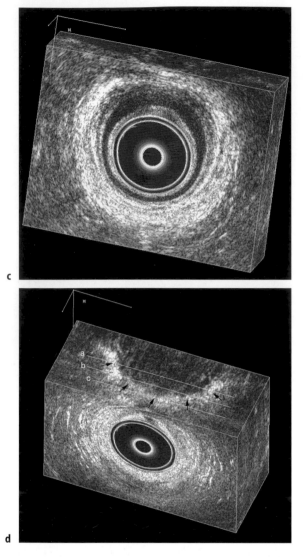

c

d

FIGURE 10.4. *Continued*

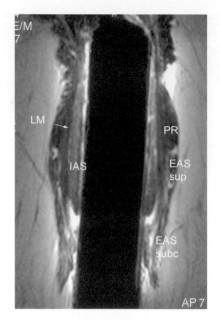

FIGURE 10.5. Endocoil magnetic resonance imaging coronal section showing the internal sphincter (*IAS*) to be of moderate signal, and the striated muscle in the longitudinal muscle (*LM*), puborectalis (*PR*) and external sphincter (*EAS*) of low signal. The deep EAS is fused with the PR, but the superficial (*sup*) and subcutaneous (*subc*) parts are clearly separate.

not compressed and closes off the canal and the internal sphincter is thicker than during endosonography.[13] High quality pelvic MRI with a phased array also gives detailed images of the

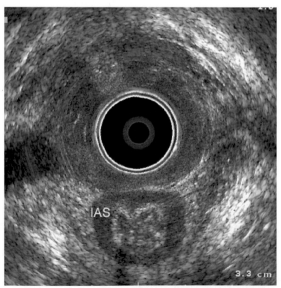

FIGURE 10.6. Transvaginal endosonography with the internal sphincter (*IAS*) in its resting state and the anal cushions seen within the ring of the sphincter.

"wings" to join with (ii) the superficial part, which forms a complete ring around the anal canal, and (iii) the subcutaneous part, which starts at the termination of the internal sphincter.[12] On coronal endocoil MRI it can be seen to hook around the perianal region (Figure 10.5), whereas on axial endosonography an outer thin low reflective ring surrounds the highly reflective terminations of the longitudinal layer fibres running through the subcutaneous external sphincter into the perineal skin. If an external probe is used, such as a transvaginal transducer, the sphincter is seen in its resting state (Figure 10.6). The subepithelium is undisturbed sphincter,[14] though more detail is obtained with an endocoil.[15]

10.4   Transperineal Ultrasound

Specialised endoanal ultrasound probes are expensive and therefore unavailable in many units. In 1997, Peschers et al.[16] used a conventional convex transducer placed on the perineum to visualise the anal sphincters. In a prospective, single-blind study of 25 patients with faecal incontinence and 43 asymptomatic controls, there was 100% intraobserver agreement on internal sphincter defects that were subsequently confirmed at surgery. There was only one discordant result in terms of external sphincter defects.[16] A recent prospective study has shown that if anal sonography is taken as a reference method for diagnosing anal sphincter defects, the sensitivity of transperineal ultrasound is 50% and the specificity is 84%.[17] This method was not found to be useful in visualising the internal anal sphincter in the immediate postpartum period with perineal trauma, probably due to the presence of oedema.[18] Roche et al.[19] have suggested that perineal sonography might be useful in incontinence screening. Further evaluation of this more accessible ultrasound

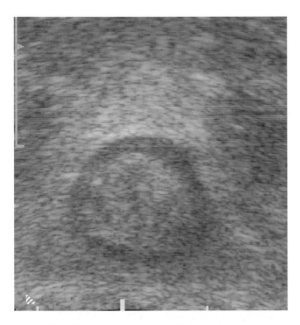

FIGURE 10.7. Transperineal ultrasound demonstrating the anal sphincter at rest.

technique (Figure 10.7) and anatomical correlation is needed before it is introduced into routine practice.

10.5   Vaginal Endosonography

Although anal sonography provides clear images of anal sphincters, the anal probe may distort the anatomy and epithelial structures and sphincter muscles, producing inaccurate muscle thickness measurements. Sultan et al.[13] first described vaginal endosonography to image the anal sphincters at rest with a rotating probe. They performed both endoanal and transvaginal scans in 20 females and found the internal sphincter to be significantly thicker on vaginal endosonography. They attributed this finding to stretching and thinning of the internal anal sphincter as a result of anal distension with the anal probe. However, there was a good correlation between the techniques in terms of detection of sphincter defects. Frudinger et al.[20] compared endoanal and transvaginal methods in 47 patients and concluded that the transvaginal approach is inaccurate because of anatomic limitations imposed on axial imaging by the transvaginal technique. However, in a prospective study of 44 consecutive females with anorectal dysfunction, Stewart and Wilson[21] found that not only was the transvaginal approach (Figure 10.6) reliable and as accurate as endoanal sonography, but also preferable for the evaluation of the perineal body and perianal inflammatory processes.[19] Sandridge and Thorpe[22] and more recently Timor-Tritsch[23] used a conventional 5–8 MHz transvaginal probe to image the anal sphincters producing good images in both the sagittal and transverse planes. However, they did not correlate their findings with anal endosonography.

10.6   Changes Following Vaginal Delivery

10.6.1   Sphincters and Perineum Intact

Niether pregnancy nor elective caesarean section appear to affect sphincter morphology. A study comparing   nulliparous   with   age-matched multiparous patients[24] suggested that vaginal delivery even without any tear might result in some thinning of the anterior external sphincter, with thickening of the longitudinal layer and the superficial external sphincter, consistent with diffuse trauma to the anus during delivery. Another study using 3D multiplanar imaging to compare pre- and post-delivery datasets[25] confirmed a change in the external sphincter, with the anterior portion becoming shorter (21.7 : 20.5 mm) and more angulated (10 : 13.8°), but with no alteration in the longitudinal layer. It would therefore seem that uncomplicated vaginal delivery may produce a minor change in the orientation of the external sphincter, with some possible thinning anteriorly, but does not cause any overall change in measurement.[26]

10.6.2   Sphincter and Perineal Disruption

A major impact of endosonography has been to image tears of the sphincters not apparent on clinical examination: so-called "occult" tears. These were initially reported in 35% of first-time vaginal deliveries.[27] Major tears are relatively easy to visualise, but minor tears can be quite subtle, and the distinction between tears of the sphincter and the support structures requires careful analysis.

Tears are often called "defects", a term that came into being when lack of striated muscle continuity was identified on single-fibre electromyography (EMG) as an electrical deficiency in activity. The term remains in common usage, but is synonymous with a tear or scar. Traumatic rupture of the external sphincter may be partial or complete. Haemorrhage becomes organised into granulation tissue, and the resulting scar is composed of avascular collagenous tissue that acoustically is homogeneous and low in reflectivity, which will be seen to cross normal tissue planes (Figure 10.8). A major tear will involve the internal sphincter as well, usually in the same quadrant (Figure 10.9).

All obstetric trauma affects the sphincters anterior to a horizontal line through the mid canal. Any tear of the internal or external sphincter posterior to this line is due to some other aetiology. The internal sphincter may be distorted by the shearing forces during vaginal delivery but does

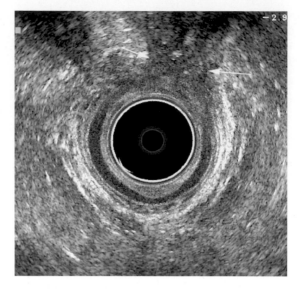

FIGURE 10.8. Endosonography of a tear involving the external and internal sphincter between 12 and 2 o'clock (*arrows*). The granulation tissue is of uniform low reflectivity.

not appear to tear without an accompanying external sphincter tear; an isolated anterior internal sphincter defect may therefore not be clinically significant[27] or may indicate an aetiology other than childbirth. Tears of the internal sphincter may extend about 1 cm above the anterior ring

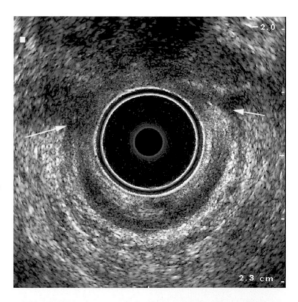

FIGURE 10.9. Endosonography of an extensive tear following vaginal delivery involving both the internal and external sphincters between 9 and 2 o'clock (*arrows*).

of the external sphincter.[28] The internal sphincter exhibits a slow rhythmic contractility and may not be exactly symmetric in thickness. Pronounced thinning of the anterior internal sphincter without actual disruption may be seen after vaginal delivery. The termination of the internal sphincter is often slightly asymmetric, so that a ragged end is not significant. The internal sphincter is best measured in the mid coronal plane at 3 and 9 o'clock in the mid canal, just after the level when the external sphincter becomes a complete ring.

External sphincter tears from obstetric trauma always involve the upper sphincter, and may extend down throughout the length of the sphincter. A complete tear of the perineum, causing a cloacal type defect, will show only the posterior half of the internal sphincter and anterior reflections from the posterior vaginal wall.

Minor tears produce a less homogeneous area of low reflectivity within the upper external sphincter with loss of symmetry and failure to meet anteriorly in the midline.

Tears of the support structures are more common than actual tears of the sphincter. In a review of 45 first deliveries pre- and postpartum, 3D endosonography showed that the puboanalis was torn in 20% of the women, the transverse perineii in 7%, and the external sphincter in only 11%.[29] Tears of the puboanalis create asymmetry of the low reflective triangular area just inside the puborectalis that extends down into the longitudinal layer, sometimes widening this quite dramatically (Figure 10.10). Tears of the transverse perineii are seen as asymmetrical to these structures just below and lateral to the puborectalis. Distinguishing isolated tears of the transverse perineii from those involving the external sphincter is difficult as the transverse perineii are an integral part of the sphincter. Multiplanar imaging may help by revealing if the upper curve of the external sphincter is intact or not (Figure 10.11). Magnetic resonance imaging confirms a 20% incidence of levator ani tears, mainly of the pubovisceral portion.[30] Endocoil MRI has been claimed to be more accurate in the detection of sphincter damage,[31] though this was mainly in showing atrophy. Internal sphincter tears are easier to appreciate on endosonography and scarring is more conspicuous, as the signal on MRI is similar

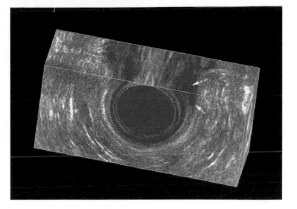

FIGURE 10.10. Tear of the left puboanalis seen in the upper coronal section as a low reflective widened area just above the puborectalis level, extending down into the longitudinal layer and widening, also in the front axial view (arrows).

to that of striated muscle, making scarring more difficult to differentiate (Figure 10.12).

A healthy perineum on clinical examination does not exclude a sphincter tear, though with the combination of episiotomy and perineal scars, an underlying tear is more likely.[32] The perineal body thickness may be measured by applying very gentle digital pressure to the posterior vaginal wall and measuring from the interface reflection. A thickness of <10 mm is considered abnormal

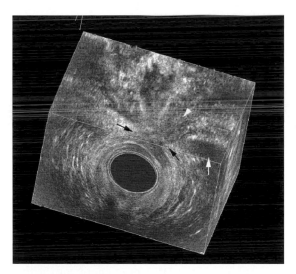

FIGURE 10.11. Endosonographic three-dimensional view of a major obstetric tear with scarring in the anterior ring of the external sphincter (black arrows), in the left puboanalis (arrowhead) and the left transverse perineii (white arrow).

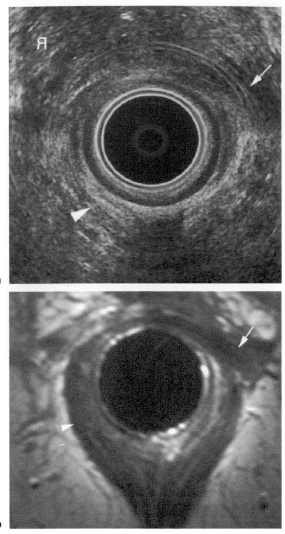

structures are damaged more frequently, and do not seem to affect anal sphincter function,[29] it is important to differentiate these from sphincteric tears. The precise understanding of the sonographic anatomy for making such a distinction is relatively recent. In reviewing the literature, it is often difficult to be certain of the criteria used to diagnose an external sphincter tear, and if tears of the support structures have been included or excluded. This could obviously have a significant effect on the reported incidence of external sphincter tears. A recent meta-analysis of tears shown on endosonography after 717 vaginal deliveries[36] revealed an overall incidence of 26.9% for nulliparous and 8.5% for subsequent deliveries. The incidences ranged from 11.5% to 35% and from 3.4% to 12.1%, respectively. Obstetric interpretation and observer error obviously have a bearing on these variations. In one study[37] from a review of hard copy, tears were reported in 13–28% of women, with an intraobserver agreement kappa of 0.63, and interobserver agreement of 0.34. Even allowing for all these variations, a significant proportion (probably 10–20%) of first-time vaginal deliveries will be associated with an "occult" tear.

10.7 Striated Muscle Atrophy

Various age-related changes occur in the sphincters. Thinning of the external sphincter with age has been recorded sonographically[38] on endocoil MRI in men,[15] whereas the longitudinal layer becomes thinner in both sexes. An external sphincter <2 mm in thickness is abnormal irrespective of age. A visual assessment of thinning on MRI has a sensitivity of 89%[39] for histologically proven atrophy. In comparison to single-fibre EMG, a visual score based on muscle thinning and/or fat replacement is also quite accurate.[40]

Atrophy on endosonography remains a difficult diagnosis. This is because it is usually not possible to measure the thickness of the external sphincter when it is atrophic. The reason for this is that fat replacement and muscle fibre loss reduce the clarity of the outer interface reflection, so that the outer border of the external sphincter is not visible. It is therefore impossible to measure its

Figure 10.12. a Endosonography showing an extensive obstetric tear with a small defect of the internal anal sphincter and scarring extending out into the left transverse perineii (*arrow*). The right side of the external anal sphincter is quite difficult to see (*arrowhead*); **b** the endocoil magnetic resonance image demonstrates the external anal sphincter clearly (*arrowhead*) but the left-sided scarring (*arrow*) is difficult to differentiate from striated muscle on signal content.

and associated with faecal incontinence[33–35] and external sphincter tears.

In major trauma it is common to see tears of both sphincteric and support components, so that it is obvious that the external sphincter has been damaged. Minor trauma is both more common and more difficult to interpret. As the support thickness. Poor definition of the external sphincter may in itself therefore be a sign of atrophy, and combined with an internal sphincter of <2 mm thickness has a positive predictive value for external sphincter atrophy of 74%.[40] In practical terms, if a patient has a tear but a good squeeze pressure, external sphincter atrophy is unlikely. However, if the squeeze pressure is poor, an endocoil MRI study is the only way to image atrophy reliably.

10.8   Conclusion

Endosonography yields highly detailed images of the sphincter and perineum, and has shown that a substantial number of vaginal deliveries result in "occult" sphincter tears (see Chapter 2 on diagnosis of obstetric anal sphincter injuries). Atrophy of striated muscle is evaluated better by MRI. Imaging has become essential in the assessment and management of faecal incontinence particularly related to obstetric trauma.

References

1. Williams AB, Bartram CI, Halligan S, Marshall MM, Nicholls RJ, Kmiot WA. Multiplanar anal endosonography – normal anal canal anatomy. Colorectal Dis 2001;3:169–74.

2. Bartram CI, DeLancey JO. Imaging pelvic floor disorders. Berlin: Springer-Verlag, 2003.

3. deSouza NM, Puni R, Kmiot WA, Bartram CI, Hall AS, Bydder GM. MRI of the anal sphincter. J Comput Assist Tomogr 1995;19(5):745–51.

4. Law PJ, Bartram CI. Anal endosonography: technique and normal anatomy. Gastrointest Radiol 1989;14(4):349–53.

5. Sultan AH, Nicholls RJ, Kamm MA, Hudson CN, Beynon J, Bartram CI. Anal endosonography and correlation with in vitro and in vivo anatomy. Br J Surg 1993;80(4):508–11.

6. Sultan AH, Kamm MA, Hudson CN, Nicholls RJ, Bartram CI. Endosonography of the anal sphincters: normal anatomy and comparison with manometry. Clin Rad 1994;49:368–74.

7. Stewart LK, McGee J, Wilson SR. Transperineal and transvaginal sonography of perianal inflammatory disease. AJR Am J Roentgenol 2001;177(3):627–32.

8. Tunn R, Petri E. Introital and transvaginal ultrasound as the main tool in the assessment of urogenital and pelvic floor dysfunction: an imaging panel and practical approach. Ultrasound Obstet Gynecol 2003;22(2):205–13.

9. Dietz HP. Ultrasound imaging of the pelvic floor. Part II: three-dimensional or volume imaging. Ultrasound Obstet Gynecol 2004;23(6):615–25.

10. Frudinger A, Bartram CI, Halligan S, Kamm M. Examination techniques for endosonography of the anal canal. Abdominal Imaging 1998;23(3):301–3.

11. Williams AB, Cheetham MJ, Bartram CI, Halligan S, Kamm MA, Nicholls RJ et al. Gender differences in the longitudinal pressure profile of the anal canal related to anatomical structure as demonstrated on three-dimensional anal endosonography. Br J Surg 2000;87(12):1674–9.

12. Hsu Y, Fenner DE, Weadock WJ, DeLancey JOL. Magnetic resonance imaging and 3-dimensional analysis of external anal sphincter anatomy. Obstet Gynecol 2005;106:1259–65.

13. Sultan AH, Loder PB, Bartram CI, Kamm MA, Hudson CN. Vaginal endosonography. New approach to image the undisturbed anal sphincter. Dis Colon Rectum 1994;37(12):1296–9.

14. Beets-Tan RG, Beets GL, van der Hoop AG, Borstlap AC, van Boven H, Rongen MJ et al. High-resolution magnetic resonance imaging of the anorectal region without an endocoil. Abdom Imaging 1999;24(6):576–81.

15. Rociu E, Stoker J, Eijkemans MJ, Lameris JS. Normal anal sphincter anatomy and age- and sex-related variations at high-spatial-resolution endoanal MR imaging. Radiology 2000;217(2):395–401.

16. Peschers UM, DeLancey JOL, Schaer GN, Schuessler B. Exoanal ultrasound of the anal sphincter. Br J Obstet Gynaecol 1997;104:999–1003.

17. Lohse C, Bretones S, Boulvain M, Weil A, Krauer F. Trans-perineal versus endo anal ultrasound in the detection of anal sphincter defects. Eur J Obstet Gynaecol 2002;103:79–82.

18. Shobeiri SA, Nolan TE, Yordan-Jovet R, Echols KT, Chesson RR. Digital examination compared to trans-perineal ultrasound for the evaluation of anal sphincter repair. Int J Gynaecol Obstet 2002;78:31–6.

19. Roche B, Deleaval J, Fransioli A, Marti MC. Comparison of transanal and external perineal ultrasound. Eur Radiol 2002;11:1165–70.

20. Frudinger A, Bartram CI, Kamm MA. Transvaginal versus anal endosonography for detecting damage to the anal sphincter. AJR Am J Roentgenol 1997;168:1435–8.

21. Stewart LK, Wilson SR. Transvaginal sonography of the anal sphincter: reliable or not? AJR Am J Roentgenol 1999;173:179–85.

22. Sandridge DA, Thorpe JM. Vaginal endosonography in the assessment of the anorectum. Obstet Gynecol 1995;86:1007–9.

23. Timor-Tritsch IE, Monteagudo SW, Smilen SW, Proges RF, Avizova E. Simple ultrasound evaluation of the anal sphincter in female patients using a transvaginal transducer. Ultrasound Obstet Gynecol 2005;25:177–83.

24. Frudinger A, Halligan S, Bartram CI, Spencer JA, Kamm MA. Changes in anal anatomy following vaginal delivery revealed by anal endosonography. Br J Obstet Gynaecol 1999;106(3):233–7.

25. Williams AB, Bartram CI, Halligan S, Marshall MM, Spencer JA, Nicholls RJ et al. Alteration of anal sphincter morphology following vaginal delivery revealed by multiplanar anal endosonography. BJOG 2002;109(8):942–6.

26. Starck M, Bohe M, Fortling B, Valentin L. Endosonography of the anal sphincter in women of different ages and parity. Ultrasound Obstet Gynecol 2005;25(2):169–76.

27. Sultan AH, Kamm MA, Hudson CN, Thomas JM, Bartram CI. Anal-sphincter disruption during vaginal delivery. N Engl J Med 1993;329(26):1905–11.

28. DeLancey JO, Toglia MR, Perucchini D. Internal and external anal sphincter anatomy as it relates to midline obstetric lacerations. Obstet Gynecol 1997;90(6):924–7.

29. Williams AB, Bartram CI, Halligan S, Spencer JA, Nicholls RJ, Kmiot WA. Anal sphincter damage after vaginal delivery using three-dimensional endosonography. Obstet Gynecol 2001;97(5 Pt 1):770–5.

30. DeLancey JO, Kearney R, Chou Q, Speights S, Binno S. The appearance of levator ani muscle abnormalities in magnetic resonance images after vaginal delivery. Obstet Gynecol 2003;101(1):46–53.

31. Rociu E, Stoker J, Eijkemans MJ, Schouten WR, Lameris JS. Fecal incontinence: endoanal US versus endoanal MR imaging. Radiology 1999;212(2):453–8.

32. Frudinger A, Bartram CI, Spencer JA, Kamm MA. Perineal examination as a predictor of underlying external anal sphincter damage. Br J Obstet Gynaecol 1997;104(9):1009–13.

33. Zetterstrom JP, Mellgren A, Madoff RD, Kim DG, Wong WD. Perineal body measurement improves evaluation of anterior sphincter lesions during endoanal ultrasonography. Dis Colon Rectum 1998;41(6):705–13.

34. Oberwalder M, Thaler K, Baig MK, Dinnewitzer A, Efron J, Weiss EG et al. Anal ultrasound and endosonographic measurement of perineal body thickness: a new evaluation for fecal incontinence in females. Surg Endosc 2004;18(4):650–4.

35. Fornell EU, Matthiesen L, Sjodahl R, Berg G. Obstetric anal sphincter injury ten years after: subjective and objective long term effects. BJOG 2005;112(3):312–16.

36. Oberwalder M, Connor J, Wexner SD. Meta-analysis to determine the incidence of obstetric anal sphincter damage. Br J Surg 2003;90(11):1333–7.

37. Faltin DL, Boulvain M, Stan C, Epiney M, Weil A, Irion O. Intraobserver and interobserver agreement in the diagnosis of anal sphincter tears by postpartum endosonography. Ultrasound Obstet Gynecol 2003;21(4):375–7.

38. Frudinger A, Halligan S, Bartram CI, Price AB, Kamm MA, Winter R. Female anal sphincter: age-related differences in asymptomatic volunteers with high-frequency endoanal US. Radiology 2002;224(2):417–23.

39. Briel JW, Zimmerman DD, Stoker J, Rociu E, Lameris JS, Mooi WJ et al. Relationship between sphincter morphology on endoanal MRI and histopathological aspects of the external anal sphincter. Int J Colorectal Dis 2000;15(2):87–90.

40. Williams AB, Bartram CI, Modhwadia D, Nicholls T, Halligan S, Kamm MA et al. Endocoil magnetic resonance imaging quantification of external anal sphincter atrophy. Br J Surg 2001;88(6):853–9.

11

Conservative Management of Anal Incontinence

Christine Norton

11.1 Background

Anal incontinence (AI) may be defined as any involuntary loss of stool or gas via the anus.[1] Specifically, faecal incontinence (FI) is loss of stool, whether liquid or solid.

Anal incontinence is an under-reported symptom.[2,3] There are many possible reasons for this, including lack of awareness among health professionals and patient embarrassment. For some, symptoms may not be bothersome enough to seek help. Other women may assume that symptoms will resolve with time, or that AI is an inevitable consequence of childbearing, or be so busy with the demands of a new baby that there is little time to concentrate on her own health. Whatever the reason, there can be little doubt that this is a difficult symptom to talk about, therefore necessitating active case-finding by health professionals who will increase awareness that help is available.

It must always be remembered that factors other than anal sphincter trauma may contribute to symptoms of AI. It is often a combination of anal sphincter damage and another bowel problem that precipitates frank incontinence. Other disorders such as haemorrhoids, irritable bowel syndrome and inflammatory bowel disease need to be considered and managed appropriately. This variety of possibilities makes comprehensive assessment crucial to identifying all elements of an often multifactorial symptom.[4] Assessment will include detailed consideration of symptoms, medical history, medications, psychosocial factors, diet, lifestyle and the impact of symptoms on the patient and her desire for interventions.

This chapter will cover conservative and pharmacological options for women with anal incontinence. The next chapter will explore surgical options. These are not mutually exclusive interventions, and many of the options discussed here can be combined with surgery. For many patients surgical options are either not appropriate, or not totally successful. Expert opinion agrees that conservative management is appropriate for almost all patients exhibiting the first signs of anal incontinence.[1] Figure 11.1 gives an algorithm for decision-making based on an international consensus. However, the evidence base for this pathway and most interventions is extremely sparse. Unfortunately, much advice given to patients is based on clinical experience rather than good quality research. Instead, the treatment (if treated at all) offered to a patient will often depend on local expertise and availability.

11.2 "Lifestyle" Interventions

11.2.1 Body Mass Index

There is an association between obesity and FI.[5] This could be a directly causative association via increased pressure or impaired blood flow, or could be mediated via a general lack of health awareness, lack of exercise and muscle tone and poorer diet in the obese patient. It is not known whether weight reduction has a role in treating symptoms in women following perineal trauma. If weight loss does help, it is not clear if this is a direct effect, or the effect of a change in diet and

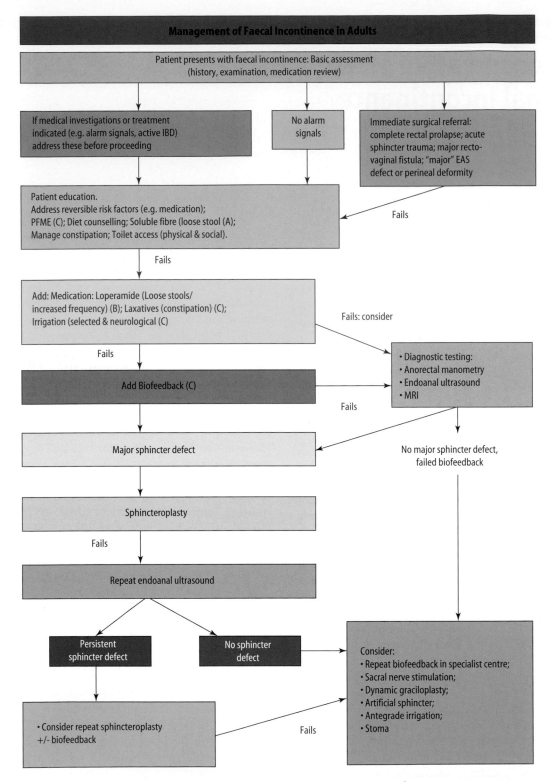

FIGURE 11.1. Management of faecal incontinence in adults.[1]

general fitness that is usually associated with weight reduction. It is not known if women who regain their normal body mass index most rapidly following childbirth are less prone to symptoms of AI, or if those who have a permanent weight increase following childbirth are at higher risk of AI. Some modern diets promoted for weight loss, such as low carbohydrate diets, have a known constipating effect and any effect on AI may simply be the result of constipation.

11.2.2 Smoking

Nicotine is a known distal colonic stimulant[6] and smoking a cigarette anecdotally promotes the urge to defaecate in some individuals. No association has been found between antenatal smoking and postnatal FI[7] and no study has assessed the role of smoking or smoking cessation in patients with AI or bowel urgency.

11.2.3 Physical Exercise and Work

There have been no studies on the impact of physical exercise on FI or bowel habit in non-institutionalised adults. The epidemiological literature is consistent in showing less constipation in people who report that they exercise. It is known that endurance running is associated with diarrhoea and FI in over 10% of individuals,[8] but there are no studies on treatment.

Excessive exercise may also be a factor in rectal prolapse. This is seen in young women with anorexia nervosa who combine excessive exercise with extreme nutritional impairment, presumably thus compromising tissue quality. Women whose jobs involve a lot of heavy lifting are more likely to need vaginal prolapse surgery than the general population (odds ratio [OR] = 1.6),[9] but it is not known if this is also true of FI.

11.3 Patient Education

Most people have little notion of how the bowel works and how to control its function. From the time of acquisition of continence, control usually functions at a subconscious, albeit voluntary, level.[10] This means that if an injury is sustained

and control is impaired, it can be difficult to regain as there is little conscious awareness of how control was previously maintained.

There is some evidence that patient education may be helpful for AI. Simple explanations and diagrams can be used to teach people about normal and disordered function[11] (www.bowel-control.org.uk; www.iffgd.org). One study has found that patient education, when combined with simple strategies such as modifying diet and urge resistance (see below) is as effective as performing pelvic muscle exercise or biofeedback.[12] Other support for the benefits of patient education comes from a study[13] showing that education and standard medical care, when provided systematically to a group of FI patients who had failed prior attempts at medical management, led to a successful outcome in 38%. Success in this trial was defined as a patient's report that they had experienced adequate relief of bowel symptoms.

Emotional support is an important element of this education. Patients with AI tend to feel very isolated, and because people seldom discuss bowel symptoms there is a tendency for each patient to feel that she is the only one.[10,14] Simply giving the opportunity to talk and express feelings seems to be therapeutic for some.

11.4 Bowel Routines

Expert opinion supports the importance of attempting to establish a regular predictable pattern of bowel evacuation by patient teaching and adherence to a routine.[15,16] Because peristaltic contractions of the colon that are associated with defaecation increase in frequency following awakening from sleep and following meals,[17,18] the period after breakfast is the best time for scheduled defaecation, but no studies have evaluated the effectiveness of this in adults.

11.5 Diet and Fluids

Modifying the diet will often have a direct effect on bowel function, stool consistency and motility. It is known that fibre softens stool, increases stool weight and speeds transit, particularly in the colon. Fibre retains intralumenal fluid and can also form a matrix binding together otherwise loose stool.

Many patients with both urge and passive FI find that they have more incontinent episodes when the stool is loose. Firmer stool seems to leak less and it may be easier to achieve complete evacuation when stool is formed. Fibre seems to act in different ways for different patients. Some derive clinical benefit from moderating the fibre content of diet, particularly restricting unrefined cereal fibres such as bran and wholewheat.[11] One small randomised controlled trial (RCT) has found less FI in patients who add fibre supplements to their diet, with gum Arabic and psyllium both improving FI when compared to placebo.[19] Other patients find that particular foods cause a problem and are best avoided, but there is no way to discover which foods have an effect other than trial and error. It does not seem that people with FI have a different diet from other people,[20] but rather that those prone to FI are less able to cope with some foodstuffs.

Inability to digest cows' milk products because of lactase deficiency is common, particularly in non-Caucasian populations. In the large intestine, fermentation of lactose by colonic bacteria typically results in flatulence, distension, diarrhoea and cramps. However, the majority of adults who have lactase deficiency can tolerate a small amount of lactose in foods.[21] Due to its prevalence in approximately 25% of the population, lactose maldigestion is currently regarded as a normal physiological pattern rather than a disease.[22] It occurs in 6–19% of whites, 53% of Mexican Americans, 62–100% of native Americans, 80% of African Americans and 90% of Asian Americans.[22,23] If the patient suspects that milk worsens symptoms, a dairy-free diet for 2 weeks can be tried, but care needs to be taken to avoid all milk products, including milk solids, which are often used in commercially prepared foods.

Malabsorption of fructose and sorbitol results in osmotic diarrhoea and adverse symptoms, similar to lactose intolerance. A diet reduced in fructose and sorbitol content is suggested for some patients with irritable bowel syndrome to reduce adverse gastrointestinal symptoms[24] and may help patients with urgency and flatulence associated with loose stool. Artificial sweeteners in low calorie drinks or chewing gum and diabetic foods are often found to worsen symptoms.[11]

Caffeine is known to stimulate colonic motility[25] and can increase urgency in susceptible individuals. This can be useful to enable evacuation at a chosen time, such as before leaving the house in the morning, but some patients find that restricting the amount or timing of caffeine is useful.[26] Coffee, tea and colas, especially when combined with artificial sweeteners, may all worsen symptoms. Excessive alcohol can also lead to loose stool.

Some foods seem to promote flatus production or an offensive odour from flatus for some people. Common culprits are onions, spicy food, excessive alcohol, brassicas and other green vegetables, beans and pulses. Although there is no way to stop flatus production completely, being careful with some foods may help, but this seems to be very individual.

There is increasing interest in the potential of probiotics to influence gut flora and health. In patients with inflammatory bowel disease, ingesting these "beneficial bacteria" has been found to restrict relapse and reduce symptoms. However, as yet there are no reports in people with AI or FI.

11.6   Anal Sphincter Exercises

There have been surprisingly few studies of exercises as a sole treatment for faecal incontinence. Almost all protocols that have included exercises (variations of pelvic floor muscle training, but more usually referred to as anal sphincter exercises) have been in combination with biofeedback (see below). One study in women recruited because of postnatal urinary incontinence has found that women performing pelvic muscle training had less FI at 1 year than controls who did not exercise (4% vs 10%).[27] However, the focus of this study was not on FI and this result was an incidental finding. Also, the results do not persist in the long term.[28] Another small study found that women who did exercises after a repaired third degree tear had minimal symptoms of AI (7%) and increased ability to hold a voluntary squeeze at 1 year,[29] suggesting that there may be a preventive value.

There is no research or consensus on what might be the optimum exercise regimen to enhance external anal sphincter strength. As with urinary incontinence, vastly different protocols have been suggested (with between five and several hundred squeezes per day), with the mode around 50. Some have recommended, in addition to maximal contractions, sub-maximal and fast-twitch contractions[30] (Figure 11.2). It is unclear whether the aim of exercises should be to enhance strength, speed of reaction or endurance of contraction, or if improving any of these necessarily improves symptoms. It has been suggested that fatigue rate is more important than absolute strength,[31] but this observation has yet to be validated.

Some groups have suggested that the addition of electrical stimulation as an external skin electrode or via an anal plug will enhance the effect of exercises alone. There are several case series reported, but the evidence base from RCTs for the efficacy of this does not exist at present.[32] One randomised study in women with obstetric-related FI did find better results with electrical

Patient instructions for anal sphincter exercises

Sit comfortably with your knees slightly apart. Now imagine that you are trying to stop yourself passing wind from the bowel. To do this you must squeeze the muscle around the back passage. Try squeezing and lifting that muscle as tightly as you can, as if you are really worried that you are about to leak. You should be able to feel the muscle move. Your buttocks, tummy and legs should not move much at all. You should be aware of the skin around the back passage tightening and being pulled up and away from your chair. Some people find it helpful to imagine that they are trying to pick up a penny from the chair with their anal sphincter muscles. You are now exercising your anal sphincter. You should not need to hold your breath when you tighten the muscles!

Now imagine that the sphincter muscle is a lift. When you squeeze as tightly as you can your lift goes up to the 4th floor. But you cannot hold it there for very long, and it will not get you safely to the toilet, as it will get tired very quickly. So now squeeze more gently, take your lift only up to the 2nd floor. Feel how much longer you can hold it than at the maximum squeeze.

Practising your exercises
1. Sit, stand or lie with your knees slightly apart. Tighten and pull up the sphincter muscles as tightly as you can. Hold tightened for at least (5) seconds, and then relax for at least 10 seconds to allow the muscle to recover.

Repeat at least (5) times. This will work on the strength of your muscles.

2. Next, pull the muscles up to about half of their maximum squeeze. See how long you can hold this for. Then relax for at least 10 seconds.

Repeat at least (5) times. This will work on the endurance, or staying power, of your muscles.

3. Pull up the muscles as quickly and tightly as you can and then relax and then pull up again, and see how many times you can do this before you get tired. Try for at least (5) quick pull-ups.

4. Do these exercises – (5) as hard as you can, (5) as long as you can and as many quick pull-ups as you can – at least (10) times every day.

5. As the muscles get stronger, you will find that you can hold for longer than 5 seconds, and that you can do more pull-ups each time without the muscle getting tired.

6. It takes time for exercise to make muscle stronger. You may need to exercise regularly for several months before the muscles gain their full strength.

FIGURE 11.2. Patient instructions for anal sphincter exercises. Note: length of squeeze and number of repetitions is individualised (figures in brackets), depending on what is achieved at the initial assessment.

stimulation than exercises and biofeedback alone, but the results were compounded by different methods and therapists for the two groups.[33] In another study, randomising women to exercise or exercises plus anal electrical stimulation following repair of a third degree tear, the stimulation was abandoned because of reported discomfort.[34] This was possibly because stimulation was commenced too soon after delivery.

If there is a clinical effect from electrical stimulation, it is unclear whether this is via direct muscle strengthening, or via sensitisation of the anal area, enabling better recognition of rectal contents or enhanced ability to perform exercises. One study has compared anal stimulation at 35 Hz, which should produce a tonic muscle contraction, with stimulation at 1 Hz, which produces sensation but no contraction: no difference in outcome was found after 8 weeks of stimulation, with two-thirds of patients completing the protocol finding that FI improved to at least some extent.[35]

11.7 Resisting Urgency

In contrast to urinary incontinence, where a body of knowledge has developed on the efficacy of bladder training techniques, particularly in relation to the overactive bladder syndrome, the possibility of bowel retraining for resisting urgency to defaecate is almost unexplored. Some biofeedback protocols focus on altering rectal sensory thresholds (see below). One RCT compared patients who received education, including urge resistance techniques, and dietary advice, to a group of patients who received the same training plus anal sphincter exercises with or without home or clinic biofeedback. There were no significant difference in outcomes.[12] However, this study did not assess the effectiveness of the behavioural training compared to an appropriate control group.

11.8 Biofeedback

"Biofeedback" has dominated the colorectal literature as the first-line conservative intervention for FI in adults. However, "biofeedback" is a term

that has been applied to many different interventions, and some groups have not described the intervention at all. Three broad approaches may be distinguished:

1. Use of anal pressure or electromyography feedback to teach the patient voluntarily to contract the anal sphincter and then utilising feedback to monitor and enhance the performance of anal sphincter exercises.

2. Use of a rectal distension balloon to "train" the patient to lower the threshold of sensation of rectal contents. A rectal balloon is inflated until the patient can feel it: it is then deflated and subsequent inflations are at progressively lower volumes. The rationale is that the sooner rectal contents are felt, the sooner the appropriate action of contraction of the anal sphincter can be made to avoid FI occurring.

3. Coordination training. This is usually performed with a three-balloon system, allowing simultaneous rectal distension and monitoring of anal pressures. Protocols often involve showing the patient the normal rectoanal inhibitory reflex consequent upon rectal distension and "teaching" the patient to counteract this fall in anal pressure with a voluntary anal squeeze.

Within these three broad categories, there has been huge variation in terms of frequency and length of sessions, instructions given to patients, and practice expected between sessions. The three modalities have also been combined with each other, and with a variety of the other interventions mentioned in this chapter[30] (Table 11.1).

From the first report of biofeedback in the early 1970s, there have been numerous case series published with positive outcomes, usually in well over a half of all patients treated.[1,36,37] As with any other

TABLE 11.1. Possible elements of a biofeedback programme.[30]

Diary and symptom questionnaire
Structured assessment
Patient teaching
Emotional support
Lifestyle modifications
Management of faecal incontinence
Urge resistance programme
Anal sphincter exercises
Clinic computer biofeedback
Home biofeedback unit

intervention, positive case reports do not constitute evidence that the treatment is effective, as there is a widely recognised and large placebo response to intervening per se in patients with functional gut disorders.[38] Evidence from a few RCTs is equivocal about the benefit of biofeedback.[39] Different modes of biofeedback seem to yield similar results.[40] Patient education and/or exercises may be as effective as adding biofeedback to either.[12,41] As a way of structuring a consultation and delivering patient education, biofeedback seems to be clinically useful: there must be some doubt on current evidence as to whether giving patients direct feedback is crucial or adds anything over and above a well-structured and individually tailored advice package.[1]

11.9 Drug Management

There have been very few good quality studies of drug treatment for FI.[42]

11.9.1 Modifying Existing Medication

A large number of prescription and over-the-counter medications can affect bowel function, either increasing constipation or loosening the stool. These are far too numerous to mention here, but it is important that all patients with AI have their medications reviewed in detail and any modifications made if possible.

11.9.2 Diarrhoea and Constipating Agents

There is a reported association between loose stools and FI.[43,44] This is consistent with reports that FI is more prevalent in patients with irritable bowel syndrome,[45] in those with illnesses that produce diarrhoea,[46-48] and in people who run long distances for exercise.[49]

If AI is secondary to soft or loose stool, using medication to firm or bulk the stool is often recommended. Loperamide is usually the drug of first choice as it has multiple potentially beneficial effects and seems to have minimal side-effects in most people. It increases colonic water reabsorption, dampens the gastrocolic response and colonic motility, and raises resting tone in the anal sphincter.[50,51] It can routinely be used in doses up to 16 mg per day and clinical reports suggest that even higher doses are safe in chronic diarrhoea. Patients who find that even low doses result in unacceptable constipation may find the liquid formulation easier to titrate to achieve the desired response. Other constipating agents such as codeine phosphate and anticholinergics are also used clinically, although there are no studies on efficacy and side-effects may be troublesome.

11.9.3 Laxatives and Evacuants

Patients with FI secondary to rectal loading or incomplete evacuation may use an oral or rectal laxative in an attempt to produce more effective emptying. While this approach is well established in encopretic children,[52] evidence in adults is lacking except in a nursing home population.[53] Some patients with FI that is difficult to regulate may choose artificially to constipate themselves and then use a suppository or micro-enema to evacuate at a chosen time. While not ideal, many find this preferable to uncontrolled incontinence. Suppositories may be useful in achieving complete evacuation in those patients with post-defaecation soiling.

11.9.4 Sphincter-modifying Drugs

As with urinary incontinence, there has recently been interest in attempting to modify the function of the anal sphincters pharmacologically. Alpha-adrenergic agonists have been found to raise the resting anal sphincter pressure in normal volunteers by up to 30% for up to 8 hours by using a topical formulation of phenylephrine.[54] This translates into a clinical benefit for patients with anal leakage secondary to ileoanal pouch formation, especially improving symptoms of nocturnal leakage.[55] However, it seems to be less effective in patients with impaired sphincter function:[56] presumably the pouch patients who benefit have essentially normal sphincters and leakage is secondary to liquid stool or altered sensation rather than internal sphincter dysfunction. Newer preparations and different compounds are under investigation but none has reached the commercial market to date.

11.10 Living with Anal Incontinence

11.10.1 Products

There are very few products designed specifically for managing FI. Generally, the same absorbent products are used as for urinary incontinence, but with limited ability to disguise the smell or protect the skin following an episode of FI. Many patients report that pads or diapers are very unsatisfactory. For minor leakage the pad is in the wrong place and it is difficult to secure a product between the buttocks where it is needed. For more major FI, particularly if the stool is diarrhoea, no pad will reliably control the incontinence.

An anal plug has been designed to control FI. This is useful for a minority of patients, particularly those with limited sensation. The majority cannot tolerate the plug because of discomfort or because it stimulates the desire to defaecate.[57,58]

11.10.2 Skin Care

Most people with FI do not report problems with anal skin soreness, as long as they are able to deal with episodes promptly. When FI is combined with urinary incontinence, there is an increased propensity for soreness. There is no evidence on the best approach to managing sore skin, but clinically many baby care and stoma care barrier creams are helpful, as is meticulous personal hygiene.

11.11 Prevention of Anal Incontinence

There has been almost no research on conservative options for preventing symptoms of anal incontinence after childbirth. One option is pelvic muscle exercises before or after delivery. These are often recommended by obstetricians and midwives and promoted in antenatal and postnatal education. However, no published study has evaluated the efficacy of this advice on subsequent anal symptoms.

In a small number of studies, pelvic floor muscle training and education have been evaluated as a secondary prevention strategy for those at high risk of incontinence. Glazener and colleagues[27] compared nurse assessment plus reinforcement of pelvic floor muscle training and bladder training to standard management (no specific intervention) in 747 women with urinary incontinence 3 months following delivery. FI was present as a comorbid condition at baseline in 57/371 in the active treatment group and in 54/376 in the standard management group. At follow-up (12 months after delivery) the prevalence of FI was significantly lower in the active intervention group compared to the control group (4.4% vs 10.5%, $P = 0.012$). This suggests that exercises may have a role in reducing FI, but the primary focus of this study was urinary incontinence and FI seems to have been measured by a single question only as present or absent. Other studies have suggested no benefit for the treatment of early-onset FI after delivery with pelvic floor exercises: Meyer and colleagues[59] performed a prospective RCT in which half of 107 primiparous women received 12 weeks of pelvic floor exercises with biofeedback and electrical stimulation beginning 9 weeks after delivery; the other half received "routine care" (no specific intervention). Assessment was at 10 months after delivery. The incidence of FI was low in this study (4–5%) and was not significantly different in the group receiving biofeedback. Two other studies whose primary aim was to treat urinary incontinence with pelvic floor exercises and education, reported that these exercises did not reduce the incidence of new FI relative to the control group.[60,61]

A postal survey carried out in 7,879 women who delivered during the same year at three hospitals – one in England, one in Scotland, and another in New Zealand – showed a higher incidence of FI in Asian women than in Caucasians (OR = 3.2).[62] A higher incidence of obstetrical injury in Asian as compared to Caucasian women was reported in two other surveys.[63,64] The prevalence of obstetrical tears during spontaneous vaginal delivery was also greater in Hispanic subjects and Filipinos.

Age is a known risk factor for FI.[1] Some of the age-related increase in prevalence of FI may be attributable to age-related declines in general health, muscle strength, mobility, and the increased prevalence of other diseases that may contribute to FI. However, it is not known if older women are more likely to develop subsequent AI following childbirth. If there is an association, this could enable targeting preventive interventions to the higher-risk groups such as older mothers and certain races. It is not known whether weight reduction has a role in preventing symptom development following perineal trauma. It is not known if avoidance of heavy lifting would prevent AI development in an at-risk population.

11.12 Conclusions

Anal or faecal incontinence is a difficult and demoralising problem for many women following anal sphincter trauma. Even if symptoms are relatively rare, the fear or uncertainty of their occurrence can lead to anxiety and even isolation. There have been remarkably few intervention or prevention studies. Clinically, it is often a combination of measures that improves symptoms, rather than a single intervention. As public awareness of the problem grows, it is to be hoped that more women will summon the courage to report symptoms and more health professionals will take an interest in finding solutions.

References

1. Norton C, Whitehead WE, Bliss DZ, Metsola P, Tries J. Conservative and pharmacological management of faecal incontinence in adults. In: Abrams P, Khoury S, Wein A, Cardozo L, eds. Incontinence (proceedings of the third International Consultation on Incontinence). Plymouth: Health Books, 2005.
2. Johanson JF, Lafferty J. Epidemiology of fecal incontinence: the silent affliction. Am J Gastroenterol 1996;91(1):33–6.
3. Leigh RJ, Turnberg LA. Faecal incontinence: the unvoiced symptom. Lancet 1982;1:1349–51.
4. Norton C, Chelvanayagam S. A nursing assessment tool for adults with fecal incontinence. J Wound Ostomy Continence Nurs 2000;27:279–91.
5. Fornell EU, Wingren G, Kjolhede P. Factors associated with pelvic floor dysfunction with emphasis on urinary and fecal incontinence and genital prolapse: an epidemiological study. Acta Obstet Gynecol Scand 2004;83:383–9.
6. Rausch T, Beglinger C, Alam N, Meier R. Effect of transdermal application of nicotine on colonic transit in healthy nonsmoking volunteers. Neurogastroenterol Mot 1998;10:263–70.
7. Chaliha C, Kalia V, Stanton SL, Monga AK, Sultan AH. Antenatal prediction of postpartum urinary and fecal incontinence. Obstet Gynecol 1999;94(5):689–94.
8. Sullivan S, Wong C. Runners' diarrhea. J Clin Gastroenterol 1992;14(2):101–4.
9. Jorgensen S, Hein HO, Gyntelberg F. Heavy lifting at work and risk of genital prolapse and herniated lumbar disc in assistant nurses. Occ Med 1994;44:47–9.
10. Norton C. Nurses, bowel continence, stigma and taboos. J Wound Ostomy Continence Nurs 2004;31(2):85–94.
11. Norton C, Kamm MA. Bowel control – information and practical advice. Beaconsfield: Beaconsfield Publishers, 1999.
12. Norton C, Chelvanayagam S, Wilson-Barnett J, Redfern S, Kamm MA. Randomized controlled trial of biofeedback for fecal incontinence. Gastroenterology 2003;125:1320–9.
13. Heymen S, Jones KR, Ringel Y, Scarlett Y, Drossman DA, Whitehead WE. Biofeedback for fecal incontinence and constipation: the role of medical management and education. Gastroenterology 2001;120(Suppl 1):A397.
14. Chelvanayagam S, Norton C. Quality of life with faecal continence problems. Nursing Times 2000;96(31):Suppl 15–17.
15. Doughty D. A physiologic approach to bowel training. J Wound Ostomy Continence Nurs 1996;23(1):46–56.
16. Norton C, Chelvanayagam S. Bowel continence nursing. Beaconsfield: Beaconsfield Publishers, 2004.
17. Bassotti G, Crowell MD, Cheskin LJ, Chami TN, Schuster MM, Whitehead WE. Physiological correlates of colonic motility in patients with irritable bowel syndrome. Zeitschr Gastroenterol 1998;36:811–17.
18. Narducci F, Bassotti G, Bagurri M, Morelli A. Twenty-four hour manometric recording of colonic motor activity in healthy man. Gut 1987;28:17–25.
19. Bliss DZ, Jung H, Savik K, Lowry AC, LeMoine M, Jensen L et al. Supplementation with dietary fiber improves fecal incontinence. Nursing Research 2001;50(4):203–13.
20. Bliss DZ, McLaughlin J, Jung H, Savik K, Jensen L, Lowry AC. Comparison of the nutritional composition of diets of persons with fecal incontinence and that of age and gender-matched controls. J Wound Ostomy Continence Nurs 2000;27(2):90–7.

21. Aurisicchio LN, Pitchumoni CS. Lactose intolerance. Recognizing the link between diet and discomfort. Postgrad Med 1994;95:113–20.

22. Inman-Felton AE. Overview of lactose maldigestion (lactase nonpersistence). J Am Dietetic Assoc 1999;99(4):481–9.

23. Phillips SF, Greenberger NJ. The diverse spectrum of irritable bowel syndrome. Hosp Pract 1995;30:69–78.

24. Ledochowski M, Widner B, Bair H, Probst T, Fuchs D. Fructose and sorbitol reduced diet improves mood and gastrointestinal disturbances in fructose malabsorbers. Scand J Gastroenterol 2000;35:1048–52.

25. Brown SR, Cann PA, Read NW. Effect of coffee on distal colon function. Gut 1990;31:450–3.

26. Norton C, Chelvanayagam S. Conservative management of faecal incontinence in adults. In: Norton C, Chelvanayagam S, eds. Bowel continence nursing. Beaconsfield: Beaconsfield Publishers, 2004, pp 114–31.

27. Glazener CM, Herbison P, Wilson PD, MacArthur C, Lang GD. Conservative management of persistent postnatal urinary and faecal incontinence: randomised controlled trial. Br Med J 2001;323:593–6.

28. Glazener CM, Herbison P, MacArthur C, Grant A, Wilson PD. Randomised controlled trial of conservative management of postnatal urinary and faecal incontinence: six year follow up. Br Med J 2005;330:337.

29. Sander P, Bjarnesen J, Mouritsen L, Fuglsang-Frederiksen A. Anal incontinence after obstetric third-/fourth-degree laceration. One-year follow-up after pelvic floor exercises. Int Urogynecol J Pelvic Floor Dysfunct 1999;10(3):177–81.

30. Norton C, Chelvanayagam S. Methodology of biofeedback for adults with fecal incontinence – a program of care. J Wound Ostomy Continence Nurs 2001;28:156–68.

31. Marcello PW, Barrett RC, Coller JA, Schoetz DJ, Roberts PL, Murray JJ et al. Fatigue rate index as a new measure of external sphincter function. Dis Colon Rectum 1998;41:336–43.

32. Hosker G, Norton C, Brazzelli M. Electrical stimulation for faecal incontinence in adults (Cochrane review). The Cochrane Library, Issue 2, 2004. Chichester, UK: John Wiley & Sons, Ltd.

33. Fynes MM, Marshall K, Cassidy M, Behan M, Walsh D, O'Connell PR et al. A prospective, randomized study comparing the effect of augmented biofeedback with sensory biofeedback alone on fecal incontinence after obstetric trauma. Dis Colon Rectum 1999;42(6):753–8.

34. Sander P, Bjarnesen J, Mouritsen L. Anal incontinence in women after obstetric anal sphincter rupture, treated with pelvic floor exercises and a trial of transanal electrical stimulation. Int J Proctological Perineal Dis 1997;1(1):227.

35. Norton C, Gibbs A, Kamm MA. Randomized, controlled trial of anal electrical stimulation for faecal incontinence. Dis Colon Rectum 2006;49:190–6.

36. Heymen S, Jones KR, Ringel Y, Scarlett Y, Whitehead WE. Biofeedback treatment of fecal incontinence: a critical review. Dis Colon Rectum 2001;44:728–36.

37. Norton C, Kamm MA. Anal sphincter biofeedback and pelvic floor exercises for faecal incontinence in adults – a systematic review. Aliment Pharmacol Ther 2001;15:1147–54.

38. Whitehead WE, Corazziari E, Prizont R, Senior JR, Thompson WG, Veldhuyzen van Zanten SJO. Definition of a responder in clinical trials for functional gastrointestinal disorders: report on a symposium. Gut 1999;45:1178–9.

39. Norton C, Cody J. Biofeedback and/or sphincter exercises for the treatment of faecal incontinence in adults (Cochrane review). The Cochrane Library, Issue 3, 2006. Chichester, UK: John Wiley & Sons, Ltd.

40. Heymen S, Pikarsky AJ, Weiss EG, Vickers D, Nogueras JJ, Wexner S. A prospective randomised trial comparing four biofeedback techniques for patients with faecal incontinence. Colorectal Dis 2000;2:88–92.

41. Solomon MJ, Pager CK, Rex J, Roberts R, Manning J. Randomised, controlled trial of biofeedback with anal manometry, transanal ultrasound, or pelvic floor retraining with digital guidance alone in the treatment of mild to moderate fecal incontinence. Dis Colon Rectum 2003;46(6):703–10.

42. Cheetham M, Brazzelli M, Norton C, Glazener CM. Drug treatment for faecal incontinence in adults (Cochrane review). The Cochrane Library, Issue 2, 2004. Chichester, UK: John Wiley & Sons, Ltd.

43. Kalantar JS, Howell S, Talley NJ. Prevalence of faecal incontinence and associated risk factors; an underdiagnosed problem in the Australian community? Med J Aust 2002;176(2):54–7.

44. Walter S, Hallbook O, Gotthard R, Bengmark M, Sjodahl R. A population-based study on bowel habits in a Swedish community: prevalence of faecal incontinence and constipation. Scand J Gastroenterol 2002;37(8):911–16.

45. Drossman DA, Sandler RS, Broom CM, McKee DC. Urgency and fecal soiling in people with bowel dysfunction. Dig Dis Sci 1986;31(11):1221–5.

46. Bliss DZ, Johnson S, Savik K, Clabots CR, Gerding DN. Fecal incontinence in hospitalized patients who are acutely ill. Nursing Res 2000;49(2): 101–8.

47. Mintz ED, Weber JT, Guris D, Puhr N, Wells JG, Yashuk JC. An outbreak of Brainerd diarrhea among travelers to the Galapagos Islands. J Infect Dis 1998;177(4):1041–5.

48. Kyne L, Merry C, O'Connell B, Kelly A, Keane C, O'Neill D. Factors associated with prolonged symptoms and severe disease due to Clostridium difficile. Age Ageing 1999;28(2):107–13.

49. Lustyk MK, Jarret ME, Bennett JC, Heitkemper MM. Does a physically active lifestyle improve symptoms in women with irritable bowel syndrome? Gastroenterol Nursing 2001;24(3): 129–37.

50. Read M, Read NW, Barber DC, Duthie HL. Effects of loperamide on anal sphincter function in patients complaining of chronic diarrhoea with faecal incontinence and urgency. Dig Dis Sci 1982;27: 807–14.

51. Sun WM, Read NW, Verlinden M. Effects of loperamide oxide on gastrointestinal transit time and anorectal function in patients with chronic diarrhoea and faecal incontinence. Scand J Gastroenterol 1997;32:34–8.

52. Clayden GS, Hollins G. Constipation and faecal incontinence in childhood. In: Norton C, Chelvanayagam S, eds. Bowel continence nursing. Beaconsfield: Beaconsfield Publishers, 2004, pp 217–28.

53. Chassagne P, Jego A, Gloc P, Capet C, Trivalle C, Doucet J et al. Does treatment of constipation improve faecal incontinence in institutionalized elderly patients? Age Ageing 2000;29(2): 159–64.

54. Carapeti EA, Kamm MA, Evans BK, Phillips RK. Topical phenylephrine increases anal sphincter resting pressure. Br J Surg 1999;86(2):267–70.

55. Carapeti EA, Kamm MA, Phillips RK. Randomized controlled trial of topical phenylephrine in the treatment of faecal incontinence. Br J Surg 2000;87: 38–42.

56. Cheetham M, Kamm MA, Phillips RK. Topical phenylephrine increases anal canal resting pressure in patients with faecal incontinence. Gut 2001;48: 356–9.

57. Mortensen NJ, Smilgin Humphreys M. The anal continence plug: a disposable device for patients with anorectal incontinence. Lancet 1991;338: 295–7.

58. Norton C, Kamm MA. Anal plug for faecal incontinence. Colorectal Dis 2001;3:323–7.

59. Meyer S, Hohlfield P, Achtari C, De Grandi P. Pelvic floor education after vaginal delivery. Obstet Gynecol 2001;97(5):673–7.

60. Sleep J, Grant A. Pelvic floor exercises in postnatal care. Midwifery 1987;3(4):158–64.

61. Wilson PD, Herbison P. A randomised controlled trial of pelvic floor muscle exercises to treat postnatal urinary incontinence. Int Urogynecol J 1998; 9:257–64.

62. MacArthur C, Glazener CM, Wilson PD, Herbison P, Gee H, Lang GD. Obstetric practice and faecal incontinence three months after delivery. Br J Obstet Gynaecol 2001;108(7):678–83.

63. Combs CA, Robertson PA, Laros RK. Risk factors for third-degree and fourth-degree perineal lacerations in forceps and vacuum deliveries. Am J Obstet Gynecol 1990;163(1):100–4.

64. Green JR, Soohoo SL. Factors associated with rectal injury in spontaneous deliveries. Obstet Gynecol 1989;73(5):732–8.

12a
Surgical Management of Anal Incontinence Part A. Secondary Anal Sphincter Repair

Robin K. S. Phillips and Timothy J. Brown

12a.1 Introduction

As the prevalence of anal ultrasound examinations increases, so will the number of patients seen with a reported abnormality whose significance remains in doubt. Uncertainty regarding the meaning of abnormal studies in relation to long-term sequelae raises a few issues that could prove difficult: for example, the complexity of advising a woman how much improvement she can expect and how long that improvement will last. Furthermore, the actual operation of anal sphincter repair needs to be tailored to the severity of injury, whether it is simple with straightforward faecal incontinence, or a more complex case, either with an associated ano/rectovaginal fistula or with an accompanying evacuation disorder.

12a.2 Irritable Bowel Syndrome and Incontinence

Not all faecal incontinence is due to anal failure. A traveller who experiences severe gastroenteritis may be caught short; a sufferer with acute inflammatory bowel disease or even with cholera may lose bowel control; and a person with severe irritable bowel syndrome (IBS) may complain of faecal incontinence. A useful analogy to explain these situations is a hot plate on a hob; placed in the bare hands it will be dropped, yet there is nothing wrong with the strength of the grip. Similarly, in the above examples the stool can simply be "too hot to handle", leading to episodes of faecal incontinence.

Irritable bowel syndrome is extremely common, with a suggested prevalence of 9–12%;[1] postpartum women suffering with IBS demonstrate alteration of faecal continence.[2] It is also known that many women who have had a vaginal delivery, particularly an assisted delivery, have occult anal sphincter injuries.[3] How does a surgeon know whether the faecal incontinence is a consequence of severe IBS or a result of the birth injury? If the former, surgery will have no role to play, but if the latter, an operation may need to be contemplated – but, given the IBS, it would be wise to advise the woman of an unpredictable result.

When there is anal failure there is graded incontinence, first gas, next liquid, and finally a formed or solid stool. But imagine having severe travellers' diarrhoea; there is no problem controlling flatus, it is the stool itself that causes urgency and incontinence. Likewise, with IBS, some patients actually experience great difficulty breaking wind, and yet have no control over a bowel motion itself. This means that an irritable rectum and anal failure can be distinguished from each other by analysing patient history: if there is graded incontinence, flatus > liquid stool > formed stool, it is highly likely to be a problem in the anal sphincter; but if there is continence to gas and only incontinence to stool, the problem is not likely to lie within the anal sphincter. Anorectal physiology testing can help minimally, with a reduced maximal tolerable volume to balloon distension being indicative of an irritable rectum.

12a.3 Extent of Anorectal Injury

Examine Figure12a.1[4] and imagine the rectovaginal septum being continuous with the anal sphincter complex in its inferior part. This figure depicts the usual mechanism of obstetric anal sphincter injury and the resulting scenarios that arise from it. Injury in the proximal part of the rectovaginal septum (Figure 12a.1A) can result in a rectocele; an anal sphincter injury (Figure 12a.1C) can result in faecal incontinence; Figure 12a.1B depicts injury throughout the rectovaginal septum/anal sphincter, leading potentially to combined faecal incontinence and a rectocele, possibly with an evacuation disorder. It is this last injury that may at its midpoint then necrose, resulting in one of the three types of postobstetric rectovaginal fistulas (see Chapter 13).

Preoperative investigations cannot easily discern the difference between these three types of injury, largely because current imaging does not depict the rectovaginal septum and therefore cannot show tears in it. It might be argued that a proctogram would show the rectocele bulge, but proctography falls short as it depends on anal sphincter function for contrast during bearing down at defaecation, which is not possible when

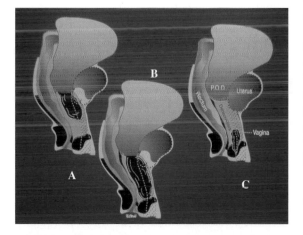

Figure 12a.1. The resultant injury to the rectovaginal septum may be in its upper part, resulting in a rectocele (**A**), in the lower part, resulting in incontinence (**C**), or throughout, resulting in both incontinence and an evacuation disorder (**B**). (Reprinted from Phillips,[4] with permission from Elsevier.)

the anus is incontinent. Furthermore, up to 80% of normal women can be shown on proctography to have a rectocele.[5] Therefore, what actually matters is the functionality, rather than the anatomy per se.

Again, the key is in the history. An incontinent woman with a simple anal sphincter injury (Figure 12a.1A) should have a low fibre diet and constipating agents such as loperamide, as this leads to a firmer stool that is easier for her weakened anus to grip. On the other hand, a woman with an injury throughout the entire length of the rectovaginal septum (Figure 12a.1B) avoids constipation. On closer questioning, the clinician will elicit that the woman prefers incontinence because of her inability to evacuate a firm stool.

This differentiation is infrequently made by colorectal surgeons, who generally are unaware of these differences, even though the injuries require different operations. In my practice, those patients with an associated rectovaginal septal injury along with an anal sphincter injury (Figure 12a.1B) undergo a more extended anal sphincter repair. The purpose of this operation is not only to perform an overlap of the anal sphincter itself, but also to enter the rectovaginal septum to the pouch of Douglas and perform a sutured repair of the rectovaginal septum with a non-absorbable material such as nylon.[4] The intention is to perform a synchronous rectocele repair. Isolated injury to the anal sphincter (Figure 12a.1C) would involve only a standard anal sphincter repair.

This failure to identify the different groups means that some who should have had more complex surgery to repair the associated rectovaginal septal tear instead are left with an evacuation disorder for which biofeedback is recommended. The authors believe this to be an avoidable problem through more focused history-taking and by tailoring the repair to the predicted injury type.

12a.4 Role of Neuropathy

Pudendal neuropathy is a useful concept but fraught with difficulty when it comes to evaluation. The gold-standard anorectal physiology test is the fibre density. This is rarely used now as it involves inserting needles into the anal sphincter, which causes patient discomfort. Instead, the pudendal nerve terminal motor latency is used (as described in Chapter 9). The problem with this test is that it is not always reliable. An investigator is able to produce widely varying results on different occasions, just as several investigators can produce widely varying results on the same occasion. Because of these differences, doctors are able to continue testing until they receive a desired result.

What this means in practice is that pudendal neuropathy and the quality of the anal sphincter are largely clinical impressions rather than anorectal physiology issues. First, the pudendal nerve supplies more than just the anal sphincter. More global pelvic floor problems (for example associated urinary incontinence) suggest more than a simple tear in the anal sphincter. There may also be a mechanical problem in the anterior compartment caused through the same mechanisms that led to the anal sphincter tear, or it could be due to pudendal nerve injury.

Second, the pudendal nerve is a mixed motor and sensory nerve. A woman with associated vaginal numbness or who feels no need to defaecate until she has been faecally incontinent may well have nerve damage. Anorectal physiology testing that shows sensory change helps diagnosis, although anal canal scarring after a fourth degree tear may equally be responsible if the abnormality is observed when testing electrical sensation in the anal canal.

Third, anal sphincter quality may feel abnormal. Imagine an intact anal sphincter as the capital letter "O" and the divided anal sphincter as a "U". Feeling in the bend of the "U" should identify normal, vigorous muscle activity, but when examining a woman with damaged nerves, little or no activity may be felt.

It is hard to determine from the literature the impact of pudendal neuropathy on subsequent outcome of anal sphincter repair, probably because much of the literature depends on measured pudendal nerve terminal motor latency. There are articles that show that reduced pudendal nerve terminal motor latency is a poor prognostic indicator to outcome of external anal sphincter repair,[6,7] and others even within the same institution that state it makes no difference to outcome.[8]

12a.5   The Extent of the Injury versus the Degree of the Symptoms

As a generality, surgeons are not able to repair a damaged and scarred internal anal sphincter. Although there are occasional reports of a separated plication or repair having been incorporated at the time of external anal sphincter repair,[9] these have not been validated as having been successful by post-repair anal ultrasonography. As the internal anal sphincter largely controls resting anal pressure, an internal anal sphincter defect is going to be responsible for minor passive soiling. This would usually amount to flatus incontinence and anal "dribbling" of up to a teaspoonful of mucus/stool each day, depending on stool consistency.

There are scant data in the literature reporting on secondary repair of isolated internal sphincter defects. Leroi et al. reported on five patients who had overlapping repair performed on their internal sphincter.[10] Of these five patients, there was a slight symptomatic improvement in two, but three felt that their symptoms had deteriorated. Objective measurement of outcome (endoanal ultrasound and manometry) was disappointing. Morgan et al. looked at 15 patients with internal sphincter incontinence.[11] Two of these patients underwent direct isolated repair of the internal sphincter. They reported no improvement in symptoms. Although in a methods paper reporting on anal ultrasound using endoscopic ultrasound, Meyenberger et al. remark that internal anal sphincter repair seems to have worked clinically in their hands, there was no post-repair anal ultrasound validation.[12]

12a.6   What Are the Best Results Achievable?

The result will depend on the extent of the anal sphincter injury itself (and in particular, whether the internal anal sphincter is divided), the quality of the anal muscle remote from the injury (pudendal neuropathy), the patient's natural bowel frequency (the anus needs to be of better quality in order to cope with two or three soft stools each day than it does to cope with two or three firm motions each week), and the presence or absence of IBS.

Take as an example a woman who on an anal ultrasound shows a full-length defect involving both the internal anal sphincter and the external anal sphincter. There is perhaps an 80%[13] chance that an anal sphincter repair will result in a complete circle of external anal sphincter around the anus afterwards. However, if the preoperative complaint is of flatus incontinence and mild mucus leakage, the clinician can reasonably deduce that as far as her symptoms are concerned, they are almost certainly arising as a consequence of the internal sphincter injury. Given that it is generally accepted that the internal anal sphincter is difficult if not impossible to repair, her best anticipated clinical result will be no better than her preoperative symptoms. At the same time she runs the general risks of surgery along with an approximately 20% chance of breakdown of the external anal sphincter component[13] (the consequences of this are hard to predict – preoperatively they did not seem to be contributing to her symptoms of faecal incontinence, but the anal surgical disturbance along with a less than adequate repair runs some risk of causing actual deterioration in her continence). Such a woman should not be advised to have anal sphincter repair. It has been postulated that ageing/the menopause have an effect on anal sphincter musculature[14] and, while it is true that as the woman ages and menopause approaches, so continence may decline, there is no evidence that a delayed anal sphincter repair is any the worse than one performed much earlier. A "wait-and-see" policy along with dietary advice, the use of loperamide, and perhaps biofeedback would seem wisest. For those postmenopausal women who have faecal incontinence, there is some early evidence that hormone replacement therapy may be helpful.[14]

There are women with a deficient perineum who have an injury to both the external anal sphincter and the internal anal sphincter, but whose level of incontinence is slight, as in the case above. Where reconstruction of the perineum is being performed on cosmetic/sexual grounds, rather than on the grounds of faecal incontinence, it does seem sensible to repair the anal sphincter at the same time – if only to give some added bulk to the perineum. However, the woman should know that there would be at least a slight risk of continence deterioration were this to be done (offset by an anticipated prevention of continence deterioration at the time of the menopause).

As another example, a woman with an external anal sphincter defect but with an intact internal anal sphincter should anticipate achieving a perfect outcome from external anal sphincter reconstruction, within certain limitations:

1. There are always the risks of surgery. The wound could break down and there could be anaesthetic problems or other problems of a more general nature.

2. The operating surgeon must not damage the internal anal sphincter during the operation. Many surgeons perform a standardised repair of the anal sphincter, which involves dividing the entire, full-thickness length of the anal sphincter complex followed by overlapping repair. Such a technique, if employed in a case such as this, would be expected to result in an unrepaired internal anal sphincter with the consequence of flatus incontinence and mild passive soiling. It is not uncommon for a woman in this predicament to have complained of urge faecal incontinence preoperatively, but not to have had much in the way of flatus incontinence or minor soiling. This woman may perceive herself to have gained little from surgery and be quite unhappy with the result. The message is to image the sphincter complex preoperatively and if the internal anal sphincter is shown to be intact, it is imperative at surgery to ensure that only the external anal sphincter is mobilised and repaired.

3. Anal muscle quality must be good on clinical grounds (feeling in the "U" bend for vigorous muscle activity).

The most common injury is a combined injury to the external anal sphincter and the internal anal sphincter with flatus and faecal incontinence, with the associated social inconveniences.

In these circumstances, anal sphincter repair should produce an 80%[13] chance of avoiding accidents in the street or at home, but should not be anticipated to result in perfect continence afterwards, for the reason that the internal anal sphincter is highly unlikely to be improved (Figure 12a.2). Women should also be counselled that, just as immediate repair of a third degree

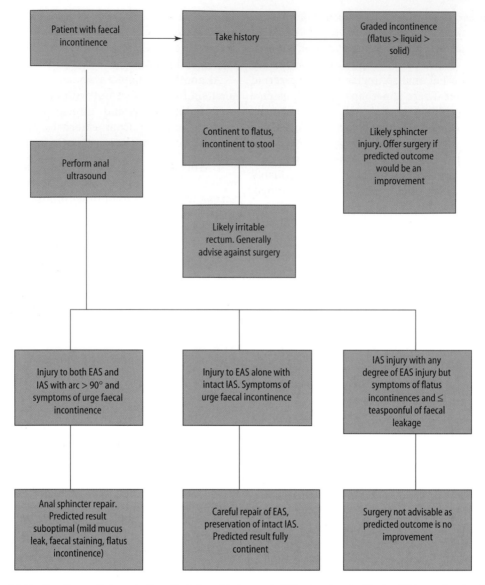

Figure 12a.2. Algorithm outlining selection criteria for sphincter repair. *EAS* external anal sphincter, *IAS* internal anal sphincter.

tear may deteriorate with time,[15] so do delayed repairs.[16]

12a.7 When Is a Stoma Necessary?

Most surgeons now agree that for a straightforward anal sphincter injury, a colostomy is not required. But not all injuries are straightforward and many surgeons still consider using a stoma in the following circumstances:

1. When there is a cloacal injury. Some injuries are so extensive that the anterior half of the anus and the lower third of the vagina are one common cavity. The repair is precarious in the thin area of the distal remaining rectovaginal septum with a serious possibility of postoperative fistulation over the top of an otherwise successful sphincter reconstruction.

2. When there is an associated rectovaginal fistula. Fistulas to the vagina can be extremely hard to treat; the published overall results of about

80% success often overlook both the short-term failure in about half of the patients and the need for multiple reoperations before success is achieved.[17] Whereas it is hard to accrue evidence that a colostomy will make a difference, most surgeons confronted by multiple failed attempts will finally resort to the use of a stoma as an adjunct to re-repair. Probably more importantly, given the high known rate of initial failure, many women find it easier to cope with failure if they feel they have already done everything possible.

3. In the presence of Crohn's disease or prior radiation therapy.

12a.8   When to Avoid Surgery

Women with gross pudendal neuropathy (that is to say, those who are numb perineally, or those who do not exhibit anal sphincter contraction in the bend of the "U" of the divided anal sphincter) are unlikely to benefit from anal sphincter repair. A wasted attempt may even compromise some of the other surgical options described in the next chapter.

12a.9   Anal Sphincter Surgery

12a.9.1   Historical Perspective

This has been extensively reviewed by Baig and Wexner.[18] Sir Alan Parks was responsible for the current form of overlapping sphincter repair, initially employing stainless steel wire as the suture.[19] Given the technical difficulties of operating with wire, many surgeons subsequently adopted nylon or prolene, later changing again to polydioxanone (PDS) or Vicryl to avoid the occasional stitch sinuses seen with the former. Slade modified Parks' overlapping repair[20] by leaving the scar tissue to aid the anchoring of sutures. Many early anal sphincter repairs were performed with a covering stoma, but when Thomson described a series of 31 patients undergoing sphincter repair and showed that success was independent of diversion of the faecal stream, most surgeons abandoned the use of a stoma as a routine.[21]

Comparison of the original method of end-to-end apposition with overlapping repair was subject to a recent, rather small randomised controlled trial in elective cases ($n = 23$)[22] that reported no difference between the methods after only a fairly short follow-up.

12a.9.2   Operative Steps for Anal Sphincter Repair

Personal practice is to use full preoperative bowel preparation with sodium picosulphate and one dose of perioperative gentamicin (120 mg) and metronidazole (500 mg) intravenously. After catheterisation, positioning (lithotomy or prone jack-knife) is according to surgeon preference. A hemicircumferential incision along the line of anal sphincter pigmentation (which is the cutaneous sign of the boundary of the external anal sphincter) is made. Next, the incision is deepened into the ischioanal fat on either side and the vagina is separated from the anal scar tissue. If there is a history of an associated evacuation disorder, the operation will be extended to incorporate repair of the rectovaginal septum, instead of a more confined and simple sphincter repair. No attempt is made to separate external from internal sphincter unless the internal sphincter has not been damaged, in which case every attempt should be made to preserve it.

The midline anal scar tissue is then split down its entire length and the anal sphincter muscle is dissected off the underlying anal canal in one block making no attempt to separate the external and internal anal sphincter muscles from each other (Figure 12a.3).

The leading edge of one side of the divided scar tissue is sutured to the underside of the opposing edge, usually using a monofilament absorbable suture. This commences the overlap (Figure 12a.4).

Having tied these initial sutures, the other leading edge is sutured over the top of the first layer of sutures depicted in Figure 12a.4, thereby obscuring the first layer of sutures and completing the overlap (Figure 12a.5). Finally, a decision is made whether to close the wound primarily or leave the central part open to heal by secondary intention.

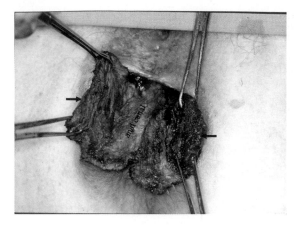

Figure 12a.3. The two divided ends of the anal sphincter muscle (*arrows*) are grasped, ready for overlapping repair.

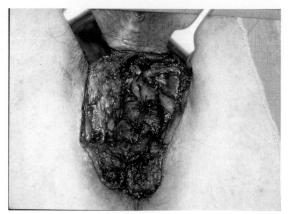

Figure 12a.5. Having tied the sutures depicted in Figure 12a.4, the overlap is completed, suturing the right hand side of muscle (depicted on the left of the image) over the first layer of sutures, thereby obscuring them from sight.

Management of internal anal sphincter injury is more complicated. Overlapping repair and imbrication repair of isolated internal sphincter injuries is described but seems to be unsuccessful.[11] Other techniques designed to improve internal sphincter function have been employed with varying success (e.g. anoplasty, injection of bulking agents). Expert opinion among colorectal surgeons confronted by patients with internal sphincter injuries is that they cannot be repaired surgically.

Frequently at the end of the operation there is not enough available skin to perform a primary

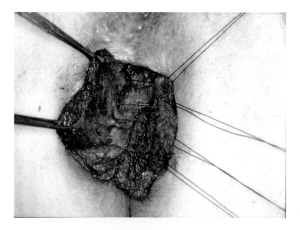

Figure 12a.4. The leading edge of the patient's left side of the anal sphincter (pictured to the right) is sutured to the deep surface of the opposing sphincter muscle usually using an absorbable suture.

skin closure. Whereas there are various surgical flap techniques that can be employed to obtain primary skin cover, many surgeons only partially close the wound, leaving the centre open. After surgery, the patient can be allowed to eat and drink normally. A mild laxative is encouraged to prevent a faecal impaction, and the woman should be advised that this may initially falsely disappoint her as to the outcome of her surgery. There no longer seems to be a case for bowel confinement.[23] When comfortable and the bowels are working, the woman is allowed home, which is commonly within 5 days of surgery.

12a.9.3   Results of Surgery

As stated, it may be considered unproductive to examine in any detail the results in the literature, as there are so many confounding factors involved (but see Tables 12a.1 and 12a.2 as supplied by the editorial team). Not only do these include all those mentioned (sphincter quality, the state of the internal anal sphincter, whether or not there is an extended injury into the rectovaginal septum), but many reports also include patients with incontinence after fistula surgery, patients who are not immediately postpartum, and patients who have had surgery on multiple occasions unsuccessfully. There have been no publications that compare

TABLE 12a.1. Short-term (<5 years) outcomes after sphincteroplasty.

Author, year	N	Follow-up period Mean (range) months	Success (%)	Improved (%)
Fang et al. 1984[24]	76	35 (2–62)	82	89
Browning and Motson 1984[25]	83	39.2 (4–116)	78	91
Ctercteko et al. 1988[26]	44	50	75	–
Laurberg et al. 1988[6]	19	18 (median; 9–36)	47	79
Yoshioka and Keighley 1989[27]	27	48 (median; 16–108)	–	74.1
Wexner et al. 1991[28]	16	10 (3–16)	76	87.5
Fleshman et al. 1991[29]	55	0 (12–24)	72	87
Engel et al. 1994[13]	55	15 (6–36)	60.4	–
Engel et al. 1994[30]	28	46 (median; 15–116)	75	–
Londono-Schimmer et al. 1994[31]	94	58.5 (median; 12–98)	50	75
Sitzler and Thomson 1996[21]	31	(1–36)	74	–
Oliveira et al. 1996[32]	55	29 (3–61)	70.1	80
Nikiteas et al. 1996[33]	42	38 (median; 12–66)	60	–
Gilliland et al. 1998[7]	100	24 (median; 2–96)	55	69

preoperative predictions of expected success to observed success. In general, most colorectal surgeons agree that:

1. A perfect result can be achieved only if the internal anal sphincter is initially intact and both anal sphincters are of good quality.

2. About 80% of patients receiving surgery for a combined injury to the internal and external anal sphincters will become continent to solid stool, but will still suffer from flatus incontinence and mild mucus leakage.

3. Those with a worse result should receive an anal ultrasound scan to determine whether or not the sphincter repair has achieved a complete ring of external anal sphincter. If it has not, repeat repair should be offered with an approximately equivalent chance of success.

4. Continence deteriorates with age. This deterioration happens not only to women who have had a secondary repair[8] or to those who have had primary repair of a third degree tear,[15] but to all women.

TABLE 12a.2. Long-term results following overlapping sphincteroplasty reported by continence type.

Author	Patients with follow-up/total (%)	Length follow-up Mean (range)	Outcomes
Malouf et al. 2000[8]	46/55 (84)	77 months (60–96)	0% continent 10% incontinent flatus only 79% soiling 21% incontinent solid stool 8/46 other surgery
Karoui et al. 2000[34]	74/86 (86)	40 months	28% continent 23% incontinent flatus only 49% incontinent stool
Halverson et al. 2002[35]	49/71 (69)	69 months (48–141)	14% continent 54% incontinent stool 7/49 other surgery
Gutierrez et al. 2004[36]	135/191 (71)	10 years (7–16)	6% continent 16% incontinent flatus only 19% soiling 57% incontinent stool 5/135 other surgery

12a.10   Conclusion

Accurate patient selection is essential, along with a realistic explanation of the likely outcome. Outcome depends on the extent of the injury, the quality of the residual muscle and the presence or absence of IBS.[37] Repair of an isolated external sphincter injury seems to give the most successful surgical outcome, while a patient with an additional injury to the internal sphincter is unlikely to gain complete continence. An accurate history should be combined with up-to-date imaging.

References

1. Guidelines for the management of irritable bowel syndrome. Gut 2000;47(Suppl II):1–19.
2. Donnelly VS, O'Herlihy C, Campbell DM, O'Connell PR. Postpartum fecal incontinence is more common in women with irritable bowel syndrome. Dis Colon Rectum 1998;41(5):586–9.
3. Sultan AH, Kamm MA, Hudson CN, Thomas JM, Bartram CI. Anal-sphincter disruption during vaginal delivery. N Engl J Med 1993;329(26):1956–7.
4. Phillips RKS. Progress in the management of anal disorders. In: Taylor I, Johnson CD, eds. Recent advances in surgery, vol. 22. Edinburgh: Churchill Livingstone, 1999, pp 123–33.
5. Shorvon PJ, McHugh S, Diamant NE, Somers S, Stevenson GW. Defaecography in normal volunteers: results and implications. Gut 1989;30:1737–49.
6. Laurberg S, Swash M, Henry MM. Delayed external sphincter repair for obstetric tear. Br J Surg 1988;75:786–8.
7. Gilliland R, Altomare DF, Moreira H Jr, Oliveira L, Gilliland JE, Wexner SD. Pudendal neuropathy is predictive of failure following anterior overlapping sphincteroplasty. Dis Colon Rectum 1998;41:1516–22.
8. Malouf AJ, Norton CS, Engel AF, Nicholls RJ, Kamm MA. Long term results of overlapping anterior anal sphincter repair for obstetric trauma. Lancet 2000;355:260–5.
9. Briel JW, de Boer LM, Hop WC, Schouten WR. Clinical outcome of anterior overlapping external anal sphincter repair with internal anal sphincter imbrication. Dis Colon Rectum 1998;41:209–14.
10. Leroi AM, Kamm MA, Weber J, Denis P, Hawley PR. Internal anal sphincter repair. Int J Colorectal Dis 1997;12:243–5.
11. Morgan R, Patel B, Beynon J, Carr ND. Surgical management of anorectal incontinence due to internal anal sphincter deficiency. Br J Surg 1997;84(2):226–30.
12. Meyenberger C, Bertschinger P, Zala GF, Buchmann P. Anal sphincter defects in fecal incontinence: correlation between endosonography and surgery. Endoscopy 1996;28:217–24.
13. Engel AF, Kamm MA, Sultan AH, Bartram CI, Nicholls RJ. Anterior anal sphincter repair in patients with obstetric trauma. Br J Surg 1994;81(8):1231–4.
14. Donnelly V, O'Connell PR, O'Herlihy C. The influence of oestrogen replacement on faecal incontinence in postmenopausal women. Br J Obstet Gynaecol 1997;104(3):311–15.
15. Tetzschner T, Sorensen M, Lose G, Christiansen J. Anal and urinary incontinence in women with obstetric anal sphincter rupture. Br J Obstet Gynaecol 1996;103(10):1034–40.
16. Malouf AJ, Norton CS, Engel AF, Nicholls RJ, Kamm MA. Long-term results of overlapping anterior anal-sphincter repair for obstetric trauma. Lancet 2000;355(9200):260–5.
17. Watson SJ, Phillips RKS. Non-inflammatory rectovaginal fistula. Br J Surg 1995;82:1641–3.
18. Baig MK, Wexner SD. Factors predictive of outcome after surgery for faecal incontinence. Br J Surg 2000;87(10):1316–30.
19. Parks AG, McPartlin JF. Late repair of injuries of the anal sphincter. Proc R Soc Med 1971;64(12):1187–9.
20. Slade MS, Goldberg SM, Schottler JL, Balcos EG, Christenson CE. Sphincteroplasty for acquired anal incontinence. Dis Colon Rectum 1977;20(1):33–5.
21. Sitzler PJ, Thomson JP. Overlap repair of damaged anal sphincter. A single surgeon's series. Dis Colon Rectum 1996;39(12):1356–60.
22. Tjandra JJ, Han WR, Goh J, Carey M, Dwyer P. Direct repair vs. overlapping sphincter repair: a randomized, controlled trial. Dis Colon Rectum 2003;46(7):937–42.
23. Nessim A, Wexner SD, Agachan F, Alabaz O, Weiss EG, Nogueras JJ, Daniel N, Lee Billotti V. Is bowel confinement necessary after anorectal reconstructive surgery? A prospective, randomised, surgeon-blinded trial. Dis Colon Rectum 1999;42:16–23.
24. Fang DT, Nivatvongs S, Vermeulen FD, Herman Fn, Goldberg SM, Rothenberger DA. Overlapping sphincteroplasty for acquired anal incontinence. Dis Colon Rectum 1984;27:720–2.
25. Browning GG, Motson RW. Anal sphincter injury: management and results of Parks sphincter repair. Anal Surg 1984;58:703–10.

26. Ctercteko GC, Fazio VW, Jagelman DG, Lavery IC, Weakley FL, Melia M. Anal sphincter repair: a report of 60 cases and review of the literature. Aust N Z J Surg 1988;58:703–10.

27. Yoshioka K, Keighley MR. Sphincter repair for fecal incontinence. Dis Colon Rectum 1989;32:39–42.

28. Wexner SD, Marchetti F, Jagelman DG, Lavery IC, Weakley FL, Melia M. The role of sphincteroplasty for fecal incontinence reevaluated: a prospective physiologic and functional review. Dis Colon Rectum 1991;34:222–30.

29. Fleshman JW, Dreznik Z, Fry RD, Kodner IJ. Anal sphincter repair for obstetric injury: manometric evaluation of functional results. Dis Colon Rectum 1991;34:1061–7.

30. Engel AF, van Baal SJ, Brummelkamp WH. Late results of anterior sphincter placation for traumatic faecal incontinence. Eur J Surg 1994;160:633–6.

31. Londono-Schimmer EE, Garcia-Duperly R, Nicholls RJ, Ritchie JK, Hawley PR, Thomson JP. Overlapping anal sphincter repair for faecal incontinence due to sphincter trauma: five year follow-up functional results. Int J Colorectal Dis 1994;9:110–13.

32. Oliveira L, Pfeifer J, Wexner SD. Physiological and clinical outcome of anterior sphincteroplasty. Br J Surg 1996;83:502–5.

33. Nikiteas N, Korsgen S, Kumar D, Keighley MR. Audit of sphincter repair: factors associated with poor outcome. Dis Colon Rectum 1996;39:1164–70.

34. Karoui S, Leroi AM, Koning E, Menard JF, Michot F, Denis P. Results of sphincteroplasty in 86 patients with anal incontinence. Dis Colon Rectum 2000;43(6):813–20.

35. Halverson AL, Hull TL. Long-term outcome of overlapping anal sphincter repair. Dis Colon Rectum 2002;45(3):345–8.

36. Gutierrez A, Madoff RD, Lowry AC, Parker SC, Buie WD, Baxter NN. Long-term results of anterior sphincteroplasty. Dis Colon Rectum 2004;47:727–32.

37. Vaizey CJ, Phillips RKS. A twisted tale. Clinical Risk 2005;11:53–6.

12b
Surgical Management of Anal Incontinence Part B. Advanced Surgical Techniques

Steven D. Wexner and Susan M. Cera

12b.1   Introduction

Patients with severe faecal incontinence from anal trauma who are unresponsive to conservative measures can be divided into two broad categories of surgical approach. The first group includes those patients with an identifiable and isolated anatomic sphincter defect who can expect 70–80% short-term surgical success with overlapping sphincteroplasty.[1] However, the effects of overlapping sphincteroplasty appear to deteriorate with time. Five-year follow-up in 47 patients undergoing sphincteroplasty for obstetric-related trauma revealed a success rate of 57% with no need for further therapy, while 14% required further intervention.[2] In a second study involving 6 years of follow-up for sphincteroplasty patients, only 46% were continent of solid, liquid or gas, with only 14% admitting to complete continence.[3] Ten-year follow-up of 191 patients revealed 40% with some continence and only 6% with complete continence.[4] In this study, risk factors identified for long-term failure of overlapping sphincteroplasty included older age and those with poor results in the short term.

The second group is those patients without an isolated sphincter defect who have experienced extensive sphincter damage, muscle loss, or pudendal neuropathy not amenable to direct sphincter repair. Fortunately, due to the development of newer surgical techniques, these patients are not obligated to permanent stomas.

12b.2   Historical Perspective

In the first half of the century, patients who were not candidates for sphincter repair underwent sphincter reconstruction with muscle transpositions involving either the gluteus maximus or gracilis muscles. These techniques only met with moderate success since these static, striated muscle flaps were prone to fatigue with chronic contraction. The transposed muscle did not have any involuntary tone at rest, and patients had to perform awkward movements to achieve imperfect continence.

In the mid-1960s, postanal repair was developed in which a levatorplasty was performed posteriorly to theoretically restore the anorectal angle and lengthen the anal canal. Because of poor long-term success rates, it is of historical significance, though it remains an option for those patients in whom other interventions have failed and who wish to avoid a stoma.

In the 1980s, external stimulators were applied to muscle transpositions to create dynamic neosphincters with resting muscle tone. The low-frequency electrical stimulation provided by these stimulators transforms the skeletal muscle from fast-twitch fatigue-prone (type II) muscle fibres to slow-twitch fatigue-resistant (type I) muscle fibres. However, the procedure involves many components and requires technical expertise with a steep learning curve. Short-term results included an array of complications that proved to undermine the advantages. Consequently, the stimulator used in this procedure has been removed from the US market, though the procedure remains an option in several other countries including Europe and Canada.

In the 1990s, the artificial bowel sphincter was introduced, offering an alternative option in sphincter reconstruction. In addition, the development of other techniques including injection of submucosal beads (ACYST), radiofrequency (the SECCA procedure) and sacral nerve stimulation (SNS) serve to augment the native continence mechanism in those who do not require neosphincter construction. These techniques will now be described in more detail, beginning with the simplest procedures and progressing to the more complex and invasive techniques. The procedure is commercially available and is currently in use as an option in many patients.

12b.3 Injectable Bulking Agents

Many types of materials, including polytetrafluoroethylene, collagen and autologous fat, have been injected into the submucosa of the anal canal in an attempt to augment the native sphincter mechanism. The additional bulk provided by these materials increases the resistance to the passage of stool and allows for improved sensation and discrimination. More recently, a silicone-based product (Bioplastique) was studied in ten patients with anatomically disrupted or intact but weak internal anal sphincters.[5] While short-term results were good with a 70% success rate, the effects decreased rapidly with a rate of success of only 30% at 6 months.

Injections of a solution containing carbon-coated beads (ACYST; the name was changed recently to Durasphere FI; Carbon Medical Technologies, St Paul, MN, USA) appears to be most promising with respect to this type of treatment. The beads are suspended in a carbohydrate gel that is injected circumferentially in the submucosa of the upper anal canal and distal rectum. The technique is an office-based procedure that requires no sedation or local anaesthetic. A recent prospective, open-label trial study performed at our institution on 20 patients revealed no changes in anorectal physiology testing but significant

symptomatic improvement in faecal incontinence and quality-of-life scores in 75% of cases at 2 years.[6] A single complication of bead extravasation associated with pain was noted. Another study of 18 patients and more than 2 years of follow-up also revealed an improvement in incontinence, patient satisfaction, and several quality-of-life parameters.[7] This technique has proven to be a simple, safe, inexpensive, effective and ambulatory technique for the treatment of moderate to severe faecal incontinence, particularly for those who are poor surgical candidates. Currently, a prospective randomised trial involving our institution is underway.

12b.4 Radiofrequency Energy

The SECCA procedure (Secca System; Curon Medical Inc., Sunnyvale, CA, USA) involves the delivery of radiofrequency energy to the lower rectum and anal canal through a specially manufactured anoscope (Figure 12b.1). Intravenous sedation, local anaesthesia and prophylactic antibiotics are used for this outpatient procedure, which can be performed in the endoscopy suite or the operating room. The device is positioned under direct visualisation at the dentate line and

FIGURE 12b.1. SECCA procedure. The specially manufactured anoscope is positioned under direct visualisation at the dentate line and four needle electrodes deliver the radiofrequency energy for 90 seconds.

four needle electrodes deliver the radiofrequency energy for 90 seconds. Additional applications in all four quadrants are administered in 5-mm increments proximal to the dentate line for a total of 16 application sites. Recent publication of a multicentre prospective trial revealed the procedure to be safe, minimally invasive, low risk and effective, with a significant therapeutic impact on the symptoms of faecal incontinence and quality of life.[8] Procedure-specific complications were minimal and included anoderm ulcerations and bleeding. A prospective, randomised, blinded, sham-controlled trial is currently underway.

12b.5 Artificial Bowel Sphincter

Augmentation of the sphincter with a prosthetic device was first reported for faecal incontinence in 1992[9] after the idea was borrowed from urology, where artificial sphincters are used for urinary incontinence. The current device used for faecal incontinence, the Acticon Neosphincter (American Medical Systems, MN, USA), consists of three silastic components: an inflatable cuff, a pressure-regulating balloon, and a control pump that allows activation or deactivation of the device (Figure 12b.2). The inflatable cuff is implanted around the anus and is connected by silastic tubing to the control pump placed in the scrotum of males or in the labium major of females. The control pump is also connected to the pressure-regulating balloon implanted in the space of Retzius. When activated, the cuff is distended and the anus is occluded. The pressure-regulating balloon maintains the cuff pressure. To defaecate, the patient compresses the control pump several times, and the fluid is displaced out of the cuff and into the regulating balloon.

After having undergone a mechanical and antibiotic bowel preparation and rectal irrigation with an iodine solution, the artificial sphincter is placed in the patient, who is under general anaesthesia in the lithotomy position. Attention is paid to prevention of contact of the silastic components with lint and powder as these materials tend to adhere easily, with potential for contribution to infection. Either through an anterior perineal incision or bilateral perianal incisions, blunt dissection is employed to create the circumferential tunnel

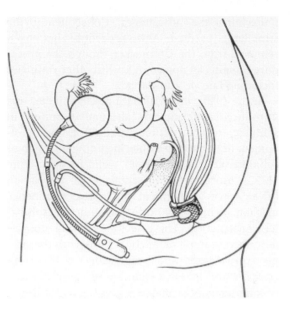

Figure 12b.2. Artificial bowel sphincter. The Acticon Neosphincter (American Medical Systems, MN, USA) consists of three silastic components: an inflatable cuff, a pressure-regulating balloon, and a control pump that allows activation or deactivation of the device. The inflatable cuff is implanted around the anus and is connected by silastic tubing to the control pump placed in the labium major of females. The control pump is also connected to the pressure-regulating balloon implanted in the space of Retzius. (The Acticon Neosphincter™ Courtesy of American Medical Systems Inc., Minnefoka Minnesota, www.AmericanMedicalSystem.com)

around the anal canal several centimetres deep in the ischiorectal fossa. The occlusive cuff is appropriately sized and placed with the connection tubing on the same side as the patent's dominant hand. A suprapubic incision is made and the pressure-regulating balloon placed in the space of Retzius. Blunt dissection creates a dependent pouch in the scrotum or labia into which the control pump is placed. The tubings are connected but the device is left deactivated for the first 6 weeks postoperatively.

The Acticon Neosphincter received Food and Drug Administration (FDA) approval in 1999. A recent, multicentre, non-randomised trial revealed the device to have a significant rate of clinical success (85%), enhancement in quality of life, and a high degree of safety.[10] Results of other studies have displayed similar good success rates of 47–90% (Table 12b.1).[11–20] However, like the stimulated graciloplasty (described below), limitations in use of this technique are related to the high rate

TABLE 12b.1. Outcome of the artificial bowel sphincter (Acticon).

Author/year	Patients	Follow-up (months)	Morbidity (%) explant/reimplant	Device	Success (%)
Wong et al. 1996[11]	12	58	33	–	75
Lehur et al. 1998[12]	13	30	18	4/2	67
Vaizey et al. 1998[13]	6	10	30	1/0	83
Christiansen et al. 1999[14]	17	84	33	7/0	47
O'Brien and Skinner 2000[15]	13	–	61	3/0	69
Lehur et al. 2000[16]	24	20	29	7/3	75
Altomare et al. 2001[17]	28	19	32	7/2	66
Devesa et al. 2002[18]	53	–	69	– 65	
Michot et al. 2003[19]	37	–	37	11/2	78
Casal et al. 2004[20]	10	29	60	3/2	90

of complications, most of which are related to infections of the foreign material with subsequent need for surgical revision. Other complications are related to erosion of the components into adjacent structures or device malfunction, with a device explant rate of 36%.[10] Morbidity related to the complications ranges from 18 to 69% (Table 12b.1).[11–20] The cost and the morbidity from this device and the stimulated graciloplasty are approximately the same. In a recent prospective comparison of eight cases of stimulated gracilo-plasty and eight implantations of the artificial bowel sphincter followed over 3 years, there was no difference in complications, wound healing problems or explantation rates, though the artificial bowel sphincter was found to be more effective in lowering the faecal incontinence score.[21] Nonetheless, this remains an important alternative for patients with end-stage faecal incontinence when no other surgical or medical options exist except stoma. At this point, long-term studies are still needed to determine the longevity of the device.

12b.6 Bilateral Unstimulated Gluteoplasty

Advantages of the gluteus maximus muscle include its large muscle bulk, single proximal innervation, and proximity to the anal canal. In addition, buttock contraction is a standard response to impending incontinence. In the prone jack-knife position, the lower 10% of both of the gluteus maximus muscles and fascia are mobil-ised from their origins on the ileum and sacrum and distally freed in two strips (Figure 12b.3). The

neurovascular bundle is preserved where it arises near the ischial tuberosity. The two strips on each side are tunnelled beneath the skin and secured to their contralateral counterparts through lateral incisions on the contralateral sides of the anus.

Although not as popular as the gracilo-plasty, this operation has been performed with variable results. Pearl and coworkers performed bilateral non-stimulated gluteoplasty without diversion in seven patients, with excellent results in six.[22] In contrast, Christiansen et al. reported poor results, as none of their seven patients were continent to liquid and only three were continent to solid.[23] Most recently, Devesa et al.[24] reported the largest

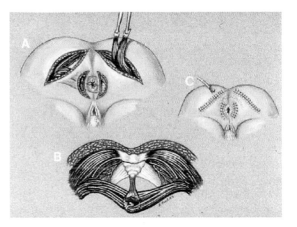

FIGURE 12b.3. Bilateral unstimulated gluteoplasty. The lower 10% of both of the gluteus maximus muscles and fascia are mobil-ised from their origins on the ileum and sacrum and distally freed in two strips. The two strips on each side are tunnelled beneath the skin and secured to their contralateral counterparts through lateral incisions on the contralateral sides of the anus. (Peat RK, Prasad ML, Nelson RL, Orsay CP, Abcarran H. Bilateral gluteus maximus transposition for anal incontinence. Dis Colon Rectum 1991; 34(6):478–81. With kind permission of Springer Science+Business Media.)

TABLE 12b.2. Outcome of bilateral unstimulated gluteoplasty.

Author/year	Patients	Good results	Fair results	Poor results
Chetwood 1902[26]	1	1	–	–
Schoemaker 1909[27]	6	6	–	–
Bistrom 1944[28]	3	2	1	–
Bruining et al. 1981[29]	1	1	–	–
Prochiantz and Gross 1982[30]	15	9	1	5
Hentz 1982[31]	5	1	–	1
Skef et al. 1983[32]	1	4	–	–
Iwai et al. 1985[33]	1	1	–	–
Chen and Zhang 1987[34]	6	3	1	2
Onishi et al. 1989[35]	1	1	–	–
Pearl et al. 1991[36]	7	4	2	1
Christiansen et al. 1995[23]	7	0	3	4
Devesa et al. 1992[25]	17	9	1	7

clinical experience to date with only moderate results. Only nine of the 17 patients who underwent bilateral non-stimulated gluteoplasty achieved normal control.[24] The morbidity of this procedure is exclusively related to wound infection of the perianal wounds.[22–24] While unilateral gluteoplasty has been described,[25] better muscle bulk and more equivalent distribution of tensile forces are created with bilateral gluteal muscle transpositions. Despite the wide variability in results, this technique continues to be an option over colostomy in patients with severe faecal incontinence. The results of unstimulated gluteoplasty are shown in Table 12b.2.

12b.7   Stimulated Graciloplasty

The technique of stimulated graciloplasty involves the transposition of the gracilis muscle from the thigh to form a skeletal muscular ring around the anus with the distal portion anchored to the contralateral ischial tuberosity (Figure 12b.4). Two phases are employed in this procedure, with the number of required operations dependent on the use of an optional stoma. Phase I consists of transposition of the muscle and implantation of the stimulator and the electrodes. Phase II involves 8 weeks of muscle conditioning with increasing levels of neuromuscular stimulation. The use of diverting stoma requires additional operative intervention for creation and closure. Upon completion of phase II, the patient is able to control continence with the use of an external magnet.

The patient can switch the neurostimulator on, causing the muscle to contract, and off, causing the muscle to relax.

The Dynamic Graciloplasty Therapy Study Group has been instrumental in providing the largest prospective multicentre data with regard to the outcome of this procedure. The initial report on the efficacy revealed improvement in continence and quality of life in the majority (60%) of patients.[37] Long-term efficacy reported in a separate study revealed the 62% success rate and improvements in functional and quality-of-life variables, which persisted for 2 years.[38]

While many studies proved the efficacy of stimulated graciloplasty, concern arose about the high rates of complications and need for reoperation. In the original study by the Dynamic Graciloplasty Therapy Study Group, the complication and reoperative rates were 74% and 40% respectively.[37] Other studies have also revealed high rates of infection, hardware failure and postoperative evacuatory dysfunction. In a single institution study of 17 patients with a mean age of 42 performed at Cleveland Clinic, Florida, complications included lead fibrosis, seroma of the thigh incision, excoriation of the skin above the stimulator, faecal impaction, anal fissure, parastomal hernia, rotation of the stimulator, premature battery discharge, fracture of the lead, perineal skin irritation, perineal sepsis, rupture of the tendon, tendon erosion, muscle fatigue during

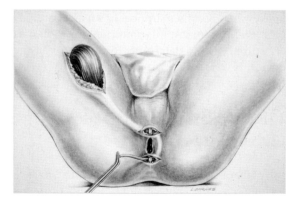

FIGURE 12b.4. Stimulated graciloplasty. The technique of stimulated graciloplasty involves the transposition of the gracilis muscle from the thigh to form a skeletal muscular ring around the anus with the distal portion anchored to the contralateral ischial tuberosity. (Cormal ML, Colon and Rectal Surgery, 3rd ed. Lippincott williams and Wilkins, 1993: 234.)

TABLE 12b.3. Outcome of stimulated graciloplasty.

Author/year	Patients	Follow-up (months)	Morbidity (%)	Revisional surgery (%)	Success (%)
Christiansen 1998[41]	13	17	–	–	84
Sielezneff et al. 1999[42]	16	20	50	44	81
Mavrantonis et al. 1999[43]	21 IM	21	–	–	93
	6 DS	12.5			10
Mander et al. 1999[44]	64	10	38	–	56
Madoff et al. 1999[45]	128	26	41	–	66
Baeten et al. 2000[37]	123	12	74	40	60
Konsten et al. 2001[46]	200 IM	–	–	3	74
	81 DS			26	57
Bresler et al. 2002[47]	24	–	42	46	79
Wexner et al. 2002[38]	129	24	–	–	62
Rongen et al. 2003[48]	200	72	–	69	72
Penninckx et al. 2004[49]	60	53	77	77	61

IM Intramuscular placement of the lead, *DS* direct stimulation of the lead on the nerve.

programming sessions, electrode displacement from the nerve and fibrosis around the nerve.[39] Some of these complications led to stoma creation or death. Consequently, the Dynamic Graciloplasty Therapy Study Group investigated the aetiology and impact of these complications.[40] In this report, 211 complications occurred in 93 cases of dynamic graciloplasty. Forty-two per cent had severe complications, though recovery was achieved in 92%. Of all the complications, only major infections adversely affected outcome, leading the authors to conclude that although the complication rate was high, most of the complications were treatable and did not adversely affect outcome. Other series report a success rate of 57–93% with a morbidity rate of 38–50% and a rate of revisional surgery of 3–69% (Table 12b.3). Because of the complexity of the procedure and the high rate of complications, the stimulator device has been removed from the US market, though it remains a viable option in other countries. Currently in the USA, gracilis transpositions are being used to augment sphincter mass prior to placement of the artificial bowel sphincter in those patients with significant muscle loss from trauma or from congenital atresia.[50]

12b.8 Sacral Nerve Stimulation

Sacral nerve stimulation (Figure 12b.5) is the most widely published "new" technique for the restoration of faecal incontinence. The technology has been adopted from urology practices in which external electrical stimulators are applied to the sacral nerve plexus for the management of urinary incontinence. Early results revealed those patients with faecal incontinence in addition to bladder dysfunction had improvement in both symptoms. The use of this technique solely for faecal incontinence was first described in 1995 by Matzel et al.[51] Since then it has been performed in several

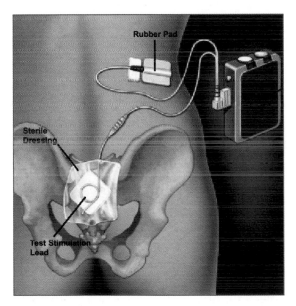

FIGURE 12b.5. Sacral nerve stimulation involves the placement of an electrical stimulator on the nerves of the sacral plexus (see text for details). (Reprinted with the permission of Medtronic Inc. © 2006.)

hundred patients in Europe but is currently under FDA investigation in the USA.

To be a candidate, a patient must have an intact sphincter without substantial defects or loss of muscle, reduced or absent sphincter function (assessed by anal manometry), and intact residual reflex function (confirmed by pudendal stimulation) demonstrating an intact nerve–muscle connection. Those patients with sphincter defects may undergo SNS after sphincteroplasty if incontinence remains problematic. In addition, candidates may also be patients with diarrhoea in whom any colidities and obstruction have been eliminated if their diarrhoea can be controlled with medical management. The procedure involves two stages separated by a 2-week period, each of which involves a visit to the operating room. The first stage consists of peripheral nerve evaluation (the diagnostic stage) and the second stage entails placement of the permanent stimulator (the therapeutic stage). Peripheral nerve evaluation (PNE) of the sacral roots (S2, S3, S4) is also divided into two phases: an acute phase to test the functional integrity of each spinal nerve to striated anal sphincter function and a chronic phase to assess the therapeutic potential of sacral spinal nerve stimulation in individual patients. For PNE, the patient is given intravenous sedation and placed in the prone position. The sacral foramina are located by identifying bony landmarks under fluoroscopy. The acute phase test is conducted by placing a 20-gauge spinal insulated needle (Medtronic Inc., Minneapolis, MN, USA) attached to an external neurostimulator (Medtronic Inc.)

into the S2-S4 foramina. An electrical current is gradually applied to the needle until a visual muscle response is obtained. Muscle responses include movement of the external sphincter and lateral rotation of the leg (S2), contraction of pelvic floor and plantar flexion of the big toe (S3), or contraction of the anus (S4). The chronic phase of PNE involves placement of a temporary stimulator lead into the same position as the testing needle. This lead is secured to a temporary stimulator placed beneath the skin of the upper buttock region and left in place for a trial period of 1–2 weeks, during which the patient records a bowel diary to allow evaluation of functional response. The decision to proceed from temporary to permanent stimulation is made on the basis of 50% functional improvement in either the number of incontinence episodes, or the number of incontinence-free days.

For placement of the permanent stimulator, the patient is again placed in the prone position. The previous scar in the upper buttocks area is opened and the temporary stimulator removed. A permanent stimulator is placed in a subcutaneous pocket and the wound reclosed. Perioperative antibiotics are continued for 24 hours for each of the procedures.

Relatively few studies have been published to date (Table 12b.4) and comparison between them is complicated by varying faecal incontinence scoring systems. However, the results reveal remarkable improvement over short and long terms. In addition, SNS clearly improved quality of life.[55,58] Failure rate is approximately 12–22%;

TABLE 12b.4. Outcome of sacral nerve stimulation.

Author	Patients	Permanent stimulator	Follow-up (months)	Score	Improvement
Malouf et al. 2000[52]	5	5	16	Wexner	16 to 2
Ganio et al. 2001[53]	16	16	16	Williams	4.1 to 1.2
Matzel et al. 2001[54]	6	6	5–66	Wexner	17 to 2
Rosen et al. 2001[55]	20	16	15	FI episodes	6 to 2
Leroi et al. 2001[56]	6	6	6	FI episodes	4.8 to 2.3
Ripetti et al. 2002[57]	4	4	15	Wexner	12.2 to 9.8
Kenefik et al. 2002[58]	15	15	24	FI episodes/week	11 to 0
Rasmussen et al. 2004[59]	45	37	6	Wexner	16 to 6
Jarrett et al. 2004[60]	46	59	12	FI episodes/week	7.4 to 1
Matzel et al. 2004[61]	37	34	24	FI episodes/week	16.4 to 2
Uludag et al. 2004[62]	75	–	12	FI episodes/week	7.5 to 0.7

FI Fecal incontinence.

and the overall complication rate of permanent implantation is 5–10%.[58] These complications consist mainly of pain at the site of the pulse generator, electrode migration and infection.

Patients with faecal incontinence from a wide variety of causes have been treated successfully, including: those with deficits resulting from anal or rectal procedures, obstetric or neurologic trauma, scleroderma, systemic sclerosis, primary internal anal sphincter degeneration, and even sphincter disruption. The exact mechanism of action is unknown; however, the sacral nerve roots are the most proximal point of the combined dual nerve supply, somatic and autonomic, to the pelvic floor and anal sphincter mechanism. External stimulation of these nerves augments the input to the native mechanical apparatus, which consists of the muscular architecture (muscles of the sphincter and pelvic floor) and its associated system of neural connections that modulate muscular contraction, reflexes and the intrinsic nervous system. The effect is not only direct efferent stimulation of the muscles of the pelvic floor and sphincter, but also modulation of the afferent neural pathways involved in the internal anal sphincter, rectal relaxation and sacral reflexes. These neural pathways are ultimately responsible for rectal sensation, motility and the smooth coordination of defaecation.

Sacral nerve stimulation has many potential advantages over sphincter repairs, reconstruction and replacement. The main advantage is that it is minimally invasive since it involves placement of electrodes at a proximal source of the nerve supply with no manipulation of the rectum, anus or pelvic floor. Consequently, it has a low complication rate, and the need for discontinuation of treatment is rare. Revisions, repeat surgeries and removal of the apparatus do not necessarily obligate the patient to a stoma since the stimulation device can be reimplanted if temporary removal is necessary. Other advantages include the ability to perform the temporary stimulation phase as a screening method prior to permanent electrode placement, the absence of required bowel preparation, the performance of procedures in an outpatient setting, the lack of decline in efficacy over an 8-year period, and the use in a variety of causes of faecal incontinence. Despite the fact that the exact mechanism of action remains to be eluci-

dated, satisfying clinical results have been achieved with this technique. It is an exciting treatment option in a population in which conservative measures have failed and traditional surgical approaches are conceptually questionable, have limited success, or are considered too high risk. The North America trial of 120 patients is nearing completion, after which the procedure will hopefully become available in the United States.

12b.9 Stoma

Severe faecal incontinence refractory to conservative management and/or previous surgical intervention may be best treated by a well-functioning stoma. A stoma may be preferentially offered as an initial procedure to patients with psychiatric disorders or who are bed-ridden to facilitate hygiene and care. The laparoscopic approach is the preferential technique used at our institution for stoma creation.

12b.10 Choosing a Technique

The recent development of multiple surgical techniques for faecal incontinence offers physicians and patients a variety of options for treatment. Choosing the appropriate therapy is based on the patient risk factors, aetiology of the incontinence, procedure-specific contraindications and associated pelvic floor deficits (Figure 12b.6).

Patient risk factors for surgery play an important role in choosing a procedure. The least invasive are the injectable procedures, which can be performed during an office visit and are ideal for those patients who are poor surgical candidates or refuse more invasive techniques. The SECCA procedure is also minimally invasive but requires anaesthesia. The ACYST and SECCA have a very low risk of complications and do not preclude the subsequent use of other techniques that can be employed in the case of their failure. The artificial bowel sphincter is an invasive procedure reserved for those in whom other techniques have failed and requires a motivated and otherwise healthy patient who is physically fit for possible multiple surgical revisions. It has a high rate of complications, is usually reserved as a last resort, and

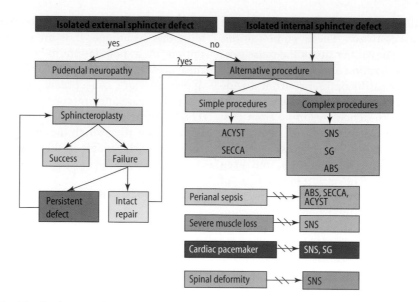

Figure 12b.6. Algorithm for the surgical approach to the management of faecal incontinence. *ACYST* Carbon-coated bead injection, *SECCA* radiofrequency procedure, *SNS* sacral nerve stimulation, *ABS* artificial bowel sphincter, *SG* stimulated graciloplasty.

failure of this technique usually obligates that patient to a stoma.

Another patient factor that needs consideration prior to choice of therapy is mental capacity with respect to the more complicated techniques. The SNS, stimulated graciloplasty and artificial bowel sphincter procedures require patients with the cognitive ability to understand the technique, incorporation into daily life, maintenance of the components, and potential complications and failure. In addition, those who undergo the stimulated graciloplasty and artificial bowel sphincter should be prepared for possible repeat surgical interventions. Therefore, those with psychiatric conditions or emotional instability may not be suitable for these high-maintenance procedures and are probably better candidates for either the ACYST or SECCA procedure, which do not require routine maintenance or follow-up.

Aetiology is important to the consideration of the type of therapy chosen. The ACYST and SECCA procedures do not attempt to correct the underlying aetiology of the incontinence. Instead, these procedures involve augmenting the resistance of faecal passage by bulking or tightening the mucosa of the anal canal and rectum. Consequently, these techniques can be employed in all

forms of faecal incontinence, but are more effective in milder forms. Sacral nerve stimulation has also been used in patients who display a variety of causes of faecal incontinence, but requires adequate neuromuscular architecture demonstrated on electromyography and pudendal nerve testing. Patients with severe neuropathy (absent bilateral pudendal motor latencies) or significant deficits/ loss of sphincter muscle may not be amenable to SNS and are better candidates for sphincter replacement with the artificial bowel sphincter.

Procedure-specific contraindications relate to the safety in performing the procedures in certain situations or in the placing of the artificial components. The presence of associated anorectal pathology precludes choice of the ACYST, SECCA and artificial bowel sphincter procedures since they all involve direct manipulation of the anus and rectum. Perianal disease (i.e. fistulas, fissures, abscesses, inflammatory bowel disease, perianal infections, anorectal carcinoma) and local radiation are contraindications to these procedures because of the inherently high risk of infectious complications. In contrast, contraindications to SNS include sacral diseases, such as spina bifida or sacral agenesis, cauda equina syndrome, or skin pathology at the site of electrode placement.

Patients with a cardiac pacemaker or an implantable defibrillator cannot undergo SNS or the stimulated graciloplasty because of the obvious interference of the electrical stimulators.

Finally, some patients with faecal incontinence have associated pelvic floor dysfunction in the form of concomitant urinary incontinence. These patients may benefit most from SNS since it has been shown to improve both of these impairments as opposed to the placement of separate urinary and bowel sphincters.

12b.11 Conclusion

Patients with faecal incontinence with an isolated, identifiable, traumatic sphincter defect are candidates for overlapping sphincteroplasty. Those patients without an isolated defect are candidates for other interventions. Simple therapies include injectable bulking agents and the SECCA procedure. More complex procedures include SNS, stimulated gracioplasty and the artificial bowel sphincter. Each offers advantages and disadvantages that can be used to tailor specific treatments to individual needs. Choice of procedure is dependent on aetiology of the incontinence, patient comorbid status, physician experience and resource availability. Fortunately, most patients with faecal incontinence can avoid a stoma.

References

1. Oliveira L, Wexner SD. Anal incontinence. In: Beck DE, Wexner SD, eds. Fundamentals of anorectal surgery, 2nd edn. Philadelphia: WB Saunders, 1998, pp 136–52.
2. Malouf AJ, Norton CS, Engel AE, Nicholls RJ, Kamm MA. Long-term results of overlapping anterior anal-sphincter repair for obstetric trauma. Lancet 2000;355:260–2.
3. Halverson AL, Hull TL. Long-term outcome of overlapping anal sphincter repair. Dis Colon Rectum 2002;45:345–8.
4. Bravo Gutierrez A, Madoff RD, Lowry AC, Parker SC, Buie WD, Baxter NN. Long-term results of anterior sphincteroplasty. Dis Colon Rectum 2004;47:727–31.
5. Kenefik NJ, Vaizey CJ, Malouf AJ et al. Injectable silicone biomaterial for fecal incontinence due to internal anal sphincter dysfunction. Gut 2002;51: 225–8.
6. Weiss EG, Effron JE, Nogueras JJ, Wexner SD. Submucosal injection of carbon coated beads is a successful and safe office-based treatment for fecal incontinence [meeting abstract]. Dis Colon Rectum 2002;45:A46–7.
7. Davis K, Kumar D, Poloniecki J. Preliminary evaluation of an injectable anal sphincter bulking agent (Durasphere) in the management of faecal incontinence. Aliment Pharmacol Ther 2003;18; 237–43.
8. Efron JE, Corman ML, Fleshman J et al. Safety and effectiveness of temperature-controlled radiofrequency energy delivery to the anal canal (Secca procedure) for the treatment of fecal incontinence. Dis Colon Rectum 2003;46:1606–18.
9. Christiansen J, Sparso B. Treatment of anal incontinence by implantable prosthetic anal sphincter. Ann Surg 1992;215:383–6.
10. Wong WD, Cogliosi SM, Spencer MP et al. The safety and efficacy of the artificial bowel sphincter for fecal incontinence: results from a multicenter cohort study. Dis Colon Rectum 2002;45:1139–53.
11. Wong WD, Jensen LL, Bartolo DC, Rothenberger DA. Artificial anal sphincter. Dis Colon Rectum 1996;39:1345–51.
12. Lehur PA, Glemain P, Bruley des Varannes S et al. Outcome of patients with an implanted artificial anal sphincter for severe fecal incontinence. A single institution report. Int J Colorectal Dis 1998; 13:88–92.
13. Vaizey CJ, Kamm MA, Gold DM et al. Clinical, physiological, and radiological study of a new purpose-designed artificial bowel sphincter. Lancet 1998;352:105–9.
14. Christiansen J, Rasmussen OO, Lindorff-Larsen K. Long-term results of the artificial anal sphincter implantation for severe anal incontinence. Ann Surg 1999;230:45–8.
15. O'Brien PE, Skinner S. Restoring control: the Acticon Neosphincter artificial bowel sphincter in the treatment of anal incontinence. Dis Colon Rectum 2000;43;1213–16.
16. Lehur PA, Roig JV, Duinslaeger M. Artificial anal sphincter: prospective clinical and manometric evaluation. Dis Colon Rectum 2000;43:1100–6.
17. Altomare DF, Dodi G, La Torre F et al. Multicentre retrospective analysis of the outcome of artificial anal sphincter implantation for severe faecal incontinence. Br J Surg 2001;88:1481–6.
18. Devesa JM, Rey A, Hervas PL et al. Artificial anal sphincter: complications and functional results of a large personal series. Dis Colon Rectum 2002;45: 1145–63.

19. Michot F, Costaglioli B, Leroi AM. Artificial anal sphincter in severe fecal incontinence: outcome of prospective experience with 37 patients in 1 institution. Ann Surg 2003;237:52–6.

20. Casal E, San Ildefonso A, Carracedo R et al. Artificial bowel sphincter in severe anal incontinence. Colorectal Dis 2004;6:180–4.

21. Ortiz H, Armendariz P, DeMiguel M et al. Prospective study of artificial anal sphincter and dynamic graciloplasty for severe anal incontinence. Int J Colorect Dis 2003;18:349–54.

22. Pearl RK, Prasad ML, Nelson RL et al. Bilateral gluteus maximus transposition for anal incontinence. Dis Colon Rectum 1991;34:478–81.

23. Christiansen J, Ronholt Hansen C et al. Bilateral gluteus maximus transposition for anal incontinence. Br J Surg 1995;82:903–5.

24. Devesa JM, Fernandez Madrid JM, Rodriguez Gallego B et al. Bilateral gluteoplasty for fecal incontinence. Dis Colon Rectum 1997;40:883–8.

25. Devesa JM, Vicente E, Enriquez JM et al. Total fecal incontinence: a new method of gluteus maximus transposition. Preliminary results and report of previous experience with similar procedures. Dis Colon Rectum 1992;35:339.

26. Chetwood CH. Plastic operation for restoration of the sphincter ani with report of a case. Med Rec 1902;61:529.

27. Schoemaker J. Un nouveau procede operatoire pour la reconstitution du sphincter anal. Sem Med 1909;29:160.

28. Bistrom O. Plastische Ersatz des M. sphincter ani. Acta Chir Scand 1944;90:431–48.

29. Bruining HA, Bos KE, Colthoff EG, Tolhurst DE. Creation of an anal sphincter mechanism by bilateral proximally based gluteal muscle transposition. Plast Reconstr Surg 1981;67:70–3.

30. Prochiantz A, Gross P. Gluteal myoplasty for sphincter replacement: principles, results and prospects. J Pediatr Surg 1982;17:25–30.

31. Hentz VR. Construction of a rectal sphincter using the origin of gluteus maximum muscle. Plast Reconstr Surg 1982;70:82–5.

32. Skef Z, Radhakrishnan J, Reyes HM. Anorectal continence following sphincter reconstruction utilizing the gluteus maximus muscle: a case report. J Pediatr Surg 1983;18:779–81.

33. Iwai N, Kaneda H, Tsuto T, Yanagihara J, Takahashi T. Objective assessment of anorectal function after sphincter reconstruction using the gluteus maximus muscle. Report of a case. Dis Colon Rectum 1985;28:973–7.

34. Chen YL, Zhang XH. Reconstruction of rectal sphincter by transposition of gluteus muscle for fetal incontinence. J Pediatr Surg 1987;22:62–4.

35. Onishi K, Maruyama Y, Shiba T. A wrap-around procedure using the gluteus maximus muscle for the functional reconstruction of the sphincter in a case of anal incontinence. Acta Chir Plast 1989; 31:56–63.

36. Pearl RK, Prasad ML, Nelson RL, Orsay CP, Abcarian H. Bilateral gluteus maximus transposition for anal incontinence. Dis Colon Rectum 1991;34: 478–81.

37. Baeten CG, Bailey HR, Bakka A et al. Safety and efficacy of dynamic graciloplasty for fecal incontinence: report of a prospective, multicenter trial. Dynamic Graciloplasty Therapy Study Group. Dis Colon Rectum 2000;43:743–51.

38. Wexner SD, Baeten CMGI, Bailey R et al. Long-term efficacy of dynamic graciloplasty for fecal incontinence. Dis Colon Rectum 2002;45:809–18.

39. Wexner SD, Gonzalez-Padron A, Rius J et al. Stimulated gracilis neosphincter operation. Initial experience, pitfalls, and complications. Dis Colon Rectum 1996;39:957–64.

40. Matzel KE, Madoff RD, LaFontaine LJ et al. Dynamic Graciloplasty Therapy Study Group. Complications of dynamic graciloplasty: incidence, management, and impact on outcome. Dis Colon Rectum 2001;44:1427–35.

41. Christiansen J. Dynamic graciloplasty. Int J Surg Invest 1999;1:267–8.

42. Sielezneff I, Malouf AJ, Bartolo DC et al. Dynamic graciloplasty in the treatment of patients with faecal incontinence. Br J Surg 1999;86:61–5.

43. Mavrantonis C, Billotti VL, Wexner SD. Stimulated graciloplasty for treatment of intractable fecal incontinence: critical influence of the method of stimulation. Dis Colon Rectum 1999;42:497–504.

44. Mander BJ, Wexner SD, Williams NS et al. Preliminary results of a multicenter trial of the electrically stimulated gracilis neoanal sphincter. Br J Surg 1999;86:1543–9.

45. Madoff RD, Rosen HR, Baeten CG et al. Safety and efficacy of dynamic muscle plasty for anal incontinence: lessons from a prospective, multicenter trial. Gastroenterology 1999;116:549–56.

46. Konsten J, Rongen MJ, Ogunbiyi OA et al. Comparison of epineural and intramuscular nerve electrodes for stimulated graciloplasty. Dis Colon Rectum 2001;44:581–6.

47. Bresler L, Reibel N, Brunaud L et al. Dynamic graciloplasty in the treatment of severe fecal incontinence. French multicentric retrospective study. Ann Chir 2002;127:520–6.

48. Rongen MJ, Uludag O, El Naggar K et al. Long-term follow-up of dynamic graciloplasty for fecal incontinence. Dis Colon Rectum 2003;46:716–21.

49. Penninckx F; Belgian Section of Colorectal Surgery. Belgian experience with dynamic graciloplasty for faecal incontinence. Br J Surg 2004;91:872–8.

50. da Silva GM, Jorge JM, Belin B et al. New surgical options for fecal incontinence in patients with imperforate anus. Dis Colon Rectum 2004;47: 204–9.

51. Matzel KE, Stadelmaier U, Hohenfellner M et al. Electrical stimulation of the sacral spinal nerves for treatment of fecal incontinence. Lancet 1995; 346:1124–7.

52. Malouf AJ, Vaizey CJ, Nicholls RJ, Kamm MA. Permanent sacral nerve stimulation for fecal incontinence. Ann Surg 2000;232:143–8.

53. Ganio E, Luc AR, Clerico G, Trompetto M. Sacral nerve stimulation for treatment of fecal incontinence: a novel approach for intractable fecal incontinence. Dis Colon Rectum 2001;44:619–31.

54. Matzel KE, Stadelmaier U, Hohenfellner M et al. Chronic sacral spinal nerve stimulation for fecal incontinence: long term results with foramen and cuff electrodes. Dis Colon Rectum 2001;44:59–66.

55. Rosen H, Urbarz C, Holzer B, Novi G, Schiessel R. Sacral nerve stimulation as a treatment for neurogenic and idiopathic fecal incontinence. Gastroenterology 2001;121:536–41.

56. Leroi AM, Michot F, Grise P et al. Effect of sacral nerve stimulation in patients with fecal and urinary incontinence. Dis Colon Rectum 2001; 44:779–89.

57. Ripetti V, Caputo D, Ausania F et al. Sacral nerve neuromodulation improves physical, psychological and social quality of life in patients with fecal incontinence. Techniques Coloproctol 2002;6: 147–52.

58. Kefenik NJ, Vaizey RCG, Cohen RJ et al. Medium-term results of permanent sacral nerve stimulation for fecal incontinence. Br J Surg 2002;89:896–901.

59. Rasmussen OO, Buntzen S, Sorensen M et al. Sacral nerve stimulation in fecal incontinence. Dis Colon Rectum 2004;47:1158–63.

60. Jarrett MED, Varma JS, Duthie GS et al. Sacral nerve stimulation for faecal incontinence in the UK. Br J Surg 2004;91:755–61.

61. Matzel KE, Kamm MA, Stosser M et al. Sacral spinal nerve stimulation for faecal incontinence: multicentre study. Lancet 2004;363:1270–6.

62. Uludag O, Koch SM, van Gemert WG et al. Sacral neuromodulation in patients with fecal incontinence: a single-center study. Dis Colon Rectum 2004;47:1350–7.

13
Rectovaginal Fistulas

Rebecca G. Rogers and Dee E. Fenner

13.1   Introduction

There are few afflictions unattended with danger to life, which give rise to greater anxiety or produce more disagreeable results than cases of rectovaginal fistula.[1]

T.H. Tanner, 1855

Rectovaginal fistula is defined as a communication between the rectum and the vagina. Although relatively rare, the impact on quality of life of patients may be profound. Causes include traumatic, congenital, inflammatory, neoplastic and iatrogenic processes (see Table 13.1). While estimates vary, the most common cause of rectovaginal fistulas is thought to be secondary obstetrical complications, followed by inflammatory and neoplastic disorders.[2-4] Fistulas that occur as a result of congenital malformations are beyond the scope of discussion in this chapter. Only the presentation and repair of acquired fistulas with particular emphasis on fistulas that occur as a result of obstetrical trauma will be presented.

The majority of fistulas are not true rectovaginal fistulas but rather inflammatory tracts from the rectum and perineum that result from either infected anal glands or inflammatory bowel disease. Collectively, rectovaginal fistulas represent less than 5% of all fistulas.[5-7]

Inflammatory anorectal fistulas that tract into the vagina can become rectovaginal fistulas once the inflammation has resolved. Processes that cause these types of rectovaginal fistulas include inflammatory bowel disease, particularly Crohn's disease, as well as infections of the anorectal region.[3] Inflammatory fistulas can also occur as a result of a vaginal delivery. Typically, these fistulas are lined with inflammatory tissue, are painful on palpation and associated with a purulent discharge.[7] These inflammatory fistulas are collectively termed fistula-in-ano.

Of particular importance to the practising obstetrician and gynaecologist are rectovaginal fistulas that occur as a complication of either vaginal birth or gynaecologic surgeries. Whenever a postpartum or post-gynaecological surgery patient presents with complaints of faecal or flatal incontinence, rectovaginal fistula should be included in the differential diagnosis. Healed fistulas of obstetrical or gynaecologic origin are epithelial lined communications between the rectum and/or anus and the vaginal canal.

13.2   Historical Background

Obstetrical fistulas have plagued women for millennia, as proven by the discovery of a large fistula in a mummy of an ancient Egyptian woman. Avicenna, an Arabo-Persian physician, was the first to describe fistulas as a result of difficult labours.[8] The history of the surgical treatment of rectovaginal fistulas lies in the evolution of the treatment of vesicovaginal fistulas. The first attempts at surgical repairs of fistulas were of vesicovaginal fistulas and made by H. van Roonhuyse in 1676, who placed patients in lithotomy, exposed the fistula with a speculum and denuded the edges of the fistula before suturing it together.[9] The first cure of a rectovaginal fistula is credited to Barton in 1840 with the use of a seton.[10] In the late nineteenth century, a number of surgeons

TABLE 13.1. Aetiology of rectovaginal fistula.

Category	Condition	Mechanism
Traumatic		
Obstetric	Prolonged second stage of labour	Pressure necrosis of rectovaginal septum
	Midline episiotomy	Extension directed into rectum
	Perineal lacerations	
Foreign body	Vaginal pessaries	Pressure necrosis
	Violent coitus	Mechanical perforation
	Sexual abuse	Mechanical perforation
Iatrogenic	Hysterectomy	Injury to anterior rectal wall
	Stapled colorectal anastomosis	Staple line includes vagina
	Transanal excision of anterior rectal tumour	Deep margin of resection into vagina
	Enemas	Mechanical perforation
	Anorectal surgery such as incision and drainage of intramural abscesses	Mechanical perforation
Inflammatory	Crohn's disease	Transmural inflammation-perforation
	Pelvic radiation	Early-tumour necrosis
	Pelvic abscess	Late-transmural inflammation
	Perirectal abscess	
Neoplastic	Rectal	Local tumour growth into neighbouring structure
	Cervical	
	Uterine	
	Vaginal	
	Primary or recurrent tumours	

From: Stenchever and Benson.[44]

Rectovaginal fistulas, which occur less commonly than vesicovaginal fistulas, are also less commonly referred to in historical reports. The first treatise on the treatment of rectovaginal fistula was probably by a student and successor of Sims, Thomas Addis Emmet, who published a book *Vesico-vaginal fistula from parturition and other causes: with cases of recto-vaginal fistula* in 1868.[11] Emmet greatly expanded the work of his mentor and introduced many surgical innovations and principles of fistula repair that are still followed today. He insisted on preoperative preparation so that "not only the vaginal walls but also the hypertrophied and indurated edges of the fistula have attained a natural color and density" prior to taking the woman to surgery. The repairs were done without anaesthesia, in the left lateral position, and began with release of tension on the scarred edges of the fistula. Repairs often required staged procedures in order to close the fistula fully. Emmet advocated the use of scissors to achieve wide dissection of the tissues surrounding the fistula, and, for vesicovaginal fistulas, continual bladder drainage following the repair. These innovations were novel. Emmet was a meticulous surgeon and scientific investigator and probably is the true father of gynaecological reconstructive surgery.[17] Further advancements in the repair of rectovaginal fistulas in the late nineteenth century include the adaptation of Tait's technique of perineorraphy at the time of repair of the fistula. Until then, repairs of the fistulas were limited to splitting apart the perineum and allowing the perineum to heal by granulation, often with poor functional results.[13] These historical reports underline the basic tenets of the repair of rectovaginal fistulas today: tissue must be free from infection and induration, repairs need to be accomplished with wide dissection of the vaginal tissues so that sutures are not under tension, and attention needs to be paid to the perineum and sphincter complex to ensure that functional outcomes are optimal.

13.3 Incidence

Although the exact incidence of rectovaginal fistulas is unknown, the most common aetiology in the developed world is still thought to be obstetri-

introduced innovations to the repair of vesicovaginal fistulas that were then popularised by James Marion Sims in a series of surgical experiments conducted from 1845 to 1849. Operating on three slave women over 6 years with more than 40 failed procedures, Sims managed surgically to close a vesicovaginal fistula. He attributed his success to the use of silver suture and the exposure of the operative site that he achieved with positioning the patient in the knee-chest position and the use of a speculum. Although he claimed credit for all of these innovations, others had utilised silver suture for the repair of fistulas prior to his publication.[8]

cal, with approximately 0.1% of vaginal births resulting in a rectovaginal fistula.[2,14] The incidence of rectovaginal fistulas in the population of women who sustain a fourth degree laceration is higher and ranges from 0.4 to 3.0%. Infection of the perineal wound following delivery may contribute to the occurrence of a fistula in these cases.[2,14–21]

Fistulas secondary to obstructed labour are rare in the developed world but common worldwide. The exact prevalence of fistulas secondary to obstructed labour is unknown: in 1989, the World Health Organization estimated that more than 2 million girls and women around the world had either rectovaginal or vesicovaginal fistulas, estimates that probably underestimate the extent of the disease because they are based on women who present for care.[22] Isolated incidence rates for rectovaginal fistula do not exist; however, rates of vesicovaginal fistula in sub-Saharan Africa may reach up to 350 women per 100,000 live births.[23] These fistulas differ from direct obstetrical trauma associated with a severe perineal laceration at the time of delivery because they are accompanied by widespread tissue destruction and necrosis. While rectovaginal fistulas occur more rarely than vesicovaginal fistulas as a result of obstructed labour, approximately 17% of fistulas seen at a large fistula centre in Addis Addaba, Ethiopia were either isolated rectovaginal fistulas or combined rectovaginal and vesicovaginal fistulas.[24] Another series by Ayhan reported that 19% of 182 vesicovaginal fistula patients also had intestinal fistulas.[25] Double fistulas (rectovaginal and vesicovaginal) in this population are indicative of a poorer prognosis for surgical cure.

13.4 Classification

Various classification schemes have been proposed for rectovaginal fistulas. No standardised system has been adopted, which has limited the ability to compare results from surgical series or to define the incidence of disease. One system divides fistulas into "simple" and "complex". Simple fistulas occur in the low or mid-vagina, are less than 2.5 cm in diameter, and are the result of trauma or infectious causes, while complex fistulas occur high in the vagina, are greater than 2.5 cm in diameter, and may occur from inflam-

TABLE 13.2. Classification of rectovaginal fistulas.

Simple rectovaginal fistula	Complex rectovaginal fistula
Low or mid vagina	High vagina
≤ 2.5 cm	>2.5 cm
Traumatic or infectious cause	Inflammatory bowel disease, irradiation, neoplastic causes, prolonged obstructed labour
	Failed prior repair

Modified from: Rothenberger and Goldberg.[6] Copyright 1983, with permission from Elsevier.

matory bowel disease, irradiation or other neoplastic causes.[6] Fistulas that have failed prior repair or result from prolonged obstructed labour should probably be added to the list of "complex fistulas" regardless of where the communication between rectum and vagina occurs[12,24] (Table 13.2). Other classification schemes divide fistulas by anatomic descriptions: high fistulas occur in the upper third of the vagina where the vagina is covered only by peritoneum, fistulas in the middle third of the vagina occur where there is only a thin septum between the vagina and rectum, and distal fistulas occur where the vagina and the anal canal are separated by the perineal body.[26]

Inflammatory fistulas are classified according to their relationship to the anal sphincter, dividing them into four main types: intersphincteric, trans-sphincteric, suprasphincteric and extra-sphincteric[27] (Figure 13.1). This classification scheme helps to dictate the approach to surgical drainage of these inflammatory fistulas. Other classification schemes have included combinations of

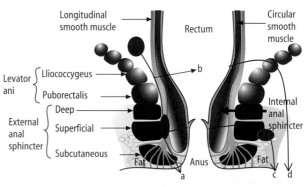

FIGURE 13.1. Diagrammatic representation of types of fistula. **a** intersphincteric, **b** suprasphincteric **c** transsphincteric, **d** extrasphincteric. (Courtesy of A. Sultan and R. Thakar.)

the above as well as the addition of horseshoe fistulas.[28] Each of the above categories for inflammatory fistulas has multiple variations; fistulas of these types may be very extensive, involving the entire pelvis.

13.5 Pathophysiology

The pathophysiology of rectovaginal fistulas varies by aetiology including obstetrical and other traumatic causes, inflammatory bowel disease, infectious aetiologies and neoplastic processes.

13.5.1 Obstetrical Fistulas

Obstetrical fistulas can occur as the result of direct trauma or as part of more global damage to the tissues of the pelvic floor. Obstetrical fistulas in the developed world are thought to occur through direct trauma to the rectovaginal septum and perineal body. Risk factors for third and fourth degree laceration of the anal sphincter are also thought to increase the risk for fistula formation and include episiotomy, operative vaginal delivery, as well as secondary infection of a repaired laceration.[4,5]

Failure to recognise injuries and inadequate repair have been implicated in the aetiology of rectovaginal fistulas.[29] Repair of obstetrical lacerations are often performed under suboptimal conditions with poor lighting, in an operative field contaminated by faecal material, and with lack of analgesia and surgical assistance. Identification and repair of severe lacerations is paramount to effective repair and may require moving a patient from the delivery room to the operating room to perform an examination under anaesthesia to determine the full extent of lacerations after a delivery. At the very least, a rectal examination with adequate lighting and analgesia is indicated, especially after an operative delivery, to detect lacerations to the rectovaginal septum. One study has determined that a second observer increased detection rates for severe lacerations by 15%, indicating that determining the extent of pelvic floor damage following delivery may be difficult under poor operative conditions with a single examiner.[30] Careful documentation of the extent

of the laceration, the repair performed, as well as the type of suture used should also be recorded. Repair of obstetrical lacerations is an operative procedure and should be documented in the medical chart as such.

Missed fourth degree lacerations with repair only of the perineum and not the sphincter or rectal mucosa may result in immediate postpartum incontinence or lead to infection followed by incontinence more remote from delivery. "Buttonhole" fistulas can also be missed at the time of delivery. These fistulas can occur above an intact perineum when a vaginal tear has extended into the rectum. Both missed fourth degree lacerations and buttonhole lacerations underline the importance of a careful rectal examination after delivery. These fistulas usually result in immediate incontinence postpartum. Any postpartum women with anal incontinence should be re-examined with adequate analgesia to ensure that a fistula is not present.

Fistulas can also occur after perineal repair of an obstetrical laceration that becomes infected or more rarely when a stitch from a repair transgresses the bowel lumen. These fistulas commonly present more remote from delivery after an infection of the wound and breakdown of the obstetrical repair. Debridement of the infected wound, removal of residual suture material and antibiotic therapy are essential prior to attempting repair of these fistulas. Although early repair of infected severe perineal lacerations has been described, repairs were only successful after daily extensive inpatient debridement of the perineal wound and antibiotic therapy until all signs of infection were resolved. More commonly, delaying repair until the inflammatory processes are completely resolved over a 2- to 3-month period is prudent.

Associated trauma to the anal sphincter complex is common in women with rectovaginal fistulas and should be evaluated by physical examination at the time of delivery as well as in the patient who presents remote from delivery with a rectovaginal fistula. Overt anal sphincter injury occurs in up to 6.4% of women after vaginal birth.[32-35] However, occult sphincter injuries are much more common and range in incidence from 6.8 to 44% of parous women. Sphincter disruption can probably be assumed to be even higher in women with rectovaginal fistulas.[36,37] The rate of preoperative anal incontinence secondary to a disrupted sphincter has been reported as high as 48% in a series of 52 patients with rectovaginal fistulas.[4,38] Further evaluation of the anal sphincter complex including ultrasound, manometry and neurological studies has been recommended for the preoperative workup for any patient who presents with an obstetrically related fistula.[4]

Fistulas that occur as the result of obstructed labour form after "sloughing" of vaginal tissue that has become necrotic from pressure of the fetal head. Typically, the sloughing follows a week after the delivery of the fetus after a prolonged labour lasting more than 2 days. A fistula "field injury" including rectovaginal and/or vesicovaginal fistula, global pelvic floor dysfunction and foot drop has been described and is indicative of widespread pelvic tissue and neurological damage. Part of the "field injury" includes the massive social displacement of the fistula patient from their families and communities.[24]

13.5.2 Other Traumatic Causes

Other traumatic causes of fistula formation include a neglected foreign body such as a pessary that has been in place for many years without removal.[39,40] Erosion of vaginal pessaries into either the rectum or the bladder is extremely rare and is documented in the literature only in the form of case reports. Violent coitus or sexual abuse is similarly reported.[41]

Fistula formation after hysterectomy can occur after injury to the anterior rectal wall, and is also rare. One large series of 3,076 women who underwent vaginal hysterectomy had a reported incidence of rectal injuries of 0.5% and all of the injuries healed without the formation of a fistula.[42] Other authors have reported a similarly low incidence of 0.07% of rectal laceration as a complication of vaginal hysterectomy; all of the injuries were repaired primarily and none resulted in the formation of a fistula.[43] Stapled colorectal anastomosis, transanal excision of anterior rectal tumour with the deep margins of the resection into vagina, anorectal surgery such as incision and drainage of intramural abscesses and mechanical perforation have also been cited as rare causes of rectovaginal fistula formation.[44] The percentages of rectovaginal fistulas resulting from "operative" or "iatrogenic" causes reported in case series of patients in the literature range from 2 to 24% and are largely dependent on the referral practice of the physician.[45-50]

13.5.3 Inflammatory Bowel Disease

Patients with Crohn's disease have a reported lifetime risk of development of an anorectal or perineal fistula that ranges from 20 to 40%, with one series reporting a risk of development of a rectovaginal fistula in 9% of Crohn's patients.[51] Rectovaginal fistulas may result from rupture of a cryptoglandular abscess or more commonly from deep ulcerations of the anterior rectal canal. Anorectal and presumably rectovaginal fistulas occur in women with colonic disease more commonly than in those with disease confined to the small intestine.[28,51,52]

13.5.4 Infectious Causes

Any infectious process contiguous with the rectovaginal septum can result in the formation of a fistula. The majority of these fistulas are thought to be the result of cryptoglandular infection; however, tuberculosis, lymphgranuloma venereum and schistosomiasis have all been reported to cause fistulas rarely. Diverticulosis is the most common cause of high rectovaginal fistulas, with women who have undergone a prior hysterectomy at higher risk.[3-5]

13.5.5 Neoplastic Causes

Fistulas can occur as a result of direct tumour extension into the rectum, or as the result of pelvic radiation, especially for endometrial and cervical cancers. The rates of rectovaginal fistula formation after irradiation for endometrial or cervical cancer range from 1 to 10%.[4-6] The development of these fistulas may occur as late as 2 years after therapy and is often preceded by the new onset of rectal bleeding. The evaluation of a fistula following treatment for neoplasm should include pathological evaluation of tissue to rule out tumour recurrence.

13.6   Diagnosis and Evaluation

Evaluation of a patient begins with a history and physical examination to determine the size, location and aetiology of the rectovaginal fistula. Women with very distal fistulas may be largely asymptomatic while women with fistulas that are large and involve the anal sphincter complex may have frank loss of stool. Women with small inflammatory fistulas may have only a purulent discharge and complain of pain without loss of bowel contents.

A thorough perineal examination, including observation of the anal opening as well as the perineal skin is warranted. Perianal dimpling and/or a "dovetail sign", which consists of perianal folds posterior to the anal opening with smooth mucosa anteriorly, may indicate a disrupted anal sphincter as well as the presence of a fistula. Observation of the perineal skin for faecal material as well as noting loss of flatus during an examination warrants further inquiry and investigation on the part of the provider. Women with loss of faecal material have proven reluctant to seek help or acknowledge the condition. In a prospective cohort study of 94 women only a few of the 38% of women with symptoms of anal incontinence had sought evaluation due to embarrassment, socioeconomic reasons or lack of knowledge of where to obtain

help.[53] An observant sensitive provider can enable a woman to seek care for this disabling condition.

Often the fistula can be visualised on rectovaginal examination, although this may be difficult with small fistula tracts (Figure 13.2). A rectal examination is also important to determine the integrity of the anal sphincters, the quality of the tissues surrounding the fistula, and to palpate for abscesses and other masses. The most likely location of the vaginal opening of the fistula is along a perineal or vaginal scar following episiotomy or laceration. On the rectal side, the most common location for the opening of the fistula is at the dentate line or superior edge of the external anal sphincter. Dimpling or retraction of the epithelium is often seen. Careful probing with a small lacrimal probe can help identify the opening (Figure 13.2). With a finger in the rectum, the probe can be passed through the fistula to the rectal side. Most patients tolerate this manipulation without pain unless there is active infection. If the fistula is not easily identified, placing methylene blue dyed lubricant in the rectum, massaging the rectovaginal septum and observing the posterior vaginal wall for extravasation can help to identify the fistula. Other techniques include the instillation of methylene blue stained fluid into the rectum via a large Foley catheter with a

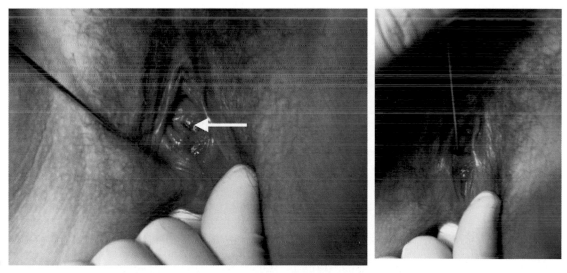

a   b

FIGURE 13.2. **a** Small rectovaginal fistula opening on posterior vaginal wall (*arrow*). **b** The rectovaginal fistula track is demonstrated by inserting a lacrimal probe through the vaginal opening. (Courtesy of A. Sultan and R. Thakar.)

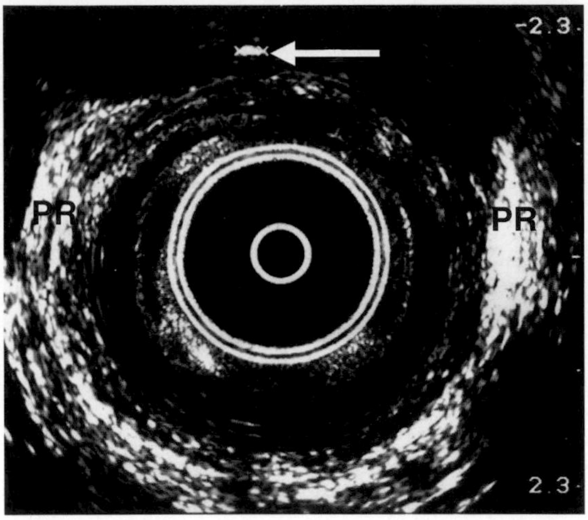

Figure 13.3. Endoanal ultrasound demonstrating the level of rectovaginal fistula track just above the level of the puborectalis (*PR*). (Courtesy of A. Sultan and R. Thakar.)

30-cc balloon that can be used to occlude the anal canal. The rectum can also be insufflated with air, while the vagina is filled with water or saline. Bubbling may indicate the site of the fistula. The use of barium enemas, contrast material placed vaginally, and hydrogen peroxide injected into the fistulous tract with an angiocath may help to define the exit or entrance to the tract.[54]

Endoanal ultrasound is indicated to identify concurrent sphincter laceration, and can also identify fistulous tracts (Figure 13.3).

In general, a mature epitheliased fistula that is not infected is not painful on digital examination. If the fistula cannot be identified or if it is too painful, an examination should be performed under anaesthesia. Office anoscopy or proctoscopy may also help to evaluate the surrounding tissues or to identify the fistula. In women where inflammatory bowel disease is suspected by history or physical examination, colonoscopy is warranted. Biopsy of the fistulous tract is indicated when neoplasia is suspected.

13.7 Repair Techniques

The approach to repair of rectovaginal fistulas should be dictated by the complexity of the fistula, its size and location as well as its cause.

For example, high fistulas are probably better addressed by abdominal procedures while distal fistulas are better addressed by transvaginal, transperineal or transrectal procedures. The tenets of repair of obstetrically related rectovaginal fistulas date back to the innovations and recommendations made nearly 135 years ago: repair without tension, an operative field free from infection or inflammation, wide mobilisation of the tissue surrounding the fistulous tract, excision of the tract if possible, and care to avoid strain on the repair in the immediate postoperative period. Most authors state that the fistula needs to be completely free from inflammation or induration, with waits as long as 3–6 months suggested before repair of obstetrical fistulas be undertaken.[53,54] However, a recent series of 1,716 obstetrical vesicovaginal fistulas reported that patients were treated with early closure of their fistula even if all induration had not resolved by the time of surgery. Twelve per cent of these women also had rectovaginal fistulas. The primary closure rate for the fistulas was 92%, with low rates of postoperative infection, indicating that early closure may be possible after debridement of necrotic tissue.[55] If the local tissues have active infection and faecal contamination that does not respond to local measures, or the patient has a complex recurring fistula, a diverting colostomy is indicated until the tissue is suitable for repair.

Mechanical and antibiotic treatments, accompanied by a restricted diet for 1–3 days prior to surgery are often recommended, although no randomised data support these practices. A recent review of six randomised trials evaluating bowel surgery compared patients undergoing mechanical bowel preparation to those with no preparation and found no difference in wound infection rates (44/595 vs 35/609, OR 1.34, 95% CI 0.85–2.13) or other parameters measured, suggesting that these practices may need to be revisited.[56]

In general, distal rectovaginal fistulas are repaired transvaginally (as preferred by gynaecologists), transrectally (as preferred by colorectal surgeons) or transperineally. All three repair methods have similar reported success rates. Adherence to the basic tenets of fistula repair is probably more important than surgical approach to the success of the intervention.

Transvaginal repair methods include conversion of the fistula to a complete fourth degree laceration followed by excision of the fistulous tract and a layered closure. In the case of a fistula that is not accompanied by anal sphincter disruption, this entails damaging an intact sphincter. Given poor rates of success with sphincteroplasty at long-term follow-up,[57–60] this practice may not be in the patient's best interest. Other transvaginal repairs include inversion of the fistulous tract, followed by a layered closure. This method will spare an intact sphincter complex. The Latzko technique is a variation of this where the anterior and posterior walls of the vagina are joined to invert the fistula into the rectum. This closes off a portion of the upper vagina and is suitable for high fistulas.

Transvaginal repair of rectovaginal fistulas secondary to obstructed labour is influenced by the size of these fistulas (on average 2.3 by 2.5 cm) and the fact that the fistulas exist in a bed of severely damaged tissue. Excision of the fistulous tract may be impossible because of the size of the fistula and most authors introduce healthier tissue in the form of a Martius graft to ensure adequate blood supply to the area.

The transperineal approach starts with a curved incision on the perineum, through which the vagina and rectum are separated. The fistula is then divided and both the vaginal and rectal sides of the fistula are closed in layers in opposing directions so that the lines of the repair do not directly overlie one another.[13]

Transrectal repairs generally involve the development of rectal mucosal flaps, mobilised to cover the excised fistula tract. In these repairs, the rectal mucosa, submucosa with or without a portion of the rectovaginal septum and internal anal sphincter is mobilised. The fistula is excised and the flap is sutured over the previous site of the fistula. Proponents of this method of repair state that the high-pressure side of the fistula is in the rectum and that this approach focuses the repair on the rectal side. The vaginal side may be closed or left open to drain.

The best suture material for repair of fistulas has not been studied. Most series report the use of a delayed-absorbable suture, such as a 3-0 polysorb, or polyglycolic acid on all layers. Permanent suture is not used. The use of either a Martius fat pad, or gracilis flap to bring well-vascularised tissue to the fistula site is widely recommended for the repair of complex fistulas.[61,62]

Abdominal approaches to high and complex fistulas secondary to radiation therapy, inflammatory bowel disease or multiple failed prior repairs include wide mobilisation of the rectovaginal septum, division of the fistula and layered closure with or without bowel resection. Usually omentum is introduced as a pedicled graft. Low anterior resections, colorectal anastomoses, and onlay patch anastomosis procedures have all been described. For women who have underlying disease not amenable to other surgical intervention, colostomy as a salvage operation may greatly improve quality of life.[4,6,38]

Postoperative management has not been studied extensively, but many surgeons recommend a restrictive diet including 3 days of clear liquids followed by a low-residue diet as well as the continuation of broad-spectrum antibiotics. A single randomised study of 54 patients undergoing other anorectal reconstructive surgery randomised patients to either a "regular" diet versus a "bowel confinement" regimen and found no benefit to dietary restriction.[63] Local care including sitz baths, followed by drying with a heat lamp or blow dryer is commonly recommended to keep the operative site clean and dry.[54]

13.8 Outcome of Surgery

Reports of success rates for rectovaginal fistula repair are largely limited to the success of closure of the fistula with little description of quality of life changes or functional outcomes. The literature is also limited by small retrospective series of patients with limited follow-up, inclusion of patients with different aetiologies for the fistula and lack of a standardised classification schema to make comparisons between reports. A thorough evaluation of the anal sphincter complex with associated sphincter repair may greatly influence surgical cure rates. If the fistula is closed, but the sphincter non-functional, the outcome may be less than desired for the patient. Reports of sexual function following fistula repair are limited to descriptions of the effect of a Martius graft on function: Elkins reported on six patients with rectovaginal fistulas who were repaired with grafts, one of whom complained of mild dyspareunia.[62] Others have reported up to a 38% incidence of pain at the site of graft harvest in small series.[64]

Medical management of fistulising Crohn's disease includes anti-inflammatory medications, antibiotics, immunomodulators and anti-tumour necrosis factor-alpha therapies. Success of these interventions varies widely.[28] Inflammatory fistulas secondary to an acute infectious process or Crohn's disease are better addressed by either seton placement (loose nylon suture along fistula tract) or fistulotomy and drainage. For the treatment of simple perianal fistulas, reported rates of healing for these interventions range from 70 to 100%, with minor incontinence reported in 10% of individuals. Recurrence may occur up to 20% of the time.[28] For more complicated fistulas, or recurrent fistulas in the face of active rectal Crohn's disease with multiple tracts, surgery including seton placement, fistulotomy or advancement flaps shows improvement in symptoms in 25–100% of patients, with fistula recurrence rates up to 67%.[28]

Repair success rates of simple (less than 2.5 cm in size located in the distal rectovaginal septum) rectovaginal fistulas range from 40 to 86%.[38] In one summary of results from repair of simple rectovaginal fistula, recurrence rates ranged from 3% for perineoproctotomy to 12% for transanal advancement flaps. As the author pointed out, many series report operating on another surgeon's failures, which is not always figured into reports of primary closure rates.[65]

Cure rates for more complex obstetrically related rectovaginal fistulas secondary to obstructed labour are lower than reported rates for vesicovaginal fistulas: 78% for either combined vesicovaginal and rectovaginal fistula or isolated rectovaginal fistula, versus a widespread reported cure (or closure) rate of 90% for isolated vesicovaginal fistula.[66] Nearly all the literature describing the treatment of these complex fistulas is retrospective in nature and because of geographical barriers, most follow-up is limited to hospital discharge. All of these reports focus on the repair of vesicovaginal fistulas. Arrowsmith reported on 98 vesicovaginal fistula patients, of

whom nine had combined fistulas. However, he does not further describe the outcomes of this small cohort of combined rectovaginal fistulas.[66] Another series by Ayhan et al. reported that 19% of 182 patients had intestinal fistulas; the overall success rate for this series of patients was reported at 91%, with no further evaluation of the effect of rectovaginal fistula on surgical cure rates. Both surgical and obstetrical fistulas were represented in this cohort; however, the majority of the fistulas (76%) were obstetrical in origin.[25] A series by Kelly reports a similar cure rate of 85%, with approximately 20% of patients with either isolated or combined rectovaginal and vesicovaginal fistulas. Again the impact of rectovaginal fistulas on the cure rate was not analysed: however, even among this series of difficult fistulas, the author did classify rectovaginal fistulas as "complex".[67]

Elkins reported a series of fistula patients that he followed for 6 months. Women with combined vesicovaginal and rectovaginal fistulas had poorer outcomes than those with vesicovaginal fistulas alone, with success rates of the former with primary closure rates of 3/6 (50%) versus an overall primary closure rate of 78/82 (95%) for vesicovaginal fistulas. Despite repair, 46/78 (59%) women were found to have serious complications following successful closure of their fistula with continued complaints of either urinary or anal incontinence. In a review of fistula repair series in the same article for papers published between 1965 and 1993, primary closure rates for vesicovaginal fistula ranged from 58 to 95%.[68] A single series has examined the outcome of future pregnancies following vesicovaginal repair and concluded that women who were repaired had better obstetrical outcomes than those who were not repaired, and that prenatal planning resulted in more of the women undergoing the recommended caesarean delivery than those who were not scheduled for delivery.[69] Presumably, the same outcomes may be applicable to women who sustain rectovaginal fistulas, given that the overall reported prognosis for these fistulas is poorer than that for vesicovaginal fistulas. Unfortunately many women who sustain fistulas secondary to obstructed labour are infertile as part of the "field injury".

13.9 Conclusions

Rectovaginal fistulas are a devastating condition for patients and although rare in the developed world, they occur commonly worldwide. Repair of the fistula with restoration of continence can be challenging and requires a detailed knowledge of the continence mechanism. Evaluation and management include locating the fistula, assessing tissue quality and timing the repair. The integrity and function of the anal sphincters should be considered in planning the fistula repair. If the anal sphincters are involved in the fistula tract or the sphincters are not intact, surgery should address both the fistula and chronic sphincter laceration. Repair without tension, an operative field free from infection or inflammation, wide mobilisation of the tissue surrounding the fistulous tract, excision of the tract if possible, and care to avoid strain on the repair in the immediate postoperative period are rules for success. Repair or other treatment of these fistulas can restore patients to a healthy productive life.

References

1. Russell TR, Gallagher DM. Low rectovaginal fistulas. Am J Surg 1977;134:13–18.
2. Venkatesh KS, Ramanujum PS, Larson DM, Haywood MA. Anorectal complications of vaginal delivery. Dis Colon Rectum 1989;32:1039–41.
3. Saclaides TJ. Surg Clin N Am 2002;82:1261–72.
4. Tsang CBS, Rothenberger DA. Rectovaginal fistulas. Therapeutic options. Surg Clin N Am 1997;77(1): 9–114.
5. Stern HS, Dreznik Z. Rectovaginal fistula. Adv Surg 1987;21:245–62.
6. Rothenberger DA, Goldberg SM. The management of rectovaginal fistulae. Surg Clin N Am 1983;63(1): 61–79.
7. Howard D, Delancey JOL, Burney RE. Fistulo in ano after episiotomy. Obstet Gynecol 1999;93(5): 800–2.
8. Rock JA. Historical development of pelvic surgery. In: Thompson J, Rock JA, eds. Telinde's operative gynecology. Philadelphia: JB Lippincott Co, 1992, pp 3–9.
9. Thompson JD. Vesicovaginal fistulas. In: Thompson J, Rock JA, eds. Telinde's operative gynecology. Philadelphia: JB Lippincott Co, 1992, p 787.
10. Barton JR. A rectovaginal fistula – cured. Am J Med Sci 1840;26:305–6.
11. Emmet TA. Vesico-vaginal fistula from parturition and other causes: with cases of recto-vaginal fistula. New York: Samuel S and William Wood, 1868.
12. Wall LL. Thomas Addis Emmet, the vesicovaginal fistula, and the origins of reconstructive gynecologic surgery. Int Urogynecol J 2002;13:145–55.
13. Wiskind AK, Thompson JD. Transverse transperineal repair of rectovaginal fistulas in the lower vagina. Am J Obstet Gynecol 1992;107(3): 694–9.
14. Goldaber KG, Wendel PJ, McIntire DD, Wendel GD. Postpartum perineal morbidity after fourth degree perineal repair. Am J Obstet Gynecol 1993; 168(2):489–93.
15. Legino LJ, Woods MP, Rayburn WF, Mcgoogan LA. Third and fourth degree perineal tears. 50 years' experience at a university hospital. J Reprod Med 1988;33:423–6.
16. Brantly JT, Burwell JC. A study of fourth degree perineal lacerations and their sequelae. Am J Obstet Gynecol 1960;80:711–14.
17. O'Leary JL, O'Leary JA. The complete episiotomy: analysis of 1224 complete lacerations, sphincterotomies and episioproctotomies. Obstet Gynecol 1965;25:235–40.
18. Mahomed K, Grant A, Ashurst H, James D. The Southmead perineal suture study. A randomised comparison of suture materials and suturing techniques for repair of perineal trauma. Br J Obstet Gynaecol 1989;96:1272–80.
19. Kammerer-Doak DN, Wesol AB, Rogers RG, Dominguez CE, Dorin MH. A prospective cohort study of women after primary repair of obstetric anal sphincter laceration. Am J Obstet Gynecol 1999;181(6):1317–22.
20. Sultan AH, Monga AK, Kumar D, Stanton SL. Primary repair of obstetric anal sphincter rupture using the overlap technique. Br J Obstet Gynaecol 1999;106:318–23.
21. Homsi R, Daikoku NH, Littlejohn J, Wheeless CR. Episiotomy: risks of dehiscence and rectovagnial fistula. Obstet Gynecol Surv 1994;49:803–8.
22. Murray C, Lopez A. Health dimensions of sex and reproduction. Geneva: WHO, 1998.
23. Donnay F, Well L. Obstetric fistula: the international response. Lancet 2004;363:71–2.
24. Arrowsmith S, Hamlin EC, Wall LL. Obstructed labor injury complex: obstetric fistula formation and the multifaceted morbidity of the maternal birth trauma in the developing world. Obstet Gynecol Survey 1996;51(9):568–74.
25. Ayhan A, Tuncer ZS, Dogan L, Pekin S, Kisnisci HA. Results of treatment in 182 consecutive patients with genital fistulas. Int J Gynecol Obstet 1995;48: 43–7.

26. Rosenshein NB, Genadry RR, Woodruff JD. An anatomic classification of rectovaginal septal defects. Am J Obstet Gynecol 1980;137(4):439–42.

27. Parks AG, Gordon PH, Hardcastle JD. A classification of fistulo in ano. Br J Surg 1976;63:1–12.

28. Judge TA, Lichtenstein GR. Treatment of fistulizing Crohn's disease. Gastroenterol Clin N Am 2004;33:421–54.

29. Thompson JD. Relaxed vaginal outlet, rectocele, faecal incontinence and rectovaginal fistula. In: Thompson J, Rock JA, eds. Telinde's operative gynecology. Philadelphia: JB Lippincott Co, 1992, pp 967–9.

30. Groom KM, Patterson-Brown S. Third degree tears: are they clinically underdiagnosed? Gastroenterology International 2000;13(2):76–8.

31. Hankins GDV, Jauth JC, Gilstrap LC. Early repair of episiotomy dehiscence. Obstet Gynecol 1990;75(1):48–51.

32. Thacker SB, Banta HD. Benefits and risks of episiotomy: an interpretative review of the English language literature, 1860–1980. Obstet Gynecol Surv 1982;38:322–38.

33. Helwig JT, Thorp JM, Bowes WA. Does midline episiotomy increase the risk of third and fourth degree lacerations in operative vaginal deliveries? Obstet Gynecol 1993;82:276–9.

34. Combs CA, Robertson PA, Laros RK. Risk factors for third-degree and fourth-degree perineal lacerations in forceps and vacuum deliveries. Am J Obstet Gynecol 1990;163:100–4.

35. Zetterstrom J, Lopez A, Anzen B, Norman M, Holmstrom B, Mellgren A. Anal sphincter tears at vaginal delivery: risk factors and clinical outcome of primary repair. Obstet Gynecol 1999;94:21–8.

36. Sultan AH, Kamm MA, Hudson CN, Thomas JM, Bartram CI. Anal-sphincter disruption during vaginal delivery. N Engl J Med 1993;329:1905–11.

37. Varma A, Gunn J, Gardiner A, Lindow S, Duthie G. Obstetrical anal sphincter injury: prospective evaluation and incidence. Dis Colon Rectum 1999;42:1537–43.

38. Tsang CBS, Madoff RD, Wong WD, Rothenberger DA, Finne CO, Singer D, Lowry AC. Anal sphincter integrity and function influences outcome in rectovaginal fistula repair. Dis Colon Rectum 1998;41(9):1141–6.

39. Kankam OK, Geraghty R. An erosive pessary. J R Soc Med 2002;95:507.

40. Russell JK. The dangerous vaginal pessary. BMJ 1961;ii:1595–7.

41. Parra JM, Kellogg ND. A rectovaginal fistula in a sexually assaulted child. Semin Perioper Nurs 1995;4(2):140–5.

42. Mathevet P, Valecia P, Cousin C, Mellier G, Dargent D. Operative injuries during vaginal hysterectomy. Eur J Obstet Gynecol 2001;97:71–5.

43. Hoffman MS, Lynch C, Lockhart J, Knapp R. Injury of the rectum during vaginal surgery. Am J Obstet Gynecol 1999;181:274–7.

44. Benson JT. Atlas of Clinical Gynecology: Ilrogynecology and Reconstructive Pelvic Surgery, Vol. 5, Philadelphia: Current Medicine, 2000.

45. Rothenberger DA, Christenson CE, Balcos EG, Schottler JL, Nemer FD, Nivatvongs S, Goldberg SM. Endorectal advancement flap for the treatment of simple rectovaginal fistula. Dis Colon Rectum 1982;25(4):297–300.

46. Given FT. Rectovaginal fistula: a review of 20 years' experience in a community hospital. Am J Obstet Gynecol 1970;108(1):41–6.

47. Jones IT, Fazio VW, Jagelman MS. The use of transanal rectal advancement flaps in the management of fistulas involving the anorectum. Dis Colon Rectum 1987;30(12):919–23.

48. Mazier WP, Senagore AJ, Schiesel EC. Operative repair of anovaginal and rectovaginal fistulas. Dis Colon Rectum 1995;38(1):4–6.

49. Kodner IJ, Mazor A, Shemesh EI, Fry RD, Fleshman JW, Birnbaum EH. Endorectal advancement flap repair of rectovaginal and other complicated anorectal fistulas. Surgery 1993;114(4):682–90.

50. Wise WE, Aguilar PS, Padmanabhan A, Meesig DM, Arnold MW, Stewart WRC. Surgical treatment of low rectovaginal fistulas. Dis Colon Rectum 1991;34(3):271–4.

51. Radcliffe A, Richie J, Hawley P, Lennard-Jones J, Northover J. Anovaginal and rectovaginal fistulas in Crohn's disease. Dis Colon Rectum 1988;31:94–9.

52. Bandy LC, Addison A, Parker RT. Surgical management of rectovaginal fistulas in Crohn's disease. Am J Obstet Gynecol 1983;147(4):359–63.

53. Tetzschner T, Sorensen M, Lose G, Christionsen J. Anal and urinary incontinence in women with obstetric anal sphincter rupture. Br J Obstet Gynaecol 1996;103(10):1034–40.

54. Song AH, Advincula AP, Fenner DE. Common gastrointestinal problems in women and pregnancy. Gastroenterology 2004;6(3):755–73.

55. Waaldijk K. The immediate management of fresh obstetrical fistulas. Am J Obstet Gynecol 2004;191:795–9.

56. Guenaga KF, Matos D, Castro AA, Atallah AN, Wille-Jorgensen P. Mechanical bowel preparation for elective colorectal surgery (Cochrane review). In: The Cochrane Library, Issue 2, 2004. Chichester, UK: John Wiley and Sons, Ltd.

57. Gutierrez AB, Madoff RD, Lowry AC, Parker SC, Buie WD, Baxter NN. Long-term results of anterior sphincteroplasty. Dis Colon Rectum 2004;47: 727–32.

58. Malouf AJ, Norton CS, Engel AF, Nicholls RJ, Kamm MA. Long-term results of overlapping anterior anal-sphincter repair for obstetric trauma. Lancet 2000;355(9200):260–5.

59. Karoui S, Leroi AM, Koning E, Menard JF, Michot F, Denis P. Results of sphincteroplasty in 86 patients with anal incontinence. Dis Colon Rectum 2000; 43(6):813–20.

60. Halverson AL, Hull TL. Long-term outcome of overlapping anal sphincter repair. Dis Colon Rectum 2002;45(3):345–8.

61. Wang YU, Hadley HR. The use of rotated vascularized pedicle flaps for complex transvaginal procedures. Urology 1993;149:590–2.

62. Elkins TE, DeLancey JO, McGuire EJ. The use of modified Martius graft as an adjunctive technique in vesicovaginal and rectovaginal fistula repair. Obstet Gynecol 1990;75(4):727–33.

63. Reissman P, Teoh TA, Cohen SM, Weiss EG, Nogueras JJ, Wexner SD. Is early oral feeding safe after elective colorectal surgery? A prospective randomised trial. Ann Surg 1995;222(1):73–7.

64. Tunuguntla HSGR, Gousse AE. Female sexual dysfunction following vaginal surgery: myth or reality? Curr Urol Reports 2004;5:403–11.

65. Watson SJ, Phillips RKS. Non-inflammatory rectovaginal fistula. Br J Surg 1995;82:1641–3.

66. Arrowsmith SD. Genitourinary reconstruction in obstetric fistulas. J Urol 1994;152:403–6.

67. Kelly J. Vesico-vaginal and recto-vaginal fistulae. J Roy Soc Med 1992;85:257–8.

68. Elkins TE. Surgery for the obstetric vesicovaginal fistula: a review of 100 operations in 82 patients. Am J Obstet Gynecol 1994;170(4): 1108–18.

69. Emembolu J. The obstetric fistula: factors associated with improved pregnancy outcome after successful repair. Int J Gynecol Obstet 1992;39: 205–12.

14
Medicolegal Considerations: The British and U.S. Perspective

Nicholas A. Peacock, Kara Jennings, and Kjell Erik Roxstrom

14.1 Introduction

This chapter is an introduction to the relevant law (both substantive and procedural) of England and Wales (the Scottish system is different) and the United States. It seeks to explain how a lawyer considers and then litigates (or defends) the scenario when a patient wishes to pursue a claim against her doctor for clinical negligence. It considers the elements that a patient must prove in order to establish a right to an award of compensation. It explains the procedure for bringing a claim and gives examples of claims and cases. In both legal systems the laws applied to malpractice claims are predominantly contract and tort law.

Most medical malpractice claims are negligence-based. That is, physicians are charged with a duty to perform as adequately as a "reasonable physician" in her or his field. Negligence claims are based on common law, and vary by jurisdiction or state. In addition to negligence claims, a patient could bring a claim based on an intentional tort, strict liability, contract law, or warranty.

14.2 English Law

14.2.1 Duty of Care

In order to bring a claim for damages, the patient must first establish that the doctor owed her a duty of care. Such a duty can come about under one or both of two main areas of law: (i) the law of contract and/or (ii) the law of tort (occasionally "torts"), by far the most important sub-category of which is the law of negligence.

Where treatment or surgery is undertaken by a doctor for reward, i.e. on behalf of a private patient, the law of contract will apply. The four principal elements that need to be established are: a binding offer (in this case, the offer to undertake treatment/surgery); acceptance of the offer; consideration (the payment of money); the intention to create legally binding relations. Strictly, the contract will usually give rise to an implied term that the doctor will treat the patient with reasonable skill and care.

Where treatment or surgery is provided under the National Health Service legislation, the law of tort applies. The law has long recognised that the relationship of a patient to a doctor is one that deserves special protection (whether as a development of that part of jurisprudence that attaches special importance to bodily integrity or as the corollary to the rights that the doctor has upon qualification is beyond the scope of this chapter) and there is in general terms no difficulty in establishing that a surgeon owes his patient a duty of care.

14.2.2 What Is the Nature of the Duty?

Whether the doctor's duty is owed to his private patient (contract) or his NHS patient (tort/negligence), the nature of the duty owed is the same: the doctor owes the patient a duty of care to treat her with reasonable skill and care so as to prevent foreseeable harm.

14.2.3 Elements of a Claim

In order to succeed in obtaining an award of compensation (usually styled "damages"), the patient has to prove three main elements: (i) that the doctor has breached his duty of care; (ii) that the breach has caused the patient to suffer (iii) injury and, if relevant, financial loss.

It is important at this stage to make clear that lawyers mean something very different from doctors as far as proof is concerned. To a lawyer, proof means only that something can be established on the balance of probabilities, i.e. it is more likely than not to have happened. Put simply, "probably" is sufficient; "possibly" is not. Contrast this with the standard of proof required in a criminal case, namely proof beyond reasonable doubt (so that the jury is sure of guilt). Doctors, by contrast, are used to scientific standards of proof, (effectively, proof beyond reasonable doubt).

Moreover, the patient who brings the claim bears what lawyers call the "burden of proof"; the patient brings the claim and she must establish every element to the requisite standard (the balance of probabilities). If at the end of the case the judge cannot say which of two explanations is more likely (both being equally likely), the patient's case will fail.

14.2.4 Breach of Duty

Medical (which for these purposes includes surgical) cases usually fall into two main categories: (i) failure to give full advice and counselling prior to undertaking surgery (relevant to the giving of consent to treatment) and (ii) failure to treat properly. For these purposes the law regards an act (doing something) in the same way as it regards an omission (failing to do something).

As stated above, the law requires that a doctor treats his patient with reasonable skill and care. A gloss on the "reasonable skill and care" test exists in medical cases, and indeed in any case where the defendant is a skilled professional. A doctor is not guilty of negligence where he acts in accordance with a standard of care that is accepted as proper by a responsible body of medical opinion skilled in that particular discipline, provided that such opinion stands up to logical scrutiny. This encapsulates the so-called "*Bolam* test", named after the

case in which the test was first expressed. The test has since been upheld by the Judicial Committee of the House of Lords (the UK's highest Court) on four occasions. It applies to both categories of claim, "advice" cases and "treatment" cases.

Much academic discussion has been devoted to the perceived iniquities of the *Bolam* test, which has been thought to favour doctors. Whilst it might be thought (and has been said) that the test permits a doctor to adduce evidence in support of his practice from a small minority of colleagues, in practice courts have always been prepared to subject medical practice to critical analysis. In the most recent of the four House of Lords cases referred to, known now only by the surname of the claimant *Bolitho*,[1] Lord Browne-Wilkinson said:

"... in cases of diagnosis and treatment there are cases where, despite a body of professional opinion sanctioning the defendant's conduct, the defendant can properly be held liable for negligence.... In my judgment that is because, in some cases, it cannot be demonstrated to the judge's satisfaction that the body of opinion relied upon is reasonable or responsible. In the vast majority of cases the fact that distinguished experts in the field are of a particular opinion will demonstrate the reasonableness of that opinion. In particular, where there are questions of assessment of the relative risks and benefits of adopting a particular medical practice, a reasonable view necessarily presupposes that the relative risks and benefits have been weighed by the experts in forming their opinions. But if, in a rare case, it can be demonstrated that the professional opinion is not capable of withstanding logical analysis, the judge is entitled to hold that the body of opinion is not reasonable or responsible. I emphasise that in my view it will very seldom be right for a judge to reach the conclusion that views genuinely held by a competent medical expert are unreasonable. The assessment of medical risks and benefits is a matter of clinical judgment which a judge would not normally be able to make without expert evidence.... it would be wrong to allow such assessment to deteriorate into seeking to persuade the judge to prefer one of two views both of which are capable of being logically supported. It is only where a judge can be satisfied that the body of expert opinion cannot be logically supported at all that such opinion will not provide the benchmark by reference to which the defendant's conduct falls to be assessed."

In practice, the trial judge will submit the expert evidence for and against the defendant doctor to careful critical analysis.

Whilst the duty is easily stated in terms of principle, it is clear that, in practice, highly qualified consultant surgeons will be more adept at discharging their duty than, for example, first-year registrars. The duty of care is formulated in such a way that the junior doctor is not required to display the same skills and ability as the consultant; the law requires that a doctor displays the requisite degree of skill and care for his particular level. However, note that the law will expect that: (i) a junior doctor will recognise when his abilities are insufficient to deal with a particular problem and a more experienced colleague is required and, conversely; (ii) the supervising consultant should always consider whether it is proper to delegate the case to a more junior colleague in the first place.

Finally, it is important to remember that a doctor is to be judged by the standards that prevailed at the time when he gave the treatment, advice, etc. (or failed to do so), and not by the standards that prevail at the time of trial.

14.2.5 Guidelines

It is worth a very quick detour into the ever-increasing world of clinical guidelines. To a lawyer, guidelines provide no more and no less than guidance; they are not a set of rules to be followed in every case.

That said, the world of medicine is subject to an increasing amount of guidance, much of it extremely useful, in particular the use of evidence-based guidance from, for example, the Royal Colleges or the National Institute for Health and Clinical Excellence (NICE). The General Medical Council publishes guidance in particular on consent.

In practice, the availability of clinical guidelines from a recognised source will be an important factor in a case; a doctor will be expected to know of the existence of relevant guidelines. A doctor who departs from relevant guidelines may have good reason, but will have to be prepared to explain his reasoning. The importance of good note-keeping in these circumstances is crucial.

14.2.6 Causation

What does "causation" mean? In a simple road traffic accident, the concept of causation (whilst it remains something that the injured party must prove) presents no difficulty; the defendant's bad driving caused the crash in which someone was injured.

In medical cases, the requirement to prove causation often presents an insuperable hurdle for patients. The breach of duty or negligence must make a difference to the outcome; put another way, it does not matter how negligent the doctor has been if the patient would have suffered the same outcome in any event.

At its simplest, the law poses the following question: but for the negligence complained of, would the outcome have been any different? Unfortunately, the "but-for" test sometimes produces an unfair result, something the law has sought to correct in ways that produce an end result that is probably understandable on the particular facts of the case, but which does not produce a statement of principle that can then be universally applied. "Hard cases" (which, in its original formulation meant "cases that produce harsh results", as opposed to "cases that are difficult to solve") do indeed produce bad law.

Two areas in which the law has struggled to cope with the difficulties thrown up by the requirement to prove causation are: (i) "advice" cases and (ii) "loss of a chance" cases.

In the former, a patient complains that she was not given sufficient advice about the treatment that the doctor recommended; she suffers an adverse outcome, usually one that is rare though recognised; she argues that had she been fully counselled in advance, she would not have elected the treatment in the first place. Until recently, such cases were defended on the basis that, the adverse outcome being so unlikely, the patient would have undertaken the risk and undergone treatment in any event. Thus the patient would be unable to prove causation; if there was any negligent failure to advise, it made no difference because the patient would have undergone the treatment in any event. There are many examples where this argument prevailed. However, the House of Lords has recently held that cases of failure to advise are in a special category of their own, the duty to advise of risks prior to undertaking treatment being an important aspect of the patient's right to choose/bodily autonomy.[2] Now, provided that the patient can demonstrate that she would not have undergone the same treatment at the same time at the hands of the same surgeon, her claim will succeed on causation.

More difficult are cases where the patient has lost the chance of a better outcome, but that chance was always less than 50%. The classic example is delayed diagnosis of cancer, where the patient argues that an earlier diagnosis would have given her a better chance of survival. At present, one function of the law's concept of proof is that, if the prospects of survival were always less than 50%, the delay has made no difference. The possible iniquity of this approach is obvious: say, for example, a patient would have had a 49% chance of survival had her cancer been diagnosed in time, but as a result of the delay, her prospects of survival have been reduced to 10%; she has plainly lost a significant chance of survival. The present law, however, holds that since her prospects were always less than 50%, she cannot prove causation. This was recently upheld by the House of Lords.[3] Many commentators expect this aspect of law to continue to develop.

14.2.7 Injury, Loss and Damage

The final element that a patient must prove is an injury. Once the hurdle of causation has been overcome, this last element usually gives rise to few problems in practice in medical cases; an adverse outcome involving physical injury can usually be established. Any harm that is more than merely minor will suffice.

Psychiatric injury that is consequent upon a physical injury also attracts compensation; psychiatric injury on its own has caused the law some problems in the past, but a full explanation is beyond the scope of this chapter.

14.2.8 Compensation

A patient who establishes that a breach of duty has caused her to suffer an injury that would not otherwise have occurred is entitled to an award of compensation. (Note that the law cannot provide any other remedy, for example an apology.)

The award of compensation is designed to put the patient in the same position as if the negligence had not occurred (or, for a private patient, as if the contract had been properly performed);

no better, no worse. This involves two main elements: (i) an award for the injury itself (the pain, suffering and "loss of amenity" and (ii) any financial loss, both past and future. As to the first, lawyers rely on, in descending order, a set of guidelines produced by the Judicial Studies Board, past cases and experience. As to the second, actuarial tables exist to enable calculation of the future element to take into account accelerated receipt.

14.2.9 Defences

Two possible defences should be mentioned. The first, and the first time in which an Act of Parliament needs to be mentioned, is limitation: the time limit within which a claim must be commenced. Pursuant to the Limitation Act 1980, a claim for damages for personal injury must be commenced within 3 years of either the date on which the cause of action accrued (when the injury was suffered) or within 3 years of the date when the patient first knew that she had suffered an injury caused by possible breach of duty by an identifiable defendant, whichever is later. Even if a case is commenced late, the Court has discretion to disapply the 3-year period.

Next, damages may be reduced in cases of contributory negligence. This is rare in cases of clinical negligence, but examples exist where a patient repeatedly fails to follow clear medical advice.[4]

14.2.10 Procedure

The commencement and continuation of proceedings is regulated by the Civil Procedure Rules 1998 (CPR); this chapter provides no more than a skeleton overview.

The patient's solicitor will first seek copies of the patient's medical records. The first formal indication that a claim is to be made is the Letter of Claim, which in the case of an NHS patient is sent to the relevant hospital trust (and thence to the National Health Service Litigation Authority) and in the case of a private patient to the relevant Medical Defence Organisation. The Letter of Claim should set out in brief the patient's case on the three main elements above (breach; causation; injury) together with an indication of the level of compensation expected.

Within 3 months the doctor's representative should send a Letter of Response, responding on each of the above points. The views of treating clinicians are important and, on behalf of hard-working lawyers everywhere, a prompt response to requests for information is invited.

Assuming this exchange of letters does not result in settlement and compromise of the claim, formal court proceedings will follow. The originating document is called a Claim Form, supported by Particulars of Claim, which spell out the facts and allegations that the patient sets out to prove. The doctor's response is called a Defence (Figure 14.1).

Thereafter the progress of the case is carefully managed by a procedural judge, who gives directions for the case until trial and sets up, and then monitors, a timetable.

Witness statements from witnesses who can give evidence as to the facts (in particular the patient and the treating doctor(s)) are exchanged.

Of more importance, expert reports are commissioned from independent experts (usually one per relevant discipline per party) who give their opinion on the case. The requirement for expert evidence necessarily flows from the *Bolam* test itself (see above): no case can succeed (whether for the patient or the doctor) without supportive expert evidence. It is crucial for an expert to recognise and adhere to the duty he owes to the Court, as set out in Part 35 of the CPR. An expert should provide independent evidence on matters within his expertise, uninfluenced by the exigencies of litigation. He is not an advocate for the party instructing him. He should be able to speak to practice generally in the relevant area over the time period under consideration. He will be expected to have reviewed the relevant literature (textbooks, articles, etc.) and to refer properly to

matters that support (and, importantly, any that detract from) his opinion. Where there is a range of opinion about a relevant issue, he is expected to state what the range is.

Before any trial the experts will almost always discuss the issues, usually without lawyers being present. The idea is to identify which issues remain for the trial judge to determine, but concerns have been raised (particularly from patients) that cases can be decided by experts alone behind closed doors.

Compromise of cases by alternative dispute resolution (ADR, usually mediation) is now encouraged in all cases; some Courts are undertaking trials of mandatory ADR before trial.

Either side may wish (at any time) to put forward a formal offer to settle the claim by making an offer pursuant to CPR Part 36; such offers are binding if accepted and, if not, can have an important impact on costs where the party who makes the offer does materially better at any subsequent trial.

Any trial will result in determination of all outstanding issues by a judge, having heard factual and expert evidence subjected to cross-examination and analysis by lawyers. At the conclusion of the trial the judge will give judgment for one party or the other, explaining his reasoning. The losing party will usually be ordered to pay the legal costs of the winning party.

14.2.11 Law in Practice

On 15th December 2000 David Foskett QC, sitting as a Deputy High Court Judge, handed down judgment in the case of *Coffey-Martin v. Royal Free Hampstead NHS Trust*.

The claimant, Mrs Coffey-Martin, gave birth to her son, Connor, on 18th September 1996. Connor was delivered by forceps, the indication for which

- Disclosure of medical records
- Letter of Claim
- Letter of Response
- Claim Form, Particulars of Claim and Initial Schedule of Loss and Damage
- Defence
- Case management conference
- Exchange of witness statements of fact

- Exchange of expert reports
- Meeting of experts
- Pre-trial review
- Updated Schedule of Loss and Damage
- Counter-Schedule of Loss and Damage
- Alternative Dispute Resolution (optional)
- CPR Part 36 offers to settle (optional)
- Trial

FIGURE 14.1. The principal steps in a legal claim in the UK.

was fetal distress on the cardiotocographic trace. The circumstances required that he was delivered in the occipito-posterior position. An episiotomy was created in the right medio-lateral position. The claimant suffered damage to her external anal sphincter, a partial tear in which the anal margin was uninvolved and the internal sphincter undamaged. The issues in the case were: (i) whether the external sphincter damage should have been observed shortly after delivery (breach of duty) and (ii) if so, whether it would have been recognised and successfully treated (causation).

As to breach of duty, the expert obstetricians agreed that examination for anal sphincter damage should have been carried out. Implicitly, the judge subjected the expert views to the requirement that they stand up to logical scrutiny, stating:

"If there did remain any lingering difference between [the experts'] two positions on the precise nature of the examination required, I would have to express my preference for [the claimant's expert's] description of it because it conveyed to me the thoroughness which logic dictates is required if the examination itself is required."

The judge found, with regret, that the treating clinician had negligently failed to examine the anal sphincter.

As to causation, the judge found that: (i) had a specific examination of the anal sphincter been carried out, the damage would probably have remained undetected. The judge placed reliance on the expert evidence of Professor Phillips, who had relied on an article by Sultan and others published in the *New England Journal of Medicine* in December 1993, which demonstrated that only one in ten women with third or fourth degree tears were seen on competent clinical examination shortly after delivery to have such damage; (ii) he could not in any event conclude that it was on balance likely that primary repair would have resulted in an uneventful recovery. Again he relied on the evidence of Professor Phillips, who had cited an article in the *British Journal of Obstetrics and Gynaecology* by Tetzschner and others in October 1996 and a further article by Sultan and others published in 1997. In the latter, Mr Sultan stated:

"Childbirth remains the major contributory factor to the development of anal incontinence. Because of recent technological advances and increased publicity, obstetricians and gynaecologists are now beginning to appreciate the true magnitude of the problem. However, even when anal sphincter trauma is recognised and repaired, the outcome is far from satisfactory."

The judge expected that further research would be carried out in this area. Accordingly, the claimant's case failed on causation.

14.3 United States Law

In the USA, nearly all claims arise under the doctrine of negligence; this will be the focus of this chapter. In general, to establish a claim of negligence, one must prove (1) a duty is owed, (2) the duty was breached, (3) the breach of that duty caused an injury, i.e. causation, and (4) an injury resulted. Each will be dealt with in turn.

14.3.1 Duty

A duty is owed when a relationship has been established. Establishment of a doctor–client relationship has many facets; only the most straightforward example of an obstetric–gynaecological doctor–patient relationship will be examined here, although all doctor–client relationships – for purposes of the law – are very similar in nature.

A relationship, usually voluntary or consensual, is established when the physician agrees to treat the patient, often directly implied based on the services rendered. When a consensual relationship is impossible, i.e. the patient is unconscious, the court may still hold a physician liable based on an implied-in-fact or an implied-in-law conception. For example, when another person such as a relative acts on the patient's behalf, an implied-in-fact relationship is created. Conversely, when an emergency worker treats a patient, the court will find that an implied-at-law relationship has been established.[5]

Once a relationship is established, the physician owes a duty to the client. The duty owed is proportional to the expertise of the provider. In *Pike v. Honsinger*, 155 NY 201, 49 NE 760 (Ct App NY, 1898), the court held that:

The rule requiring [the physician] to use his best judgment does not hold him liable for a mere error of judgment, provided [the physician] does what [the physician] thinks is best after careful examination. [The physician's] implied engagement with the patient does not guarantee a good result, but [the doctor] promises by implication to use the skill and learning of the average physician, to exercise reasonable care, and to exert his best judgment in the effort to bring about a good result.

Throughout the last century, the courts have vacillated on the degree of duty owed a patient from the physician. Historically, courts have held that the standards should be of a local nature, based upon the practices of those physicians in the area. More recently, however, most jurisdictions or states have adopted the position of a national standard:

Ever-increasing emphasis on medical specialisation has accelerated the erosion of the locality rules and the concomitant emergence of the so-called national standard. Even within the framework of the locality rules, it has been generally accepted that where a physician holds himself out as a specialist, he is held to a higher standard of knowledge and skill than a general practitioner. Some courts, therefore, have abandoned the locality rules for a national standard only as to specialists ... This is consistent with the American Law Institute, which otherwise adopts the similar locality rules. We align ourselves with [other courts] and hold that a physician is under a duty to use that degree of care and skill which is expected of a reasonably competent practitioner in the same class to which [the physician] belongs, acting in the same or similar circumstances. Under this standard, advances in the profession, availability of facilities, specialisation of general practice, proximity of specialists and special facilities, together with all other relevant considerations, are to be taken into account. Here, there was evidence that there is a national standard of care for accredited hospitals in the prenatal, intrapartum and perinatal periods of pregnancy. Similarly, the evidence proffered by appellants showed national standards of care for child delivery [and] infant care ... that are observed by specialists and general practitioners alike. *Shilkret v. Annapolis Emergency Hosp. Assn,* 276 MD 187, 349 A.2d 245, 999 ALR.3d 1119 (Ct App MD, 1975).

Hence, while it varies among states, the degree of one's specialisation is generally taken into account when determining the duty owed to the patient.

14.3.2   Breach of Duty

Once a duty – and its degree – is established, a client must also establish a breach of that duty to prove liability. A physician, like any individual subject to a tort, must act in a "reasonable" manner. The standard of due care is based upon what a reasonable practitioner would do under the circumstances at hand. Hence, a physician is not held to a standard of excellence or superior practice, but only that which would be expected of the average qualified practitioner. Further, the breach must be established by objective standards; a physician's good faith is not relevant.

Similarly, if one or more alternative procedures could have been used, the issue is whether a competent or reasonable physician would have employed it, even if another would not.

While [one physician] might well prefer [a particular] technique, at least an equal number of ... fellow surgeons throughout the country apparently prefer the so-called standard technique. Since both are recognised as acceptable, if follows that the choice by [the defendant] of one of the two acceptable techniques was not a negligent act on his part. *DiFilippo v. Preston,* Supreme Court of Delaware 53 DE (3 Storey) 539, 173 A.2d 333, 1961.

To establish whether a breach has occurred, it is common to use expert testimony; in fact, to go without such evidence is almost fatal to a plaintiff's claim (*Evanstone Hosp. v. Crane* [Ill App 1993]; whether a patient should be referred to a specialist is not common knowledge). Who may be called as an expert depends somewhat on the state or jurisdiction one finds oneself; however, generally only a physician with like knowledge and expertise may be used as an expert.

14.3.3   Causation

An essential element of a plaintiff's cause of action for medical negligence is a reasonably close connection between the substandard level of care and an identifiable harm. The question of legal cause in medical malpractice cases involves two different inquiries. The first inquiry is concerned with whether a physician's negligent conduct was a cause of the injury. The second inquiry, that of "proximate cause" or "remoteness", deals with a distinctly different question: assuming that the defendant's conduct did cause the injury, what legal consequences should the law attach to the defendant's conduct? Both of these concepts, "causation-in-fact" and "proximate cause", engender a great deal of confusion and headache among lawyers and defendant physicians alike.[6]

14.3.3.1 Cause-in-fact

The commonest way to establish causation *in fact* is by posing the counterfactual question "but for agent A's conduct(s) would outcome (x) have occurred?" This test is commonly referred to as the "but-for" test. Another way of formulating this test is by asking if the defendant's conduct was a substantial factor causing the plaintiff's injury. Thus, according to the "but-for" test, the plaintiff's conduct is a cause in fact of the complained harm if the harm would not have occurred without it.

14.3.3.2 Proximate Cause

For liability to incur, it is not sufficient that the conduct was a cause in fact of the harm, i.e. an affirmative application of the but-for test, it is also required that the act be the proximate cause.

The proximate-cause inquiry is not a causal inquiry but rather is a policy inquiry that deals with reasons for absolving a defendant from liability, even though the conduct attributed to her was a cause of the injury. The question becomes not whether the conduct was a cause – that question has already been answered. Rather, the question is whether the provider, whose tortuous conduct caused the injury, should be absolved of liability for reasons such as the unforeseeable causes of the result.

In *Madigan Christensen v. Gleason*, 2000, US Dist LEXIS 1029 (DC KS, 2000), for example, the court analysed the theory of proximate cause in the context of expert testimony, where forceps were necessary to complete the birth process, and – as a result of the delivery – the plaintiff-mother suffered urinary incontinence.

Expert testimony is also required to show that the physician breached the duty owed, or in other words that he or she failed to use reasonable care in the diagnosis and treatment of the patient. [Further,] expert testimony is necessary to establish that there is a causal connection between the breach and the injuries sustained. *This causal connection is equated with the term proximate cause, which is a cause that in the natural and continuous sequence of events produces the injury, and without which the injury would not have occurred.* Sharples, 249 KS at 295, 816 P.2d at 397. [Emphasis added.]

The concept is useful as it may seem unfair to hold a defendant liable where the actual result of the defendant's conduct varies from the result that was foreseeable. In other words, only when a physician's conduct creates a foreseeable risk will liability be imputed to the physician. To put this differently, one may find proximate cause lacking, e.g. if an intervening act of the plaintiff, a third person, or some unlikely or extraordinary non-human event results in the injury.

Proximate cause is a confusing concept in part because there is no accepted and common understanding of its meaning. Instead, commentators and courts sometimes apply different standards. The observant reader might note that proximate cause is oftentimes indistinguishable from the concept of duty.

14.3.4 Injury or Damages

In some sense, the issue of injury or damages (terms often used interchangeably in the legal arena) is rather straightforward. A plaintiff must present proof of some type of injury, i.e. that the plaintiff patient suffered some kind of compensable harm as a result of the defendant physician's wrongful act.

Having provided sufficient proof, i.e. proof of injury by a preponderance of the evidence, a patient can recover out-of-pocket expenses (including future medical costs), loss of income and temporary or permanent impairment of earning capacity, et al. Reimbursement for pain and suffering may also be had, with certain limitations imposed by both state and federal law, infra. The most legislatively regulated area tort law is in the area of punitive or "exemplary" damages, which often serve to punish the tortfeasor. Regulation has generally been found necessary by many jurisdictions in light of a jury's unpredictable and/or unreasonable damage awards.

In the context of obstetrics, the issue of injury can be rather interesting. Does an injury exist, for example, in the context of a wrongful birth, i.e. where a couple is faced with an unexpected pregnancy? Courts have varied in their response to this type of injury, but most have concluded that such claims are not viable. In wrongful conception claims, for example, damages may be had for child-rearing expenses, but such damages are usually offset by the courts due to the "benefits" of having a health child. Also see *Lininger v. Eisenbaum*, 764 P.2d 1202 (CO 1988); *Kassama v. Magat*, 773 A.2d 513 (MD Ct. Spec. App. 2001), in refusing to recognise claims for wrongful life when it is difficult if not impossible to "calculate damages based on a comparison between life in an impaired state and no life at all".

14.3.5 Affirmative Defences

Affirmative defences limit liability. Such defences include, among others, statutes of limitations (which limit the time in which an individual can bring a malpractice claim) and contributory and comparative negligence. If a jurisdiction has adopted the traditional contributory negligence doctrine, a patient must be free of any fault in order to recover damages. Those jurisdictions that have adopted the comparative negligence doctrine permit a claimant to recover as long as the claimant is no more than 50% responsible for the injury. An example might include a scenario where a patient had the ability to mitigate the damage or injury, but did not.

Although there are any number of defences, one worth particular mention is the "assumption of risk" doctrine. Under this rule, a patient informed of certain risks and who proceeds in spite of those risks cannot later hold a physician liable for negligence. This doctrine may be expressed by having the patient sign an explicit form. Alternatively, the assumption of risk doctrine may be implied by the circumstances.

14.3.6 Procedural Aspects

The procedural requirements of a medical malpractice claim vary widely by state. Most states have now implemented some sort of legislation regulating such claims. In Michigan, for example, both statutes and court rules have been adopted

that require more stringent procedures for medical malpractice torts, e.g. those who allege medical malpractice have a shortened period of time in which to file the initial claims. Generally speaking, an injured individual files a claim of action, which is followed by a period of discovery (wherein parties exchange relevant information in order to create a claim or defence).

Discovery may include medical records and other documents, depositions (recorded interviews of relevant individuals), and the exchange of expert reports. Most courts require pre-trial conferences in order to facilitate settlement. Settling claims before trial, which is most often the case, may be facilitated by arbitration (oftentimes required by law or by contract) and mediation. Failing that, a trial will by held, most often with a jury, which decides on the facts of the case (matters of law are determined by the court).

14.3.7 Application of the Law

To illustrate the workings of the law in a medical context, *Bolt v. Hickok*, 887 F. Supp. 709 (D DE 1995) will be examined in some depth. In *Bolt*, the plaintiff patient brought suit against her gynaecologist for medical malpractice. The defendant physician determined that a vaginal birth would create less risk than a caesarean section. Unfortunately, complications resulted.

During the birth, the defendant physician performed an episiotomy, after which the area became infected. Several months later, the patient started experiencing manifestations of cystocele and rectocele: urinary incontinence, flatus and stool incontinence.

The plaintiff claimed that the physician violated the relevant medical standard of care and should have delivered the child by caesarean section. The plaintiff's experts testified to the appropriate standard of care in the field. In contrast, two physician experts testified that the defendant's decision to deliver the plaintiff's baby vaginally was "within the appropriate medical standard of care for obstetricians". *Bolt*, supra at 713. The jurors found the defendant physician was not liable for malpractice.

While the court's legal analysis is focused on the debate concerning the neutrality of jurors, the case is useful to illustrate both the standard of care a physician owes her or his patient and the importance of experts in establishing the standard of care.

Here, the duty owed was one of a specialist in the field of obstetrics and gynaecology. The plaintiff patient claimed that duty was breached by the physician's failure to perform a caesarean section, and that the decision caused an injury, creating uterine and rectal incontinence. Under such circumstances, both the plaintiff's and defendant's experts, who presented most of the evidence to the jury, were pivotal in the jury's decision to rule in favour of the defendant physician.

14.4 Conclusion

The role of tort law in medical malpractice claims cannot be understated. While issues of duty, breach, and causation in particular may be thorny philosophical and legal terms of art, each is an element of a malpractice claim and is therefore quite relevant to the medical profession. Hence, this area of law makes legislative and administrative policies concerning malpractice – often subject to the winds of current politics and political leaders – particularly important.

References

1. *Bolitho v. City & Hackney HA* (1998) AC 232, HL.
2. *Chester v. Afshar* (2005) 1 AC 134, HL.
3. *Gregg v. Scott* (2005) 2 AC 176, HL.
4. *Pidgeon v. Doncaster HA* (2002) Lloyd's Rep Med 130.
5. When a physician acts as a consultant, courts have found the nature of the relationship to be very fact-based. For example, it has been found that when a physician is consulted by phone, a relationship has been established. *O'Neill v. Montefiore Hospital*, 11 AD.2d 132 (NY AD 1960). On the other hand, informal opinions are unlikely to result in a duty of care. *Oliver v. Brock*, 342 So.2d 1 (AL 1976) (informal conversation recorded in patient's record did not result in physician–client relationship).
6. There is a distinction between medical and legal causation illustrated well in *Hawkinson v. A.H. Robins Co., Inc.* 595 F. Supp. 1290, 1315 (D CO 1984): [A] distinction must be made between fact finding in the courts and in the scientific community. In the courts, cases are decided according to probabilities. Probabilities may, in turn, be based upon fair inferences from circumstantial evidence. It is not necessary to exclude all other possible explanations, or to avoid all apparent inconsistencies.

Index